Practical Liver Biopsy Interpretation: Diagnostic Algorithms

Practical Liver Biopsy Interpretation: Diagnostic Algorithms

Jurgen Ludwig, MD

Professor of Pathology
Head, Section of Medical Pathology
Department of Laboratory Medicine and Pathology
Mayo Clinic and Mayo Medical School
Rochester, Minnesota

With contributions by:
Kenneth P. Batts, MD
Assistant Professor of Pathology and Senior Associate Consultant
Department of Laboratory Medicine and Pathology
Mayo Clinic and Mayo Medical School
Rochester, Minnesota

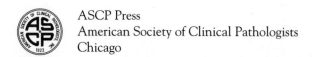

ASCP Press
American Society of Clinical Pathologists
Chicago

Acquisition & Development: Joshua Weikersheimer
Editor: Philip Rogers
Production Manager: Lisa Pollak
Designer: Ophelia M. Chambliss-Jones
Production Coordinator: Jeffrey L. Carlson

Printed on recycled paper

Notice
Trade names and equipment and supplies described herein are included as suggestions only. In no way does their inclusion constitute an endorsement or preference by the American Society of Clinical Pathologists. The ASCP did not test the equipment, supplies, or procedures and, therefore, urges all readers to read and follow all manufacturer's instructions and package insert warnings concerning the proper and safe use of all products.

Library of Congress Cataloging-in-Publication Data

Ludwig, Jurgen, 1931-
  Practical liver biopsy interpretation : diagnostic algorithms/
Jurgen Ludwig, with contributions by Kenneth P. Batts.
      p. cm.
  Includes bibliographical references and index.
  ISBN 0-89189-347-4
  1. Liver—Biopsy—Tables. 2. Liver—Histopathology—Tables.
3. Liver—Diseases—Diagnosis—Tables. 4. Diagnosis, Differential—
Tables. I. Batts, Kenneth P. II. Title.
  [DNLM: 1. Biopsy—handbooks. 2. Diagnosis, Differential—handbooks. 3. Liver—pathology—
handbooks. 4. Liver Diseases—diagnosis—handbooks. 5. Liver Diseases—pathology—handbooks.
WI 39 L948p]
RC847.5.B56L84 1992
616.3'620758—dc20
DNLM/DLC
for Library of Congress   91-41443
                                                                                                                                        CIP

Printed in the United States of America.

96   95   94   93   92   5   4   3   2   1

Contents

Preface xvii
Introduction xix

Chapter 1: Portal Hepatitis 1

Morphologic Definition 1
Clinical Conditions 2
Cellular (Acute) Hepatic Allograft Rejection 2
Chronic Active Hepatitis in Remission 2
Chronic Hepatitis, Stage 1, Associated With Primary Sclerosing Cholangitis 2
Chronic Nonsuppurative Destructive Cholangitis, Stage 1
    (Syndrome of Primary Biliary Cirrhosis) 3
Chronic Persistent Hepatitis 4
Drug-Induced Hepatitis 5
Graft-Versus-Host Disease 5
Incomplete Obstruction of Large (Extrahepatic or
    Perihilar Intrahepatic) Bile Ducts 5
Lymphoproliferative and Myeloproliferative Diseases 6
Nonspecific Reactive Hepatitis 6
Systemic Diseases 7
Tumor-Associated Change 7
Unresolved Viral Hepatitis 7
References 8

Chapter 2: Periportal Hepatitis 9

Morphologic Definition 9
Clinical Conditions 10
Acute Viral Hepatitis A 10
Alpha-1-Antitrypsin Deficiency 10

Cellular (Acute) Allograft Rejection   10
Chronic Active Hepatitis   11
Chronic Hepatitis, Stage 2, Associated With Primary Sclerosing Cholangitis   12
Chronic Nonsuppurative Destructive Cholangitis, Stage 2
    (Syndrome of Primary Biliary Cirrhosis)   13
Drug-Induced Hepatitis   14
Incomplete Obstruction of Large (Extrahepatic or Perihilar Intrahepatic)
    Bile Ducts   14
Lymphoproliferative and Myeloproliferative Diseases   15
Nonspecific Reactive Hepatitis   16
Systemic Diseases   16
Unresolved Viral Hepatitis   16
Wilson's Disease   17
References   19

Chapter 3: Lobular Hepatitis   21

Morphologic Definition   21
Clinical Conditions   22
Acute Viral Hepatitis   22
Chronic Active Hepatitis (With Lobular Inflammation)   22
Chronic Lobular Hepatitis   23
Drug-Induced Hepatitis   24
Lymphoproliferative and Myeloproliferative Diseases   24
Nonspecific Reactive Hepatitis   25
Surgery-Associated Hepatitis ("Surgical Hepatitis")   25
Systemic Diseases (Bacterial, Fungal, Protozoal, and Viral Infections)   26
Unresolved Viral Hepatitis   27
References   29

Chapter 4: Cholestatic Hepatitis   31

Morphologic Definition   31
Clinical Conditions   32
Acute Alcoholic Cholestasis   32
Acute or Unresolved Viral Hepatitis   32
Alcoholic Hepatitis   33
Cholestatic Hepatitis Associated With Total Parenteral Nutrition   34
Cholestatic Steatohepatitis Associated With Total Parenteral Nutrition   34
Chronic Active Hepatitis   34
Chronic Hepatitis Associated With Primary Sclerosing Cholangitis   35
Chronic Lobular Hepatitis   36
Chronic Nonsuppurative Destructive Cholangitis
    (Syndrome of Primary Biliary Cirrhosis)   37
Congenital Hepatic Fibrosis and Related Conditions   38

Cystic Fibrosis (Mucoviscidosis)   38
Drug-Induced Hepatitis   38
Fibrosing Cholestatic Hepatitis   38
Genetic (Familial) Liver Diseases   38
Graft-Versus-Host Disease   38
Hepatic Allograft Dysfunction   39
Infantile Obstructive Cholangiopathy   39
Massive or Submassive Hepatic Necrosis (Any Cause)   41
Obstruction of Large (Extrahepatic or Perihilar Intrahepatic) Bile Ducts   41
Recurrent Intrahepatic Cholestasis   42
Sarcoidosis   42
Sepsis, Hemolysis, and Shock   43
Wilson's Disease   43
References   45

Chapter 5: Pure Cholestasis   49

Morphologic Definition   49
Clinical Conditions   50
Amyloidosis   50
Benign Postoperative Intrahepatic Cholestasis   50
Cholestasis Associated With Total Parenteral Nutrition   51
Cholestasis of Pregnancy   51
Congenital Hepatic Fibrosis   51
Drug-Induced Cholestasis   51
Hepatocellular Tumors   51
Inspissated Bile Syndrome   51
Lymphoma   51
Progressive Intrahepatic Cholestasis (Byler's Disease) and Other Familial
    Intrahepatic Cholestatic Syndromes   52
Recurrent Intrahepatic Cholestasis   53
Sepsis, Hemolysis, and Shock   53
References   54

Chapter 6: Fatty Changes   55

Morphologic Definition   55
Clinical Conditions   56
Acute Fatty Liver of Pregnancy   56
Alcoholic Fatty Liver   57
Alcoholic Foamy Degeneration   58
Drug Effects   58
Focal Fatty Change (Nonalcoholic)   59
Heatstroke   59
Jamaican Vomiting Sickness   60

Medium-Chain and Long-Chain Acyl Coenzyme A Dehydrogenase Deficiency 60
Nonalcoholic Fatty Liver (Nonalcoholic Steatosis of the Liver) 61
Phospholipidoses 63
Poisoning by Toxic Chemicals and Bacterial Toxins 63
Reye's Syndrome 64
Sudden Childhood Death 64
Toxic Shock Syndrome 64
Viral Hepatitis D 64
References 66

Chapter 7: Steatohepatitis 69

Morphologic Definition 69
Clinical Conditions 70
Alcoholic Hepatitis (Alcoholic Steatohepatitis) 70
Nonalcoholic Steatohepatitis (Fatty Liver Hepatitis; Steatonecrosis) 71
References 77

Chapter 8: Granulomas and Granulomatous Hepatitis 79

Morphologic Definition 79
Clinical Conditions 80
Chronic Nonsuppurative Destructive Cholangitis
    (Syndrome of Primary Biliary Cirrhosis) 80
Drug-Induced Hepatitis or Exposure to Occupational or Domestic Hepatotoxic
    Chemicals 80
Extrahepatic Malignant Tumors 81
Foreign Body Reactions 82
Immune Diseases and BCG Injection 83
Lipogranulomas Caused by Endogenous Fat Mobilization 83
Lipogranulomas Caused by Mineral Oil 84
Sarcoidosis 84
Systemic Bacterial and Mycobacterial, Fungal, Parasitic, Rickettsial, and Viral
    Infections 86
Unknown Causes 89
References 91

Chapter 9: Necrosis and Postnecrotic States 93

Morphologic Definition 93
Piecemeal Necrosis 94
Bridging Necrosis 95
Multilobular (Confluent) Necrosis 95
Zonal Necrosis 95

Focal Necrosis   95
Spotty Necrosis   95
Clinical Conditions   97
Acute Hepatic Allograft Failure   97
Acute or Unresolved Viral Hepatitis   97
Anemic Infarcts   98
Chronic Active Hepatitis   98
Circulatory Failure: Heart Disease and Shock   99
Cocaine Hepatitis   99
Cytomegalovirus Hepatitis   100
Drug-Induced Hepatitis   100
Eclampsia (Toxemia of Pregnancy)   101
Halothane Hepatitis   102
Hepatic Allograft Rejection   102
Herpes Simplex Hepatitis (Herpes Simplex Necrosis)   102
Idiopathic Neonatal Hemochromatosis   103
Labetalol Hepatitis   103
Lobular Hepatitis   104
Massive or Submassive Hepatic Necrosis of Unknown Cause   104
Nongestational Disseminated Intravascular Coagulation   104
Oral Contraceptive–Induced Hemorrhagic Necrosis and Infarcts   104
Periportal Hepatitis   105
Phosphorus and Ferrous Sulfate Poisoning   105
Systemic Bacterial, Fungal, Protozoal, and Viral Infections   105
Toxic Hepatitis (Toxic Necrosis)   105
Tumor Necrosis   105
Yellow Fever Hepatitis   106
References   109

Chapter 10: Fibrosis   111

Morphologic Definition   111
Clinical Conditions   112
Chronic Active or Unresolved Viral Hepatitis   112
Chronic Alcoholic Hepatitis   113
Chronic Congestion   114
Chronic Nonalcoholic Steatohepatitis   115
Congenital Hepatic Fibrosis   115
Genetic (Familial) Liver Diseases   116
Healed Centrilobular Necroses in Hepatic Allografts   116
Healed Infarcts   116
Hypervitaminosis A   116
Idiopathic Portal Hypertension   117
Nonsuppurative Cholangitis, All Types   118
Obstruction of Large (Extrahepatic or Perihilar Intrahepatic) Bile Ducts   118

Primary Sclerosing Cholangitis   118
Schistosomiasis   119
Syphilis   119
Toxic Fibrosis   119
Treated Neoplasms or Postinfectious States   119
Unknown Causes   119
References   120

Chapter 11: Cirrhosis and Hepatocellular Nodules Without Cirrhosis   121

Morphologic Definition   121
Clinical Conditions   123
Alcoholic Cirrhosis   123
Cirrhosis Associated With Alpha-1-Antitrypsin Deficiency   124
Cirrhosis Associated With Hereditary Hemorrhagic
    Telangiectasia (Rendu-Osler-Weber Disease)   125
Cirrhosis Associated With Total Parenteral Nutrition   126
Cirrhosis Caused by Genetic (Familial) Liver Diseases   126
Cirrhosis Caused by Nonalcoholic Steatohepatitis
    (Nonalcoholic Steatohepatitic Cirrhosis)   128
Congestive Cirrhosis   129
Cryptogenic Cirrhosis   129
Drug-Induced Cirrhosis   129
Focal Nodular Hyperplasia   130
Indian Childhood Cirrhosis   130
Liver Cell Adenoma   131
Macroregenerative Nodules   131
Mixed Hamartoma   131
Nodular Regenerative Hyperplasia   131
Obstructive Biliary Cirrhosis (Large-Duct Biliary Cirrhosis;
    Secondary Biliary Cirrhosis)   132
Partial Nodular Transformation   133
Pigment Cirrhosis in Primary Hemochromatosis or Associated With
    Alcoholism, Erythropoietic Disorders, or Venovenous Shunts   133
Posthepatitic Cirrhosis   134
Primary Biliary Cirrhosis   135
Sarcoid Cirrhosis   136
Small-Duct Biliary Cirrhosis Other Than Primary Biliary Cirrhosis   137
Toxic Cirrhosis   137
References   139

Chapter 12: Abnormal Hepatocytes   143

Morphologic Definition   143
Degenerative Changes   144
Groundglass Hepatocytes   145
Hepatocellular Storage Cells   145
Intracytoplasmic Inclusions   145
Intranuclear Inclusions   146
Multinucleated Giant Hepatocytes   147
Clinical Conditions   149
Acute and Unresolved Viral Hepatitis (Hepatitis Virus Hepatitis)   149
Acute Fatty Liver of Pregnancy   149
Adenovirus Hepatitis   149
Alcoholic Liver Disease   150
Alpha-1-Antichymotrypsin Deficiency   151
Alpha-1-Antitrypsin Deficiency   151
Autoimmune Chronic Active Hepatitis   152
Biliary Obstruction and Other Causes of Cholestasis   153
Bone Marrow Transplantation   154
Cholesteryl Ester Storage Disease   154
Chronic Active Hepatitis, Autoimmune or Viral   154
Chronic Nonsuppurative Destructive Cholangitis   154
Cirrhosis   154
Congestion   154
Cytomegalovirus Hepatitis   155
Diabetes Mellitus   156
Drug-Induced Hepatitis or Hepatopathy   156
Fabry's Disease (Angiokeratoma Corporis Diffusum)   157
Fibrinogen Storage Disease   157
Fucosidosis   158
Glycogen Storage Disease   158
Hepatic Allografts   160
Hepatocellular Carcinoma   160
Herpes Simplex Hepatitis   160
Hyperparathyroidism   160
Hypoxia   161
I-Cell Disease (Mucolipidosis Type II)   161
Indian Childhood Cirrhosis   161
Lead Poisoning   162
Mannosidosis   162
Mauriac's Syndrome   162
Mucolipidosis   162
Mucopolysaccharidosis   162
Neonatal Liver Disease   162
Niemann-Pick Disease   163

Nonalcoholic Fatty Changes or Nonalcoholic Steatohepatitis   164
Primary Sclerosing Cholangitis   164
Progressive Familial Myoclonic Epilepsy   164
Syncytial Giant Cell Hepatitis   164
Thermal Injury   165
Toxic Hepatitis   165
Viral Hepatitis B and Non-A, Non-B (C, D)   165
Wilson's Disease   167
Wolman's Disease   167
References   168

Chapter 13: Iron-Positive Pigments   173

Morphologic and Chemical Definitions   173
Ferritin   173
Hemosiderin   174
Clinical Conditions   174
Alcoholic Liver Disease   174
Cimetidine Hemochromatosis   175
Congenital Atransferrinemia   175
Dietary or Medicinal Iron Ingestion   175
Genetic (HLA-Linked, Primary) Hemochromatosis   176
Hemochromatosis After Portacaval Shunting   177
Idiopathic Perinatal Hemochromatosis   177
Parenteral Iron Administration   177
Porphyria Cutanea Tarda   178
Sideroblastic Anemias and Thalassemia Major   179
Thalassemia Major   180
Transfusions   180
Transient Hemolytic Episodes   181
Viral Hepatitis   181
References   181

Chapter 14: Iron-Negative Pigments and Abnormal Nonpigmented Substances   183

Morphologic and Chemical Definitions   183
Amyloid   183
Anthracotic Pigment   183
Barium Sulfate   184
Bile   184
Calcium   184
Cellulose   184
Ceroid   184
Copper   184

Cystine   185
Dubin-Johnson Pigment   185
Formalin Pigment   185
Hematoidin   185
Hemozoin   185
Lipochrome   185
Lipofuscin   185
Malaria Pigment   186
Melanin   186
Povidone   186
Protoporphyrin   186
Schistosomal Pigment   186
Silica   186
Silicone   187
Silver   187
Starch   187
Talc   187
Thorotrast   187
Uroporphyrin   187
Clinical Conditions   190
Alpha-1-Antitrypsin Deficiency   190
Amyloidosis   190
Anthracosis and Anthracosilicosis   190
Argyria   190
Chronic Cholestasis, Any Type   191
Chronic Granulomatous Disease of Childhood   191
Chronic Nonsuppurative Destructive Cholangitis
    (Syndrome of Primary Biliary Cirrhosis)   191
Copper Storage Disease (Exogenous Copper Toxicosis)   191
Cystinosis   192
Drug Idiosyncrasy and Toxicity   192
Dubin-Johnson Syndrome   193
Embolization of Silicone   193
Erythropoietic Protoporphyria   193
Gilbert's Syndrome   194
Hepatic Atrophy   195
Hepatocellular Necrosis, All Types   195
Hypercalcemia   196
Idiopathic Adulthood Ductopenia   196
Idiopathic Copper Toxicosis   196
Indian Childhood Cirrhosis   196
Intravenous Substance Abuse   196
Malaria   196
Malignant Melanoma   197
Old Hemorrhages and Infarcts   197

Paucity of Intrahepatic Bile Ducts and Other Types of
    Infantile Obstructive Cholangiopathy   197
Porphyria Cutanea Tarda   197
Povidone Administration   198
Previous Radiographic Studies   198
Previous Surgery   198
Primary Sclerosing Cholangitis   198
Schistosomiasis   199
Silicosis and Anthracosilicosis   199
Total Parenteral Nutrition   199
Unresolved Viral Hepatitis and Other Types of Lobular Hepatitis   199
Tumors and Pseudotumors   200
Wilson's Disease   200
References   200

Chapter 15: Abnormal Bile Ducts, Including Loss of Bile Ducts   203

Morphologic Definition   203
Proliferation of Bile Ducts (Ductal Proliferation)   203
Proliferation of Bile Ductules (Ductular Proliferation;
    Cholangiolar Proliferation)   204
Cholangiectases and Biliary Cysts   204
Inflammation of Ducts and Ductules (Cholangitis and Cholangiolitis)   204
Postinflammatory States, Degeneration, and Loss of Bile Ducts   205
Clinical Conditions   207
Alcoholic Hepatitis   207
Biliary Cystadenoma, Cystadenocarcinoma, and Cholangiocarcinoma   207
Biliary Microhamartomas and Other Fibropolycystic Liver Diseases;
    Bile Duct Adenomas   208
Cholangiocarcinoma   210
Chronic Active Hepatitis and Other Types of Periportal Hepatitis   210
Chronic Intrahepatic Cholestasis of Sarcoidosis   211
Chronic or Healing Stage of Nonsuppurative Cholangitis   212
Cystic Fibrosis (Mucoviscidosis) of the Liver   212
Drug-Induced and Toxic Hepatitis   212
Graft-Versus-Host Disease   212
Heatstroke   213
Hepatic Allograft Rejection   213
Idiopathic Adulthood Ductopenia   214
Infective Intra-abdominal Conditions   216
Lymphoproliferative Disorders   216
Mucocutaneous Lymph Node Syndrome   217
Obstruction of Large (Extrahepatic and Perihilar Intrahepatic) Bile Ducts   217
Paucity of Intrahepatic Bile Ducts (Infantile Obstructive Cholangiopathy)   218

Primary Sclerosing Cholangitis 219
Recurrent Pyogenic Cholangitis 220
Schistosomiasis 221
Solitary Hepatic Cyst 221
Syndrome of Primary Biliary Cirrhosis (Chronic Nonsuppurative Destructive
    Cholangitis) 222
Systemic Bacterial Infections, Including the Toxic Shock Syndrome, and Systemic
    Viral Diseases 223
Toxic Oil Syndrome 225
Tumor-Associated Changes 226
Viral Hepatitis and Idiopathic (Autoimmune) Chronic Active Hepatitis 227
References 229

Chapter 16: Abnormal Blood Vessels and Hemorrhages 233

Morphologic Definition 233
Clinical Conditions 236
Acquired Immune Deficiency Syndrome 236
Acute, Unresolved, or Chronic Active Hepatitis; Syndromes of Primary Biliary
    Cirrhosis and Primary Sclerosing Cholangitis 236
Alcoholic Liver Disease 237
Amyloidosis 238
Angioimmunoblastic Lymphadenopathy 238
Arsenic Poisoning 238
Arteriosclerosis 238
Arteritis 239
Bacterial Endocarditis 239
Budd-Chiari Syndrome 239
Congenital Hepatic Fibrosis 240
Congestive Heart Failure 240
Diabetes Mellitus 240
Disseminated Intravascular Coagulation (Nongestational) 241
Drug Effects 241
Eclampsia 242
Graft-Versus-Host Disease 242
Granulomatous Diseases 242
Hepatic Allograft Rejection 242
Hepatic Venous Outflow Obstruction of Unknown Cause 244
Hepatotoxins 244
Hodgkin's Disease 245
Hyperparathyroidism 245
Hypervitaminosis A 245
Idiopathic Arterial Calcification of Infancy 246
Idiopathic Portal Hypertension 246
Infarcts of Zahn 247

Infectious Intra-abdominal Processes   247
Liver Cell Adenoma, Hepatocellular Carcinoma, and Regenerative Nodules   247
Malignant Lymphoma   248
Marasmus   248
Nonalcoholic Steatohepatitis   249
Normal Specimens   249
Preeclampsia and Eclampsia (Toxemia of Pregnancy)   249
Pregnancy   250
Renal Cell Carcinoma   250
Renal Transplantation and Chronic Hemodialysis   250
Rheumatoid Arthritis   250
Sarcoidosis   250
Schistosomiasis   250
Sprue   250
Streptokinase Administration   250
Thorotrast Administration   251
Thrombi and Emboli   251
Toxic Shock Syndrome   251
Trauma   251
Tumor-Associated Change   251
Vascular Tumors and Pseudotumors   252
Veno-occlusive Disease   252
Vinyl Chloride Poisoning   252
Waldenström's Macroglobulinemia and Multiple Myeloma   252
References   254

Appendix   259

Normal Test Values for the Evaluation of Liver Diseases   260
Serologic Findings in Viral Hepatitis   265
Reference   266

Index   267

Preface

A typewritten version of this diagnostic manual has been used during the last 8 years by Mayo Clinic residents and fellows. Many of these physicians did not know that they owed most of what they learned to Archie H. Baggenstoss, MD, a giant in his field and long-time chairman of Mayo's Department of Anatomic Pathology. He instituted a course in liver biopsy interpretation in the 1950s and conducted it until he retired in 1975. I have continued these diagnostic exercises and finally decided to organize my remarks and explanations in a handout. The result was this manual, which appeared to satisfy a real need. Although I have composed these diagnostic algorithms and bear the responsibility for their contents, the guiding principles evolved from Dr Baggenstoss' approach to liver biopsy diagnosis. In contradistinction to prevailing opinion, he eschewed clinical information prior to studying submitted specimens. The fear of becoming biased was one of the many expressions of intellectual honesty that I learned to admire in this unassuming scientist and gifted teacher. Dr Baggenstoss' many contributions to the pathologic and hepatologic literature attest to the merits of his approach, which he himself scrutinized in a study entitled, "Morphologic and Etiologic Diagnoses From Hepatic Biopsies Without Clinical Data" (*Medicine* 45:435-443, 1966). One can summarize the method that led to this study as follows: First, a morphologic diagnosis is made, based solely on descriptive histologic findings; second, possible etiologies are considered, based on personal experience and evidence from the literature; and last, the pathologist correlates the choices with all available clinical and laboratory information and formulates the final diagnosis. Of course, all diagnosticians go through these steps, at least subconsciously and in an abbreviated form, but if clinical information is obtained first, the chances of compounding errors in clinical judgment undoubtedly are increased. I have found the discipline required by Dr Baggenstoss' approach most beneficial.

The history of this manual makes it clear why no attempt has been made to compete with the many excellent textbooks and atlases that currently are on the market; they are indispensable for learning about liver diseases and their morphologic features. However, the purpose of these publications differs and they may be of little use if a morphologic finding does not fit the clinical data. For example, if a slide is interpreted as showing alcoholic hepatitis but the patient is a teetotaler, appropriate book chapters may be cumbersome to find. Thus, the need for a manual that in essence provides clinical differential diagnoses of biopsy findings becomes evident. Shortcomings, inherent to such a working manual, must be accepted; lists of diagnoses rarely can be truly complete and no information can be obtained from them about pathogenetic relationships or the natural history of diseases. The diagnostic algorithms presented herein have only one purpose: to provide residents and practicing histopathologists who encounter unexplained liver biopsy findings with likely clinical diagnoses. Used to this end in my own laboratory, this manual, despite its limitations, has stood the test of time. I hope that it will do the same for my fellow pathologists elsewhere.

Finally, it gives me great pleasure to acknowledge the contributions of my colleague, Kenneth P. Batts, MD, who has selected and prepared most of the illustrations and who also has provided editorial assistance. We both are indebted to Thomas V. Colby, MD, for allowing us to use his extensive slide collection for many illustrations shown here. Piet C. de Groen, MD, was most helpful in the preparation of the Appendix. Additionally, I thank Randi J. Carlson, who helped prepare and proofread the manuscript.

Jurgen Ludwig, MD

Introduction

How to Use the Algorithms

To avoid bias, liver biopsy slides generally should be studied *before* clinical information is obtained. In all instances, a morphologic diagnosis should be made first (eg, "macrovesicular fatty change" or "pure cholestasis"). By definition, such a diagnosis should not need change because of subsequent biochemical, clinical, or other nonmorphologic information.

Each chapter heading in this manual represents a morphologic diagnosis or abnormal morphologic finding. Thus, after a slide has been studied, the reader should consult the Table of Contents to find the appropriate matching section headings—for instance, "Periportal Hepatitis" and "Abnormal Bile Ducts." The organization of each section is the same throughout this manual.

Under each heading, the histologic features that constitute the morphologic diagnosis are defined and illustrated. Each chapter begins with a morphologic definition, followed by a table listing the clinical diagnoses that must be considered. This table is then followed by diagnostic criteria and helpful morphologic signs for each clinical diagnosis; in this section, all clinical conditions shown in the preceding table are listed alphabetically. This algorithm should allow users to rank the clinical diagnoses and to identify the most likely choice, based primarily on additional morphologic features that might be present. After this has been accomplished, all available clinical and laboratory data should be obtained. The reader should now be able to formulate the final diagnosis or, at least, a short list of diagnoses that can be incorporated into the biopsy report.

In most instances, drug-induced hepatitis or a noninflammatory adverse drug effect is among the possible clinical diagnoses; for these cases, a final set of tables has been provided in which the generic names of drugs are listed that might have caused the lesion, based on available evidence in the literature.

Example for Slide Analysis

Step 1 A needle biopsy specimen of the liver shows dense portal and periportal inflammatory infiltrates consisting of lymphocytes, plasma cells, other mononuclear cells, and a few segmented neutrophils. Moderately severe piecemeal necrosis is present. The lobules show only minimal changes, including a slight increase in the number of sinusoidal mononuclear cells and presence of a few Councilman bodies. Cholestasis, fatty change, or duct abnormalities are not present.

Step 2 Consult the Table of Contents. The only fitting morphologic diagnosis is "Periportal Hepatitis" (Chapter 2).

Step 3 The morphologic definition shows that the correct section of the manual has been found; however, the list of possible clinical diagnoses in Table 2.1 is rather long.

Step 4 A review of Chapter 2 suggests that the patient probably has one of four diseases, namely, chronic active hepatitis, unresolved viral hepatitis, Wilson's disease, or drug-induced hepatitis. For most other diagnoses, the histologic features would be unusual.

Step 5 Obtain clinical information. The specimen is from a 60-year-old woman without any clinical or serologic evidence of exposure to a hepatitis virus. She had been receiving nitrofurantoin therapy for 3 years because of repeated urinary tract infections. She had become fatigued and complained about abdominal discomfort. Results of liver function tests suggested chronic active hepatitis. Ceruloplasmin levels were normal.

Step 6 Table 2.2 at the end of the chapter indicates that nitrofurantoin indeed may cause periportal hepatitis. Thus, the final diagnosis would be "suggestive of nitrofurantoin-induced chronic active hepatitis" or, depending on the preferred definition, "suggestive of nitrofurantoin-induced periportal hepatitis." The latter diagnosis makes it easier to understand that after withdrawal of the drug the prognosis should be good.

Obviously, clinical and laboratory information cannot be obtained in all instances or may not be helpful for the differential diagnosis. In such cases, the morphologic diagnosis often becomes the final diagnosis also—for instance, "Kupffer cell hemosiderosis, cause undetermined."

Some illustrations have been provided to clarify important features. Unless otherwise stated, they were prepared from sections stained with hematoxylin-eosin. Magnifications are not included because they serve no useful purpose here. Finally, a detailed index has been provided to allow access to information by key words unrelated to the organization of the chapters.

Special Stains

For correct morphologic interpretation, a connective tissue stain should be prepared in all instances. The Mallory-Heidenhain stain probably gives the best contrast but, unfortunately, the preparation is time-consuming. The van Gieson stain for collagen fibers also is acceptable, although it tends to fade; the advantage is that it also acts as a special stain for bile, which then appears green. Some authors use a stain for reticulum fibers together with, or instead of, a connective tissue stain. Reticulum stains are particularly useful for the identification of discrete nodular lesions, for instance, in nodular regenerative hyperplasia or in fragmented biopsy specimens if cirrhosis must be considered. The periodic acid-Schiff reaction with diastase digestion (PAS-D stain) is an excellent general stain that shows much cellular detail, including alpha-1-antitrypsin globules and giant lysosomes, but also shows connective tissue septa, basement membranes, and many other features. This stain can be warmly recommended, whereas the PAS stain without diastase digestion has little if any use in liver biopsy interpretation.

In addition to a connective tissue stain or the PAS-D method or both, I recommend routine use of an iron stain. Conditions such as Kupffer cell hemosiderosis and ferritin accumulations may remain undetected unless an iron stain is available. Also, iron-free pigment often cannot be distinguished from iron pigment without such a special stain.

For a limited number of liver biopsy findings or suspected liver diseases, some special purpose stains can be recommended. They include Fouchet's stain for bile, the orcein stain for copper-associated protein, and the rhodanine stain for copper. For the demonstration of hepatitis B surface antigen, Shikata's orcein stain or several other special stains, such as aldehyde thionin or Victoria blue, can be used. Immunoperoxidase stains are available for both hepatitis B surface antigen and core antigen. The delta antigen also can be stained in this manner (*Hepatology* 1:238-242, 1981). For the demonstration of bile ducts—or their absence—in conditions such as cellular hepatic allograft rejection, immunostains for cytokeratins can be very useful (*Histopathology* 15:125-135, 1989; *Arch Pathol Lab Med* 113:1135-1138, 1989). Most other staining methods and indications in liver biopsy diagnosis are the same as for any other tissue sample.

Textbooks and Atlases

Several general hepatopathologic textbooks and atlases are available, and pathologists who study liver biopsy specimens should have some of them at hand. One of the most useful general textbooks on liver pathology is that by MacSween et al.[1] The most popular book on biopsy features in liver diseases has been published by Scheuer[2]; his book is now in its fourth edition. A superb and exhaustive review of current liver pathology, particularly of rarely described conditions, has been published by Ishak.[3] An excellent *Atlas of Liver Biopsies* had been compiled by Poulsen and Christoffersen (1979, Copenhagen, Minksgaard); the quality of the illustrations was outstanding. Unfortunately, this atlas is out of print. Still available is the atlas by Wight[4] in the Current Histopathology Series. Ultrastructural features of liver diseases undoubtedly are best described and illustrated in the atlas by Phillips et al.[5] For the interpretation of hepatic tumors, the book by Okuda and Ishak[6] can be recommended and, of course, the Fascicle on Tumors of the Liver and Intrahepatic Bile Ducts from the *Atlas of Tumor Pathology* published by the Armed Forces Institute of Pathology.[7] Among the many excellent clinical textbooks on liver diseases, I would recommend the book by Sherlock[8] for a very concise version and that of Schiff and Schiff[9] for a more encyclopedic presentation. For terminology and nomenclature of liver diseases, see my publication.[10] In this coding manual, I have provided definitions, synonyms, and comments related to SNOMED and ICD-9-CM codes. This book complements *Practical Liver Biopsy Interpretation: A Manual of Diagnostic Algorithms*.

References

1. MacSween RNM, Anthony PP, Scheuer PJ (eds): *Pathology of the Liver*. 2nd edition. New York, Churchill Livingstone Inc, 1987.

2. Scheuer PJ: *Liver Biopsy Interpretation*. 4th edition. London, Baillière Tindall, 1988.

3. Ishak KG: New developments in diagnostic liver pathology. In Farber E, Phillips MJ, Kaufman N (eds): *Pathogenesis of Liver Diseases*. Baltimore, Williams & Wilkins, 1987, pp 223-373.

4. Wight DGD: *Atlas of Liver Pathology*. In Gresham GA (ed): *Current Histopathology, Vol 4*. Philadelphia, JB Lippincott Co, 1982.

5. Phillips MJ, Poucell S, Patterson J, Valencia P: *The Liver: An Atlas and Text of Ultrastructural Pathology*. New York, Raven Press, 1987.

6. Okuda K, Ishak K (eds): *Neoplasms of the Liver*. New York, Springer-Verlag New York Inc, 1987.

7. Craig JR, Peters RL, Edmondson HA: Tumors of the liver and intrahepatic bile ducts. In Hartmann WH, Sobin LH (eds): *Atlas of Tumor Pathology*, 2nd series, Fascicle 26. Washington, DC, Armed Forces Institute of Pathology, 1989.

8. Sherlock S: *Diseases of the Liver and Biliary System*. 8th edition. Cambridge, Mass, Blackwell Scientific Publications Inc, 1989.

9. Schiff L, Schiff ER (eds): *Diseases of the Liver*. 6th edition. Philadelphia, JB Lippincott Co, 1987.

10. Ludwig J: *Liver Biopsy Diagnoses and Reports: SNOMED Codes, ICD-9-CM Codes, Nomenclature and Terminology*. Basel, S Karger, 1984.

Chapter 1

Portal Hepatitis

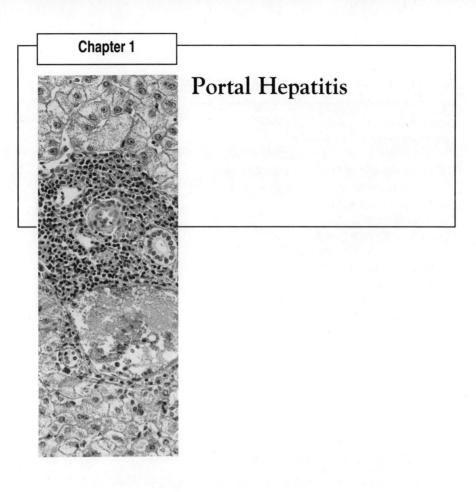

Morphologic Definition

Inflammation is largely confined to the portal tracts and is often predominantly lymphocytic, without appreciable piecemeal necrosis, prominent lobular inflammation, cholestasis, or other abnormalities that would make a different morphologic diagnosis more applicable.

Table 1.1   Clinical Conditions Associated With Portal Hepatitis

Cellular (acute) hepatic allograft rejection
Chronic active hepatitis in remission
Chronic hepatitis, stage 1, associated with primary sclerosing cholangitis
Chronic nonsuppurative destructive cholangitis, stage 1
   (syndrome of primary biliary cirrhosis)
Chronic persistent hepatitis
Drug-induced hepatitis
Incomplete obstruction of large
   (extrahepatic or perihilar intrahepatic) bile ducts
Nonspecific reactive hepatitis
Systemic diseases
Unresolved viral hepatitis
Uncommon causes:
      Graft-versus-host disease
      Lymphoproliferative and myeloproliferative diseases
      Tumor-associated change

Clinical Conditions

Cellular (Acute) Hepatic Allograft Rejection

The diagnostic criteria are nonsuppurative cholangitis and endotheliitis. If such changes are present, see Chapters 15 and 16, respectively.

Chronic Active Hepatitis in Remission

Comments: By definition, the duration of the disease is at least 6 months but generally it exceeds 1 year because this diagnosis implies that the patient had at least one previous episode of chronic active hepatitis.[1] Causative viruses are the same as in chronic persistent hepatitis.

Morphologic features: The histologic appearance of chronic persistent hepatitis (good prognosis) and of chronic active hepatitis in remission (guarded prognosis) is the same (Figure 1.1).[1] For other manifestations of chronic active hepatitis, see Chapter 2.

Chronic Hepatitis, Stage 1, Associated With Primary Sclerosing Cholangitis

Comments: Clinical and laboratory findings usually reveal chronic cholestatic liver disease. Typical cholangiographic findings confirm the diagnosis. Most patients also have chronic ulcerative colitis.[2]

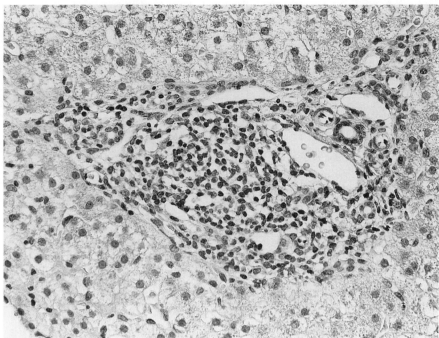

Figure 1.1
Typical example of portal hepatitis, as described in the morphologic definition. Although this specimen represents a case of chronic persistent hepatitis, its morphologic features could not be distinguished from those seen in instances such as nonspecific reactive hepatitis, chronic active hepatitis in remission, or drug-induced hepatitis. Note sharp outline of portal tract and absence of appreciable hepatocellular abnormalities.

Morphologic features: Presence of portal hepatitis defines stage 1 of this disease.[2] Changes may be indistinguishable from those in incomplete obstruction of large bile ducts (see below). Fibrous cholangitis, duct obliteration, or absence of some interlobular bile ducts (ductopenia) are important diagnostic clues. If duct changes are present, see also Chapter 15. Copper stains tend to be negative at this stage of the disease.

Chronic Nonsuppurative Destructive Cholangitis, Stage 1 (Syndrome of Primary Biliary Cirrhosis)

Comments: Clinical and laboratory findings usually reveal chronic cholestatic liver disease. High titers of antimitochondrial antibodies are characteristic.

Morphologic features: Presence of portal hepatitis defines stage 1 of this disease.[3] The diagnostic bile duct lesions and the granulomas (Figure 1.2) often are

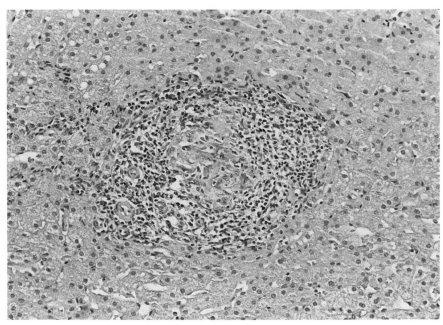

Figure 1.2
Portal hepatitis in patient with chronic nonsuppurative destructive cholangitis, stage 1 (syndrome of prima-ry biliary cirrhosis). Note poorly defined noncaseating epithelioid cell granuloma in center of lymphocytic infiltrate, and absence of interlobular bile duct. This constellation of findings is quite characteristic of chron-ic nonsuppurative destructive cholangitis, stage 1, but often the lesions are so widely spaced that they can-not be found in each specimen. Most portal tracts resemble Figure 1.1, and ducts may even be proliferated at this stage. For additional descriptions, see the Index.

---

absent; if these lesions can be found, see also Chapters 15 and 16, respectively. Copper stains tend to be negative at this stage of the disease.

Chronic Persistent Hepatitis

Comments: The duration of the disease is 6 months or longer. If previous episodes of chronic active hepatitis were noted, chronic persistent hepatitis should not be diag-nosed but the term "chronic active hepatitis in remission" should be used (see above). The prognosis of the two conditions differs.[1] Causative viruses include hepatitis viruses B and non-A, non-B (hepatitis C, D, and possibly other hitherto undescribed viruses).

Morphologic features: The portal infiltrates tend to be denser than in nonspecif-ic reactive hepatitis. The biopsy features of chronic persistent hepatitis are the proto-type of portal hepatitis (Figure 1.1). The distinction between portal hepatitis in chronic persistent hepatitis and periportal inflammation in chronic active hepatitis (see Chapter 2) is not well defined; many borderline cases are encountered.

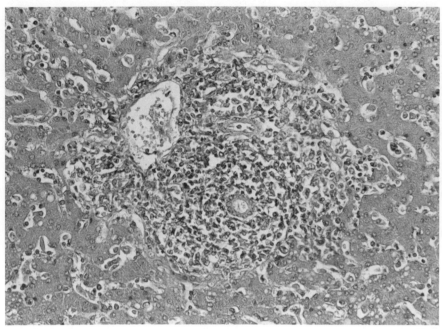

Figure 1.3
Lymphomatous infiltrate simulating portal hepatitis (from a patient with Hodgkin's disease). At this power, the nature of the malignant cells cannot be discerned. In this instance, the presence of mononuclear cells in the sinusoids associated with normal-appearing hepatocytes is diagnostically helpful.

Drug-Induced Hepatitis

The diagnosis can be suggested if an appropriate clinical history has been provided and if other possible causes cannot be found. Helpful histologic features cannot be expected.

Graft-Versus-Host Disease

The diagnostic criteria are nonsuppurative cholangitis and endotheliitis; if such changes are present, see Chapters 15 and 16, respectively.

Incomplete Obstruction of Large (Extrahepatic or Perihilar Intrahepatic) Bile Ducts

Comments: Most patients have clinical and biochemical evidence of cholestatic liver disease. Biopsy often is done because of negative cholangiographic or ultrasound studies and because parenchymal liver disease is suspected.

Morphologic features: Portal edema with proliferation of ducts and ductules is the main histologic clue (see also Chapters 2 and 15). The inflammatory infiltrate tends to be less dense than in chronic persistent hepatitis and usually contains many neutrophils.

Lymphoproliferative and Myeloproliferative Diseases

Leukemic or lymphomatous infiltrates and related neoplastic conditions may simulate portal hepatitis.[4] The infiltrates usually appear monotonous, and both neutrophils and plasma cells often are conspicuous by their absence. Clusters of neoplastic cells may also be present in sinusoids (Figure 1.3). Many specimens show hemosiderosis. Use of immunostains (pan B-cell, pan T-cell, kappa and lambda light chain stains) may be helpful.

Nonspecific Reactive Hepatitis

Comments: There is usually no evidence of primary parenchymal liver disease or biliary disorder; patients often have an extrahepatic disease or condition.

Morphologic features: In most cases, portal inflammatory infiltrates are not very dense.

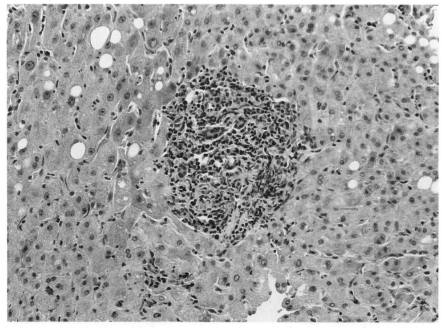

Figure 1.4
Infectious mononucleosis hepatitis with primarily portal involvement. Generally, sinusoidal infiltrates are more prominent in this condition. See also Figure 7.3.

Systemic Diseases

The features usually are those of nonspecific reactive hepatitis but they also may suggest presence of a lymphoproliferative disorder (Figure 1.4).

Tumor-Associated Change

This is occasionally found after unsuccessful attempts to obtain a specimen from a space-occupying lesion. Neutrophils in edematous portal tracts—together with abnormal bile ducts and ductules—and focal sinusoidal dilatation[5] may be present, but the condition also may resemble other types of portal hepatitis (Figure 1.5). See also Chapter 16.

Unresolved Viral Hepatitis

Comments: The duration of the disease is more than 1 month but less than 6 months. Causative viruses include hepatitis viruses A, B, and non-A, non-B (hepatitis C, D, and possibly other hitherto undescribed viruses).

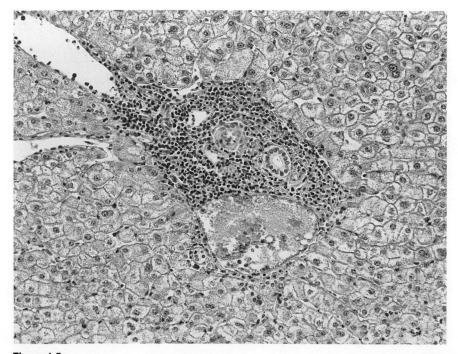

Figure 1.5
Portal hepatitis in the vicinity of metastatic adenocarcinoma. This represents nonspecific-reactive hepatitis but is indistinguishable from other types of portal hepatitis.

Morphologic features: Portal tracts often contain PAS-D–positive pigmented macrophages. In the lobules, a few spotty necroses (see Chapter 9) and some Kupffer cell proliferation may be present. Macrophages with PAS-D–positive ceroid pigment and ferritin ("diffuse iron") are common features. Both pigments may be found in the same cell. In drug addicts, portal tracts often contain birefringent embolized material.

References

1. Czaja AJ, Ludwig J, Baggenstoss AH, et al: Corticosteroid-treated chronic active hepatitis in remission: Uncertain prognosis of chronic persistent hepatitis. *N Engl J Med* 304:5-9, 1981.

2. Ludwig J: Surgical pathology of the syndrome of primary sclerosing cholangitis. *Am J Surg Pathol* 13:43-49, 1989.

3. Ludwig J, Dickson ER, McDonald GSA: Staging of chronic nonsuppurative destructive cholangitis (syndrome of primary biliary cirrhosis). *Virchows Arch [A]* 379:103-112, 1978.

4. Ludwig J, Boon SE: Liver biopsy diagnosis of unsuspected or unconfirmed lymphoproliferative or myeloproliferative disorders. *Hepatogastroenterology* 27:17-25, 1980.

5. Gerber MA, Thung SN, Bodenheimer HC Jr, et al: Characteristic histologic triad in liver adjacent to metastatic neoplasm. *Liver* 6:85-88, 1986.

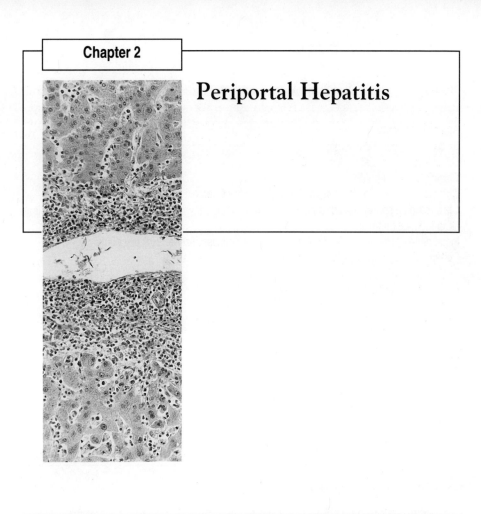

Chapter 2

Periportal Hepatitis

Morphologic Definition

Inflammation is largely confined to the portal and periportal areas and is often predominantly lymphocytic, with or without piecemeal necrosis. There is an absence of prominent midzonal or centrilobular abnormalities that would make a different morphologic diagnosis more applicable.

Table 2.1   Clinical Conditions Associated With Periportal Hepatitis

Acute viral hepatitis
Alpha-1-antitrypsin deficiency
Cellular (acute) hepatic allograft rejection
Chronic active hepatitis
Chronic hepatitis, stage 2, associated with primary sclerosing cholangitis
Chronic nonsuppurative destructive cholangitis, stage 2 (syndrome of primary biliary cirrhosis)
Drug-induced hepatitis
Incomplete obstruction of large (extrahepatic or perihilar intrahepatic) bile ducts
Nonspecific reactive hepatitis
Systemic diseases
Unresolved viral hepatitis
Uncommon causes:
    Lymphoproliferative and myeloproliferative diseases
    Wilson's disease

Clinical Conditions

Acute Viral Hepatitis A

Comments: Duration of the disease is 1 month or less, and the causative agent is the hepatitis A virus. Patients have serologic evidence of acute type A infection (IgM anti–hepatitis A virus). The condition may relapse.

Morphologic features: Some cases show prominent periportal mononuclear inflammatory cell infiltration with damage of the limiting plate and periportal necrosis. Early in the disease, centrilobular and midzonal areas are not involved.[1] This is unusual in other types of acute viral hepatitis. Cholestatic features may be present and even be severe.[2]

Alpha-1-Antitrypsin Deficiency

The morphologic findings are those of chronic active hepatitis (see entry below). For the diagnostic intracytoplasmic globules, see Chapter 12. For additional descriptions, see Index.

Cellular (Acute) Hepatic Allograft Rejection

The findings consist of periportal hepatitis associated with cholangitis and sometimes endotheliitis (Chapters 15 and Chapter 16, respectively). All cases of cellular rejection in which the inflammation spills out of the portal tracts and causes periportal hepatitis or even bridging necrosis must be considered severe.

Chronic Active Hepatitis

Comments: The duration of the disease is 6 months or longer. The condition is either idiopathic or caused by hepatitis viruses B or non-A, non-B (hepatitis C, D, and possibly other hitherto undescribed viruses). Cases of idiopathic chronic active hepatitis may represent autoimmune disease. In at least one instance, chronic hepatitis A appears to have occurred also.[3]

Morphologic features: The portal and periportal infiltrates tend to be denser than in nonspecific reactive hepatitis but they may vary in intensity from portal tract to portal tract. Lymphocytic piecemeal necrosis (see Chapter 9) is always present (Figure 2.1). This is the prototype of periportal hepatitis. Chronic active hepatitis non-A, non-B may be difficult to distinguish from the acute or chronic persistent infection.[4] This type of viral hepatitis (hepatitis C in most instances)

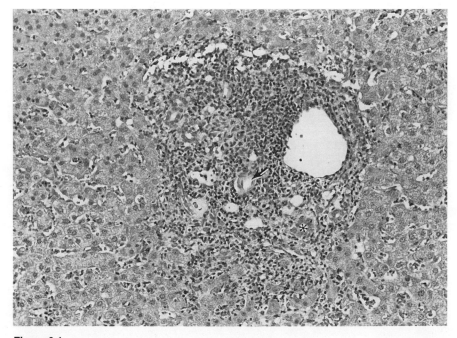

Figure 2.1
Periportal hepatitis in a patient with mild chronic active hepatitis. Note that the upper circumference of the portal tract is rather well-defined as seen in chronic persistent hepatitis (see Figure 1.2), but the lower circumference shows classic lymphocytic piecemeal necrosis. For additional descriptions, see Index. Bile duct (asterisk); hepatic artery (arrow). Mononuclear cells in sinusoids are slightly increased but hepatocytes appear normal.

should be suspected in periportal hepatitis with "naked" Councilman bodies in the lobules, portal lymphoid follicles, fatty changes, and sinusoidal lymphocytosis. For the identification of viral antigen in hepatitis B and D (delta hepatitis), immunoperoxidase techniques may be applied.

Chronic Hepatitis, Stage 2, Associated With Primary Sclerosing Cholangitis

Comments: Clinical and laboratory findings usually reveal chronic cholestatic liver disease. Typical cholangiographic findings confirm the diagnoses. Most patients also have chronic ulcerative colitis.

Morphologic features: Periportal hepatitis or periportal fibrosis or both are present in stage 2 of this disease. Changes may be indistinguishable from those in incomplete obstruction of large bile ducts (see below). Fibrous cholangitis, duct obliteration, or absence of some interlobular bile ducts (Figure 2.2) are important diagnostic clues. If duct changes are present, see also Chapter 15. Copper stains

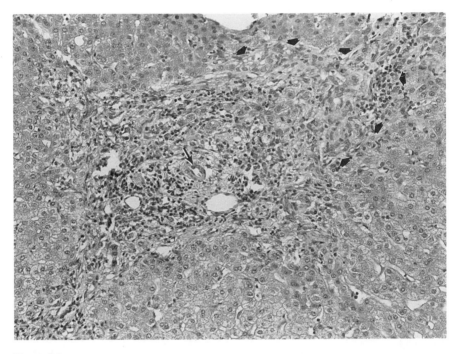

Figure 2.2
Periportal hepatitis in chronic hepatitis, stage 2, associated with primary sclerosing cholangitis. The inflammation is milder than in chronic active hepatitis (see Figure 2.1). The hepatic artery branch (long arrow) can be clearly identified, but the interlobular bile duct appears to be absent. Note tongue of connective tissue with ductular proliferation at right side of portal tract (short arrows) reaching into the lobule.

still may be negative at this stage of the disease. The distinction from the syn-drome of primary biliary cirrhosis may be difficult.[5, 6]

Chronic Nonsuppurative Destructive Cholangitis, Stage 2 (Syndrome of Primary Biliary Cirrhosis)

Comments: Clinical and laboratory findings usually reveal chronic cholestatic liver disease. High titers of antimitochondrial antibodies are characteristic.

Morphologic features: Presence of periportal hepatitis defines stage 2 of this disease.[5] Diagnostic bile duct lesions and granulomas are most commonly found during this stage of the disease (Figure 2.3A). If these lesions can be found, see also Chapters 15 and 8, respectively. Copper stains still may be negative at this stage of the disease. Some specimens closely resemble chronic active hepatitis; ductopenia may be a helpful feature in these cases (Figure 2.3B).

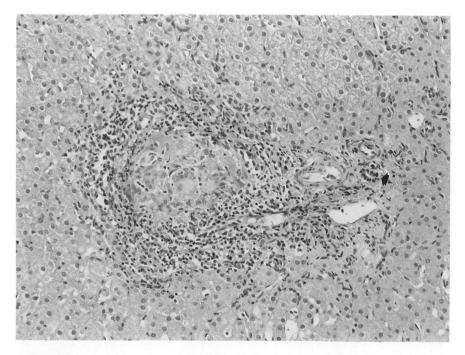

Figure 2.3A

Periportal hepatitis in chronic nonsuppurative destructive cholangitis, stage 2 (syndrome of primary biliary cirrhosis). A large noncaseating epithelioid cell granuloma with giant cells can be seen to the left of the center of the portal tract. For additional descriptions, see Index. A small bile duct is seen at the right side of the portal tract (arrow), accompanied by two artery branches. A larger duct might have been replaced by the granuloma. Mild lymphocytic piecemeal necrosis is present. Hepatocytes appear normal.

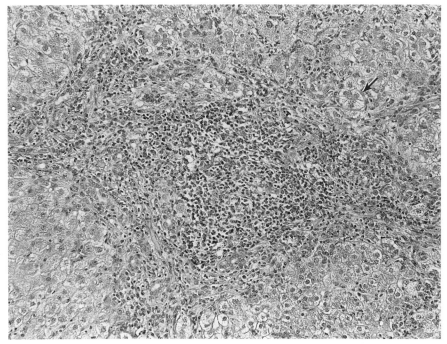

Figure 2.3B
Periportal hepatitis in chronic nonsuppurative destructive cholangitis, stage 2 (syndrome of primary biliary cirrhosis). In this instance, no bile duct and no granuloma can be seen. These features often are confused with those of chronic active hepatitis. Ductular proliferation and mild lymphocytic piecemeal necrosis can be identified; they are associated regenerative hepatocellular changes. Note hepatocellular rosette above portal tract (arrow).

Drug-Induced Hepatitis

Comments: The diagnosis can be suggested if an appropriate history has been provided. The term *drug-induced chronic active hepatitis* may not be appropriate because the condition often regresses after withdrawal of the drug. For a list of drugs that may cause periportal hepatitis, see Table 2.2.

Morphologic features: Helpful morphologic features have not been described. For an example, see Figure 2.4.

Incomplete Obstruction of Large (Extrahepatic or Perihilar Intrahepatic) Bile Ducts

Comments: Most patients have clinical and biochemical evidence of cholestatic disease. Biopsy often is done because of negative cholangiographic and ultrasound studies, and because parenchymal liver disease is suspected.

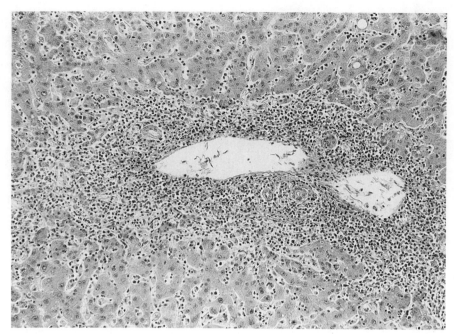

Figure 2.4
Periportal hepatitis in adverse drug reaction (phenytoin sodium [Dilantin™]). Note the monotonous appearance of the inflammatory infiltrate in the portal tract and adjacent sinusoids, resembling lymphoma (see Figure 1.3). This is characteristic for this drug.

Morphologic features: Portal enlargement with edema and proliferation of ducts and ductules is the main histologic clue (Figure 2.5). The inflammatory infiltrate tends to be less dense than in chronic active hepatitis and usually contains many neutrophils. If duct changes are present, see also Chapter 15.

Lymphoproliferative and Myeloproliferative Diseases

Comments: Hepatomegaly in a patient with known or suspected hematologic disorder is the most common presentation.

Morphologic features: Leukemic or lymphomatous infiltrates may *simulate* periportal hepatitis. The infiltrates usually appear monotonous, and both neutrophils and plasma cells often are conspicuous by their absence. Clusters of neoplastic cells may be present in sinusoids also. Many specimens show hemosiderosis. Use of immunostains (pan B-cell, pan T-cell, kappa and lambda light chain stains) may be helpful.

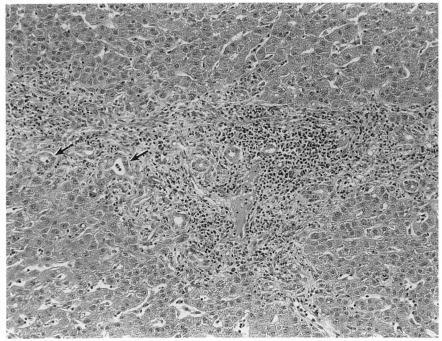

Figure 2.5
Periportal hepatitis in incomplete large duct biliary obstruction. The portal tract is enlarged and edematous, with only mild lymphocytic inflammation. In this example, ductular proliferation with neutrophilic
cholangiolitis (arrows) is prominent. Cholestasis is not present, suggesting that the obstruction is
incomplete.

Nonspecific Reactive Hepatitis

Comments: There is usually no evidence of primary parenchymal liver disease
or biliary disorder; patients often have an extrahepatic abnormality.

Morphologic features: Portal and periportal infiltrates usually are not very
dense; they spill over the limiting plate without causing piecemeal necrosis.

Systemic Diseases

The features usually are those of nonspecific-reactive hepatitis but they also
may suggest presence of a lymphoproliferative disorder (Figure 2.6).

Unresolved Viral Hepatitis

Comments: The duration of the disease is more than 1 month but less than 6

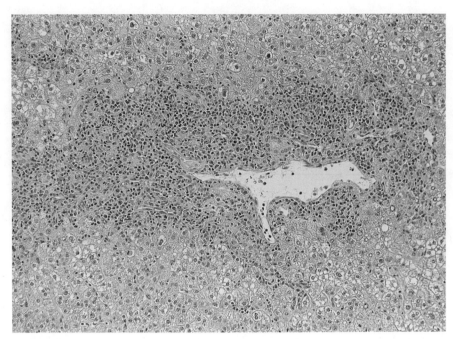

Figure 2.6
Periportal hepatitis in systemic infectious disease. The patient had infectious mononucleosis. The infiltrate consists of mononuclear cells and is rather monotonous. Note resemblance of infiltrate with lymphoma (see Figure 1.3) and with that in phenytoin hepatitis (see Figure 2.4). Although the infiltrate spills into the parenchyma, hepatocytes appear unaffected.

months. Causative viruses include hepatitis viruses A, B, and non-A, non-B (hepatitis C, D, and possibly other hitherto undescribed viruses).

Morphologic features: Portal tracts often contain PAS-D–positive pigmented macrophages. In the lobules, a few spotty necroses (see Chapter 9) and some Kupffer cell proliferation may be present. Macrophages with PAS-D–positive lipochrome pigment (ceroid) and ferritin ("diffuse iron") are common features. Both pigments may be found in the same cell. In drug addicts, portal tracts often contain birefringent embolized material.

Wilson's Disease

Comments: This hereditary disorder of copper metabolism can be confused with chronic active hepatitis. Therefore, all patients under 40 years of age need a clinical workup to exclude Wilson's disease. Onset of the disease in older patients is quite uncommon.

Morphologic features: The histologic changes also may be indistinguishable from chronic active hepatitis.[7] The most important diagnostic feature is the high hepatic copper level. However, copper stains may be negative,[8] and therefore fresh tissue or tissue from paraffin blocks should be submitted for quantitative copper determination by flameless atomic absorption spectrometry (several major centers, including Mayo Medical Laboratories, will do these studies on request). Fatty changes, periportal Mallory bodies, and vacuolated nuclei may be important diagnostic clues but these features often are absent.

Table 2.2   Drugs That May Cause Periportal Hepatitis*

Generic or Chemical Name	Product Classification
Acetaminophen	Analgesic and antipyretic
Aminosalicylic acid	Antituberculotic
Aspirin	Analgesic, anti-inflammatory, and antipyretic
Captopril[10]	Antihypertensive
Chlorothiazide	Diuretic
Chlorpromazine	Tranquilizer: phenothiazine
Clometacin	Analgesic
Danthron	Laxative
Dantrolene sodium	Skeletal muscle relaxant
Diclofenac[11]	Anti-inflammatory
Erythromycin	Antibiotic
Halothane	Inhalation anesthetic
Interferon[12]	Immune modulator
Isoniazid	Antituberculotic
Methyldopa	Antihypertensive
Nicotinic acid	Nutrient vitamin
Nitrofurantoin	Urinary antibiotic
Oxacillin	Antibiotic
Oxyphenbutazone	Anti-inflammatory
Papaverine hydrochloride[13]	Vasodilator
Penicillin	Antibiotic
Perphenazine	Tranquilizer: phenothiazine
Phenytoin sodium	Anticonvulsant (see Figure 2.4)
Propylthiouracil	Antithyroid
Sulfamethizole	Antibiotic
Sulfonamide(s), type unspecified	Antibiotic
Tolazamide	Oral hypoglycemic

*This list does not include drugs that are unavailable in the United States. For further information, see reference 9.

References

1. Abe H, Beninger PR, Ikejiri N, et al: Light microscopic findings of liver biopsy specimens from patients with hepatitis A and comparison with type B. *Gastroenterology* 82:938-947, 1982.

2. Sciot R, Van Damme B, Desmet VJ: Cholestatic features in hepatitis A. *J Hepatol* 3:172-181, 1986.

3. McDonald GSA, Courtney MG, Shattock AG, et al: Prolonged IgM antibodies and histopathological evidence of chronicity in hepatitis A. *Liver* 9:223-228, 1989.

4. Fagan EA, Williams R: Non-A, non-B hepatitis. *Semin Liver Dis* 4:314-315, 1984.

5. Ludwig J, Dickson ER, McDonald GSA: Staging of chronic nonsuppurative destructive cholangitis (syndrome of primary biliary cirrhosis). *Virchows Arch [A]* 379:103-112, 1978.

6. Wiesner RH, LaRusso NF, Ludwig J, et al: Comparison of the clinicopathologic features of primary sclerosing cholangitis and primary biliary cirrhosis. *Gastroenterology* 88:108-114, 1985.

7. Stromeyer FW, Ishak KG: Histology of the liver in Wilson's disease: A study of 34 cases. *Am J Clin Pathol* 73:12-24, 1980.

8. Jain S, Scheuer PJ, Archer B, et al: Histological demonstration of copper and copper-associated protein in chronic liver diseases. *J Clin Pathol* 31:784-790, 1978.

9. Ludwig J, Axelson R: Drug effects on the liver: An updated tabular compilation of drugs and drug-related hepatic diseases. *Dig Dis Sci* 28:651-666, 1983.

10. Bellary SV, Isaacs PET, Scott AWM: Captopril and the liver. *Lancet* 2:514, 1989.

11. Mazeika PK, Ford MJ: Chronic active hepatitis associated with diclofenac sodium therapy. *Br J Clin Pract* 43:125-126, 1989.

12. Silva MO, Reddy KR, Jeffers LJ, et al: Interferon-induced chronic active hepatitis? *Gastroenterology* 101:840-842, 1991.

13. Poncin E, Silvain C, Touchard G, et al: Papaverin-induced chronic liver disease. *Gastroenterology* 90:1051-1053, 1986.

Chapter 3

Lobular Hepatitis

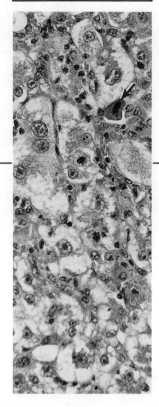

Morphologic Definition

Diffuse lobular inflammation without prominent fatty changes is present. Portal inflammation usually is present also. If hepatocanalicular cholestasis is found, the designation "cholestatic hepatitis" is preferred (see Chapter 4).

Table 3.1 Clinical Conditions Associated With Lobular Hepatitis

---

Acute viral hepatitis
Chronic active hepatitis (with lobular inflammation)
Chronic lobular hepatitis
Drug-induced hepatitis
Nonspecific reactive hepatitis
Surgery-associated hepatitis ("surgical hepatitis")
Unresolved viral hepatitis
Uncommon causes:
    Lymphoproliferative and myeloproliferative diseases
    Systemic diseases (bacterial, fungal, protozoal, and viral infections)

Clinical Conditions

Acute Viral Hepatitis

Comments: The duration of the disease is 1 month or less. Causative viruses include hepatitis viruses A, B, and non-A, non-B (hepatitis C, D, and possibly other hitherto undescribed viruses). Endemic infection with hepatitis virus E has occurred in Mexico but not yet in the United States.[1]

Morphologic features: Lobular inflammation usually is quite severe (Figures 3.1A and 3.1B). Types B and non-A, non-B are the prototypes of lobular hepatitis. For features of acute viral hepatitis A, see Chapter 2. Ballooned hepatocytes, Councilman bodies, spotty necroses, diffuse inflammatory cell infiltrates, centrilobular phlebitis (see also Chapter 16), and regenerative hepatocellular changes are common findings in acute viral hepatitis. Ferritin ("diffuse iron") and PAS-D–positive, iron-negative lipochrome pigment (ceroid) often are found in many macrophages. Bridging necrosis or multilobular (confluent) necrosis may be present, but except for zone 3 necrosis in some cases of acute viral hepatitis B, zonal necrosis is not a feature of acute viral hepatitis (see Chapter 9). Immunoperoxidase stains for viral antigen fail in most instances. Hepatitis C may be suspected if the specimen shows mild fatty changes.[2] In hepatitis D, cytotoxic and cytopathic hepatocellular damage with small-droplet vacuolar liver cell degeneration may occur.[3] Hepatitis E may be indistinguishable from other types of viral hepatitis but many specimens appear to show cholestasis.[4] Nevertheless, a reliable histologic distinction between the various types of hepatitis and some forms of drug-induced hepatitis is not possible.

Chronic Active Hepatitis (With Lobular Inflammation)

Comments: The duration of the disease is 6 months or longer. The condition

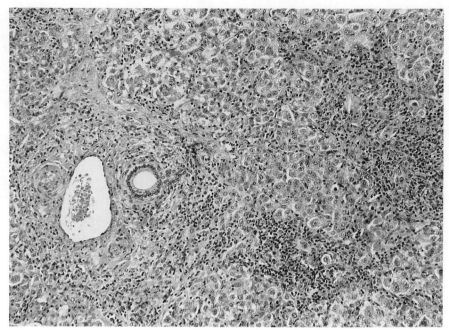

Figure 3.1A
Lobular hepatitis in acute viral hepatitis non-A, non-B. Low-power view showing lobular inflammation with only minimal involvement of the portal tract on the left. Note: Even if the portal inflammation were more severe, the morphologic diagnosis of "lobular hepatitis" would remain.

---

is either idiopathic or caused by hepatitis viruses B or non-A, non-B (hepatitis C, D, and possibly other hitherto undescribed viruses). Cases of idiopathic chronic active hepatitis may represent autoimmune disease. The presence of lobular inflammation in patients with chronic active hepatitis does not appear to affect the prognosis.[5]

Morphologic features: Portal and periportal inflammation tends to be more prominent than in acute or unresolved viral hepatitis. A clear distinction between chronic active hepatitis with lobular inflammation ("viral features") and chronic lobular hepatitis does not exist.

Chronic Lobular Hepatitis

Comments: The duration of the disease is 6 months or longer. By definition, patients have biopsy evidence of lobular inflammation. Causative viruses include hepatitis viruses B and non-A, non-B (hepatitis C and possibly other hitherto undescribed viruses; hepatitis D does not appear to occur in this setting). Many cases have a benign course and appear to be self-limited,[6] but progression to chronic active hepatitis and cirrhosis has occurred.[7]

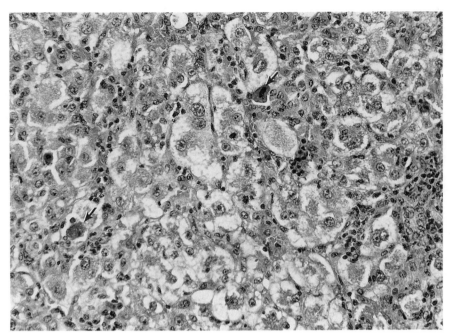

Figure 3.1B
Lobular hepatitis in acute viral hepatitis non-A, non-B. Higher-power view of the same specimen as in Figure 3.1A shows ballooned hepatocytes, Councilman bodies (arrows), and mixed inflammatory infiltrates throughout the lobule. This is the prototype of lobular hepatitis.

Morphologic features: The findings may be the same as those in acute viral hepatitis (Figure 3.2). Spotty necrosis is a common feature.[6] In other instances, the histologic features of the condition resemble nonspecific reactive hepatitis.[7]

Drug-Induced Hepatitis

Comments: The diagnosis can be suggested if an appropriate history has been provided. For a list of drugs that may cause lobular hepatitis, see Table 3.2.

Morphologic features: Principally, drug-induced lobular hepatitis cannot be distinguished morphologically from lobular viral hepatitis (Figure 3.3). Presence of eosinophils is not a distinguishing feature. If hepatocanalicular cholestasis is present, see Chapter 4.

Lymphoproliferative and Myeloproliferative Diseases

Lobular infiltrates in conditions such as lymphoma or leukemia—in particular, myelomonocytic leukemia and hairy cell leukemia—may simulate hepatitis. These diagnoses should be considered if the intrasinusoidal or perisinusoidal infiltrates of

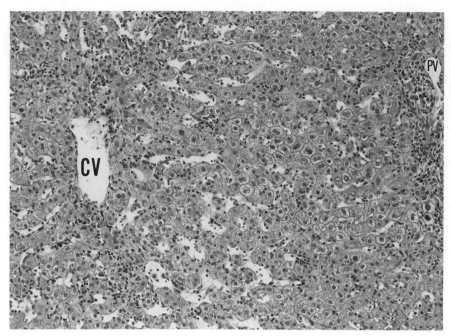

Figure 3.2
Chronic lobular hepatitis non-A, non-B. In this lower-power view, diffuse lobular inflammation with disarray ("unrest") of hepatocytes can be appreciated. However, ballooning of hepatocytes is much less than that shown in Figures 3.1A and 3.1B. Centrilobular phlebitis is present on the left side of the illustration (CV, central vein or terminal hepatic vein; PV, portal vein).

mononuclear cells appear unusually uniform and if the hepatocytes appear essentially normal. However, the diagnosis rarely can be made on this basis alone because infectious mononucleosis, hepatitis C, and chronic nonsuppurative destructive cholangitis (primary biliary cirrhosis) may show similar features. Nodular collections of mononuclear cells provide supportive evidence for a neoplastic hematologic disorder.

Nonspecific Reactive Hepatitis

In most cases, proliferation of Kupffer cells and of other sinusoidal mononuclear cells is the main abnormality. The hepatocytes remain largely uninvolved.

Surgery-Associated Hepatitis ("Surgical Hepatitis")

After surgery, particularly after prolonged procedures, liver biopsy specimens often contain multiple clusters of neutrophils in the lobules, aggregating in distended sinusoids or minute areas of necrosis (Figure 3.4). The clusters may resem-

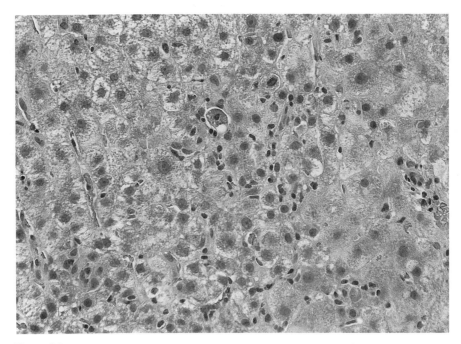

Figure 3.3
Drug-induced (nitrofurantoin) lobular hepatitis. The changes are indistinguishable from those seen in acute viral hepatitis (see Figures 3.1A and 3.1B).

---

ble microabscesses. Hepatocytes remain largely uninvolved. These findings are highly suggestive of reversible, nonspecific, surgery-related hepatitis.[8] In rare instances, this condition also can be observed in percutaneous needle biopsy specimens after prolonged anesthesia or hepatic hypoperfusion.[9]

Systemic Diseases (Bacterial, Fungal, Protozoal, and Viral Infections)

Many systemic infectious diseases in this category—in particular, tropical diseases such as the tropical splenomegaly syndrome in malaria or cases of visceral leishmaniasis—may be associated with lobular hepatitis. In the United States, toxoplasmic mononucleosis may be encountered. In conditions with septicemia and pyemia, focal necroses and microabscesses are common findings (see also Chapters 4 and 9).

Systemic viral infections such as the acquired immune deficiency syndrome, cytomegalovirus infection, or infectious mononucleosis may cause lobular hepatitis. Indeed, some cases of hepatitis C cannot be distinguished from infectious mononucleosis hepatitis. However, in most instances (eg, in herpesvirus hepatitis) focal necroses are a prominent feature (see Chapter 9). Inclusion bodies, when present, will be found at the preserved edges of these necroses. Recently, lobular and

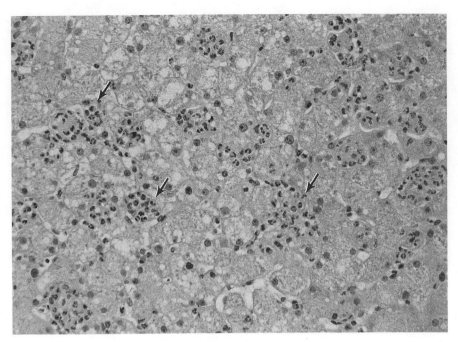

Figure 3.4
Surgery-associated hepatitis. This type of lobular hepatitis is a unique variant of nonspecific-reactive hepatitis. The characteristic spotty necroses and clusters of neutrophils (arrows) are reversible lesions and not an expression of an infectious process.

portal hepatitis with lymphocytic infiltrates and sinus histiocytosis have been observed in children with the acquired immune deficiency syndrome. Specimens also showed piecemeal necrosis, nonsuppurative cholangitis, and endotheliitis.[10] In immune-competent hosts with cytomegalovirus hepatitis, specimens often show features of mononucleosis and fail to display inclusion bodies or viral antigen.[11]

Unresolved Viral Hepatitis

Comments: The duration of the disease is more than 1 month but less than 6 months. Causative viruses are the same as in acute viral hepatitis.

Morphologic features: The findings may be the same as those in acute viral hepatitis. If the condition is resolving, the lobular inflammation tends to be milder. Presence of bridging necrosis or multilobular (confluent) necrosis suggests progressive disease, particularly in old patients. If a biopsy specimen shows severe piecemeal necrosis, tongue-shaped proliferations of periportal fibroblasts, abundant plasma cells and lymphocytes in lobules and portal tracts, formation of lymphoid follicles in portal tracts, or nonsuppurative cholangitis, one should consider possible progression to chronic active hepatitis; this appears less likely in the absence of these features. Many patients with these changes appear to have hepatitis C with early-onset chronic active hepatitis. Presence of stainable hepatitis B virus antigens also may herald chronicity. For further discussions of prognostic features, see references 12 to 16. Viral hepatitis A may relapse but generally does not become chronic. The inflammation is lobular in most protracted cases and cholestasis may be prominent.[17]

Table 3.2   Drugs That May Cause Lobular Hepatitis*

Generic or Chemical Name	Product Classification
Aminosalicylic acid	Antituberculotic
Amitriptyline hydrochloride	Antidepressant
Aspirin	Analgesic, anti-inflammatory, and antipyretic
Carbenicillin indanyl sodium	Antibiotic
Dantrolene sodium	Skeletal muscle relaxant
Diclofenac[18]	Anti-inflammatory
Disopyramide phosphate	Antiarrhythmic
Disulfiram	For the treatment of chronic alcoholism
Enflurane	Inhalation anesthetic
Halothane	Inhalation anesthetic
Hydralazine hydrochloride	Antihypertensive
Hydrochlorothiazide	Diuretic
Isoniazid	Antituberculotic
Ketoconazole	Antifungal agent
Lergotrile mesylate	Antiparkinsonian: ergot derivative
Mercaptopurine	Antineoplastic
Methimazole	Antithyroid agent
Methoxsalen	Antipsoriatic
Methoxyflurane	Inhalation anesthetic
Methyldopa	Antihypertensive
Nicotinic acid	Nutrient vitamin
Nitrofurantoin	Urinary antibiotic
Papaverine hydrochloride	Vasodilator
Penicillin	Antibiotic
Phenazopyridine hydrochloride	Urinary analgesic
Phenylbutazone	Anti-inflammatory
Phenytoin sodium	Anticonvulsant
Propranolol[19]	Antihypertensive
Sulfasalazine	Antibiotic
Sulfonamide(s), type unspecified	Antibiotic
Tranylcypromine sulfate	Antidepressant
Trimethadione	Anticonvulsant

*This list does not include drugs that are unavailable in the United States. For further information, see reference 20.

References

1. Arankalle VA, Tichehurst J, Sreenivasan MA, et al: Aetiological association of a virus-like particle with enterically transmitted non-A, non-B hepatitis. *Lancet* 1:550-553, 1988.

2. Lefkowitch JH, Apfelbaum TF: Non-A, non-B hepatitis: Characterization of liver biopsy pathology. *J Clin Gastroenterol* 11:225-232, 1989.

3. Lefkowitch JH, Goldstein H, Yatto R, et al: Cytopathic liver injury in acute delta virus hepatitis. *Gastroenterology* 92:1262-1266, 1987.

4. Fagan EA, Williams R: Non-A, non-B hepatitis. *Semin Liv Dis* 4:314-335, 1984.

5. Ludwig J: Morphology of chronic active hepatitis: Differential diagnosis and therapeutic implications. In Czaja AJ, Dickson ER (eds): *Chronic Active Hepatitis: The Mayo Clinic Experience*. New York, Marcel Dekker, Inc, 1986.

6. Liaw Y-F, Chu C-M, Chen T-J, et al: Chronic lobular hepatitis: A clinicopathological and prognostic study. *Hepatology* 2:258-262, 1982.

7. Liaw Y-F, Sheen I-S, Chu C-M, et al: Chronic hepatitis with nonspecific histological changes: Is it a distinct variant of chronic hepatitis? *Liver* 4:55-60, 1984.

8. Christoffersen P, Poulsen H, Skeie E: Focal liver cell necroses accompanied by infiltration of granulocytes arising during operation. *Acta Hepatosplenologica (Stuttgart)* 17:240-245, 1970.

9. McDonald GSA, Courtney MG: Operation-associated neutrophils in a percutaneous liver biopsy: Effect of prior transjugular procedure. *Histopathology* 10:217-222, 1986.

10. Duffy LF, Daum F, Kahn E, et al: Hepatitis in children with acquired immune deficiency syndrome: Histopathologic and immunocytologic features. *Gastroenterology* 90:173-181, 1986.

11. Snover DC, Horwitz CA: Liver disease in cytomegalovirus mononucleosis: A light microscopical and immunoperoxidase study. *Hepatology* 4:408-412, 1984.

12. Boyer JL, Klatskin G: Pattern of necrosis in acute viral hepatitis: Prognostic value of bridging (subacute hepatic necrosis). *N Engl J Med* 283:1063-1071, 1970.

13. Morphologic criteria in viral hepatitis: Review by an international group. *Lancet* 1:333-337, 1971.

14. Peters RL: Viral hepatitis: A pathologic spectrum. *Am J Med Sci* 270:17-31, 1975.

15. Dietrichson O, Juhl E, Christoffersen P, et al: Acute viral hepatitis: Factors possibly predicting chronic liver disease. *Acta Pathol Microbiol Scand (Sect A)* 8:183-188, 1975.

16. Bianchi L: Histopathology of viral hepatitis. *Prog Clin Biol Res* 143:66-76, 1983.

17. Sciot R, Van Damme B, Desmet VJ: Cholestatic features of hepatitis A. *J Hepatol* 3:172-181, 1986.

18. Iveson TJ, Ryley NG, Kelly PMA, et al: Diclofenac associated hepatitis. *J Hepatol* 10:85-89, 1990.

19. Roschlau G, Baumgarten R, Binus R: Arzneimittelhepatitis durch Propranolol (Obsidan®): Ein Bericht über 3 Fälle. *Z Klin Med* 42, 1985.

20. Ludwig J, Axelson R: Drug effects on the liver: An updated tabular compilation of drugs and drug-related hepatic diseases. *Dig Dis Sci* 28:651-666, 1983.

Chapter 4

Cholestatic Hepatitis

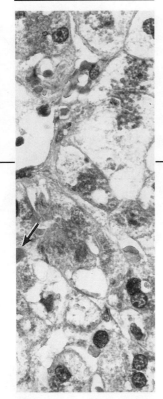

Morphologic Definition

Portal, periportal, or lobular inflammation with much bile pigment (bilirubin) in any location, with or without fatty changes, is present (see also Chapters 5 and 7). Bile can be found in the lumens of ducts, ductules (cholangioles), or bile canaliculi; in hepatocytes or macrophages; or in extravasations (sometimes forming "bile infarcts"). Feathery degeneration and lytic necrosis of hepatocytes often are associated with extravasations of bile.

Table 4.1 Clinical Conditions Associated With Cholestatic Hepatitis*

Without Prominent Fatty Changes
  Acute or unresolved viral hepatitis
  Chronic active hepatitis
  Chronic hepatitis associated with primary sclerosing cholangitis
  Chronic lobular hepatitis
  Chronic nonsuppurative destructive cholangitis (syndrome of primary biliary cirrhosis)
  Drug-induced hepatitis
  Hepatic allograft dysfunction
  Infantile obstructive cholangiopathy
  Massive or submassive hepatic necrosis (any cause)
  Obstruction of large (extrahepatic or perihilar intrahepatic) bile ducts
  Uncommon causes:
    Acute alcoholic cholestasis
    Cholestatic hepatitis associated with total parenteral nutrition
    Congenital hepatic fibrosis and related conditions
    Cystic fibrosis (mucoviscidosis)
    Fibrosing cholestatic hepatitis
    Graft-versus-host disease
    Recurrent intrahepatic cholestasis
    Sarcoidosis
    Sepsis, hemolysis, and shock
With Prominent Fatty Changes (Cholestatic Steatohepatitis)
  Alcoholic hepatitis
  Uncommon causes:
    Cholestatic steatohepatitis associated with total parenteral nutrition
    Genetic (familial) liver diseases
    Wilson's disease

*See also Chapter 5.

Clinical Conditions

Acute Alcoholic Cholestasis

This appears to be a very uncommon disorder in alcoholic patients. The cholestasis is centrilobular. Portal inflammation is minimal and the usual signs of alcoholic liver disease are inconspicuous.[1]

Acute or Unresolved Viral Hepatitis

Comments: For definitions of "acute" vs "unresolved" and for causative viruses, see Chapter 3.

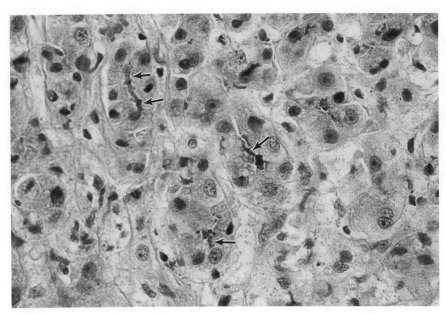

Figure 4.1
Cholestatic (lobular) hepatitis in acute viral hepatitis A. Hepatocanalicular cholestasis (arrows) with hepa-tocellular rosettes is the most prominent finding. Regenerating hepatocytes with prominent nucleoli can be seen adjacent to degenerating hepatocytes with pyknotic nuclei. Scattered inflammatory cells are present also. This is the prototype of cholestatic hepatitis. Note resemblance with Figures 3.1A and 3.1B.

Morphologic features: Cholestatic features are common in these conditions, including protracted hepatitis A (Figure 4.1).[2] Hepatocanalicular cholestasis with rosettes, zone-1 damage, as well as cholangitis and cholangiolitis with degenerative epithelial changes characterize most of hepatitis A cases. For other features of acute viral hepatitis, see Chapter 3.

Alcoholic Hepatitis

Comments: Although clinical evidence of alcohol abuse is needed to confirm the diagnosis, the morphologic features of *cholestatic* alcoholic hepatitis are nearly diagnostic for the condition. Presence of cholestasis worsens the prognosis of alcoholic hepatitis. Nonalcoholic steatohepatitis (Chapter 7) rarely is cholestatic.

Morphologic features: Lobular hepatitis with mixed microvesicular and macrovesicular fatty changes, ballooning of hepatocytes, Mallory bodies, and hepatocanalicular cholestasis (Figure 4.2) are the main features. Focal necroses, neutrophilic inflammatory infiltrates, and phlebosclerosis of hepatic venules are almost always present. Alcoholic hepatitis with cholestasis is often severe. Note: If fatty changes are minimal or absent, nonalcoholic liver diseases must be considered because bile stasis per se may induce the formation of Mallory bodies.

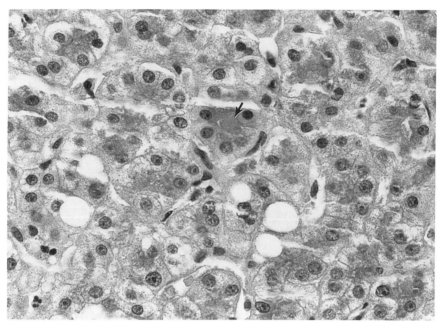

Figure 4.2
Cholestatic steatohepatitis associated with alcoholism (alcoholic hepatitis). Note bile plug in canaliculus (arrow). In severe alcoholic hepatitis, bile pigment may be found in the cytoplasm of hepatocytes, but this feature cannot be illustrated convincingly in black and white.

Cholestatic Hepatitis Associated With Total Parenteral Nutrition

Usually, hepatic abnormalities in this setting are characterized by cholestatic steatohepatitis or steatohepatitis without cholestasis.[3] However, cholestasis with mild hepatitis or pure cholestasis may occur, particularly in infants and children.

Cholestatic Steatohepatitis Associated With Total Parenteral Nutrition

See previous entry.

Chronic Active Hepatitis

Comments: For the definition of "chronic" and for causative viruses or other causes, see Chapter 2.

Morphologic features: Cholestasis is uncommon in chronic active hepatitis and if it is a prominent feature, another diagnosis should be considered. If cholestasis

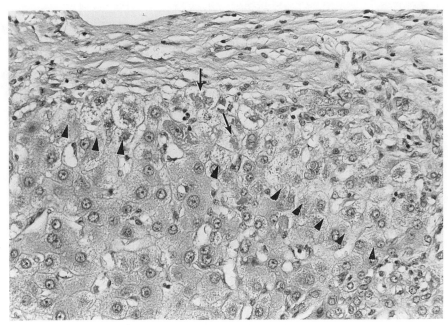

Figure 4.3
Cholestatic hepatitis and biliary cirrhosis associated with primary sclerosing cholangitis. Note hydropic swelling ("feathery degeneration") of paraseptal hepatocytes (arrowheads), which contain bile pigment and minute fragments of Mallory bodies (arrows). These hepatocytes represent cholate stasis and usually contain copper and copper-protein, demonstrable with special stains. The hepatocytes outside the area delineated by arrowheads appear normal. Compare with Figure 4.4.

indeed develops in such patients, they usually have chronic active hepatitis with lobular inflammation (see Chapter 3).

Chronic Hepatitis Associated With Primary Sclerosing Cholangitis

Comments: Clinical and laboratory findings usually reveal chronic cholestatic liver disease. Typical cholangiographic findings confirm the diagnosis. Most patients have chronic ulcerative colitis.

Morphologic features: The biopsy features may be indistinguishable from those seen in the syndrome of primary biliary cirrhosis. However, ductopenia in some portal tracts often is associated with ductal proliferation in other portal tracts. Presence of fibrous-obliterative cholangitis is very suggestive of primary sclerosing cholangitis. Unfortunately, this lesion is not commonly seen. The cholestasis associated with small-duct disease[4] tends to be periportal and paraseptal (Figure 4.3), as observed in the syndrome of primary biliary cirrhosis. If centrilobular

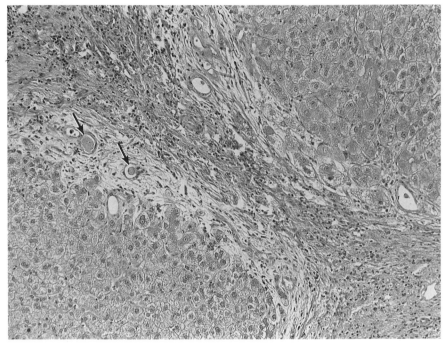

Figure 4.4
Cholestatic hepatitis and biliary cirrhosis in patient with chronic nonsuppurative destructive cholangitis, stage 4 (syndrome of primary biliary cirrhosis). The changes in the paraseptal hepatocytes resemble those seen in primary sclerosing cholangitis (see Figure 4.3). However, in this instance, fibrous and ductular piecemeal necrosis are more prominent, and ductular cholestasis (arrows) is present also.

cholestasis is the predominant feature in a patient with primary sclerosing cholangitis, large-duct disease is the most likely cause, as in patients with dominant strictures or carcinomas (see also Chapter 15).

Chronic Lobular Hepatitis

Comments: For the definition of "chronic" and for causative viruses, see Chapter 3.

Morphologic features: The morphologic changes are the same as those in acute or unresolved cholestatic viral hepatitis. Indeed, chronic lobular hepatitis with cholestasis probably represents prolonged unresolved viral hepatitis. An overlap may exist between chronic active hepatitis with cholestasis and cholestatic lobular hepatitis.

Chronic Nonsuppurative Destructive Cholangitis (Syndrome of Primary Biliary Cirrhosis)

Comments: Clinical and laboratory findings usually reveal chronic cholestatic liver disease. High titers of antimitochondrial antibodies are characteristic.

Morphologic features: Cholestasis rarely is a prominent feature in the precirrhotic stages 1 and 2 (see Chapters 1 and 2). If cholestasis does occur, bile droplets are found primarily in ballooned periportal and paraseptal hepatocytes. The ballooning (cholate stasis) often is associated with accumulation of copper (Chapter 14) and appearance of Mallory bodies (Chapter 12).[5] Ductopenia is almost always present. The changes may be indistinguishable from those seen in chronic hepatitis associated with primary sclerosing cholangitis (see that entry). In advanced cases, ductular cholestasis may be observed (Figure 4.4). Centrilobular hepatocanalicular cholestasis in patients with chronic nonsuppurative destructive cholangitis may be caused by superimposed large-duct biliary obstruction.

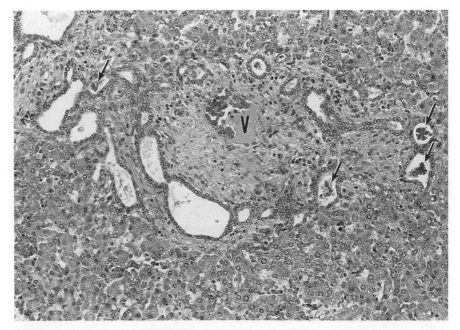

Figure 4.5
Ductular cholestasis in congenital hepatic fibrosis. Some of the hamartomatous ducts at the periphery of the fibrotic portal tract contain bile plugs (arrows). Hepatocanalicular cholestasis is not present and should not be expected in uncomplicated congenital hepatic fibrosis. Note that inflammatory changes are quite mild and that this condition also could be considered an example of pure cholestasis. In this instance, the portal vein (V) is of normal size.

Congenital Hepatic Fibrosis and Related Conditions

If cholestasis is found in this condition (see also Chapter 10), it consists of bile plugs in the cystically dilated ductules (Figure 4.5). Presence of other fibropolycystic liver diseases, for instance, focal dilatation of intrahepatic bile ducts (Caroli's disease), must be considered also. Improper remodeling of the embryonal ductal plate appears to be the common pathogenesis for these conditions.[6]

Cystic Fibrosis (Mucoviscidosis)

This condition is mentioned here only because the characteristic PAS-positive mucoid material in ductules and ducts might be misinterpreted as bile. Neither mucus plugging nor true cholestasis are common features of this condition (see also Chapter 11).[7]

Drug-Induced Hepatitis

Comments: The diagnosis can be suggested if an appropriate history has been provided. For a list of drugs that may cause cholestatic hepatitis, see Table 4.2. Cholestatic hepatitis appears to be the most common hepatic manifestation of adverse drug effects.

Morphologic features: Helpful morphologic features have not been described. Drugs such as chlorpromazine may cause histologic changes that are virtually indistinguishable from those seen in large-duct biliary obstruction.

Fibrosing Cholestatic Hepatitis

Comments: This condition represents recurrent and rapidly progressive hepatitis B infection in hepatic allografts. Host-virus interaction and immunosuppression are possible causes.[8]

Morphologic features: The lobules show prominent hepatocanalicular cholestasis, many groundglass hepatocytes, hepatocellular ballooning and dropout, mild mixed inflammatory infiltrates, and presence of abundant hepatitis B core and surface antigens in hepatocytes. In addition to the cholestasis, the name-giving feature is extensive, serpiginous periportal and perisinusoidal fibrosis with ductular transformation of hepatic cell plates.

Genetic (Familial) Liver Diseases

Cholestasis and fatty change occur in several conditions within this group of diseases (see Chapters 6 and 7).

Graft-Versus-Host Disease

Although cholestasis is not an obligatory feature of this condition, bile may be

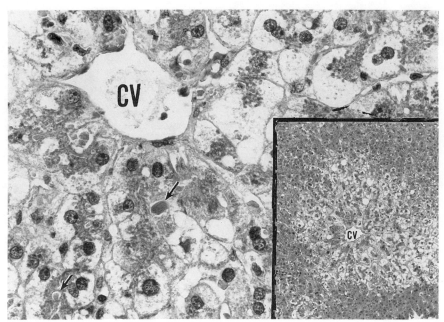

Figure 4.6
Cholestasis in hepatic allograft dysfunction ("functional cholestasis"). Note severe swelling ("feathery degeneration") of hepatocytes in zones 2 and 3, associated with hepatocanalicular cholestasis (arrows). CV, central vein or terminal hepatic vein. Inset: Low-power view of same condition. Although the degenerative changes are severe, inflammatory cells are scarce. Therefore, the condition also could be considered an example of pure cholestasis.

present in centrilobular hepatocytes, together with destructive bile duct changes (see also Chapter 15).[9]

Hepatic Allograft Dysfunction

Cholestatic hepatitis or pure cholestasis (Figure 4.6) in the first days or weeks after orthotopic liver transplantation may be an adaptive response with a good prognosis ("functional cholestasis").[10] However, most other forms of allograft damage can be associated with cholestasis. Indeed, severe cellular or ductopenic ("chronic") rejection rarely occurs without associated cholestasis.[10]

Infantile Obstructive Cholangiopathy

Comments: Conjugated hyperbilirubinemia in a neonate or infant is the lead symptom. A multitude of genetic diseases and other extrahepatic conditions may be associated with infantile obstructive cholangiopathy.[11,12] The condition includes

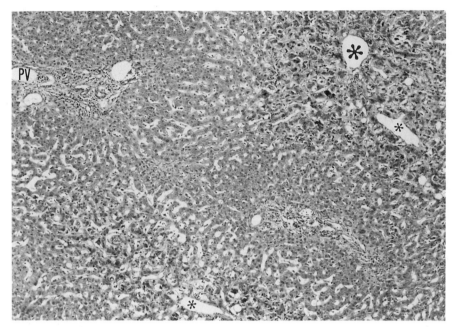

Figure 4.7A
Cholestatic hepatitis in obstruction of large bile ducts. Even in this low-power illustration, the severe hepatocanalicular cholestasis in zones 2 and 3 is clearly visible. The central veins (asterisks) can be identified in the areas of cholestasis. Two edematous portal tracts can be identified. PV, portal vein. See also Figure 2.5.

---

choledochal cysts (not all cases), biliary atresia, paucity of intrahepatic bile ducts, and neonatal hepatitis.

Morphologic features: Cholestasis may be present in ducts, ductules, bile canaliculi, or hepatocytes. In biliary atresia (large-duct disease), biopsy features are those of obstruction of large-duct bile ducts (see below). In paucity of intrahepatic bile ducts (syndromatic or nonsyndromatic[13]), ductopenia predominates, and in neonatal hepatitis, hepatocellular giant cells are the most prominent feature. However, these disease entities and the accompanying histologic features overlap, hence the name "infantile obstructive cholangiopathy."[12] For instance, hepatocellular giant cells may accompany paucity of intrahepatic bile ducts, or ductopenia may appear after the features of neonatal hepatitis ("giant cell hepatitis") have receded. Ductopenia also may complicate extrahepatic biliary atresia. Thus, in all cases of suspected infantile obstructive cholangiopathy, hepatic artery branches should be identified in portal tracts and used as landmarks for duct counts. At least 7 of 10 artery branches should be accompanied by a bile duct.[14] Ductular proliferation (Chapter 15) should be disregarded for these counts. Presence of alpha-1-antitrypsin deficiency (see also Chapter 12) also must be expected in some of these cases.

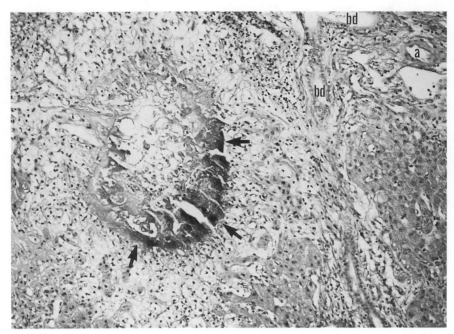

Figure 4.7B
Cholestatic hepatitis in obstruction of large bile ducts. Bile infarct is adjacent to edematous portal tract (a, artery; bd, bile duct). The "infarct" consists of pale, swollen macrophages and contains remnants of bile pigment (arrows). This pigment disappears comparatively early and many bile infarcts do not show it. See also Figures 15.5A, 15.5B, and 15.5C.

Massive or Submassive Hepatic Necrosis (Any Cause)

Regardless of cause (usually viral hepatitis or drug-induced), cholestasis may be a prominent morphologic feature (see also Chapter 9).

Obstruction of Large (Extrahepatic or Perihilar Intrahepatic) Bile Ducts

Comments: Patients have clinical and biochemical evidence of cholestatic liver disease. Biopsy often is done because of negative cholangiographic or ultrasound studies and because parenchymal liver disease is suspected.

Morphologic features: Portal edema with proliferation of ducts and ductules as well as centrilobular hepatocanalicular cholestasis (Figure 4.7A) are the most characteristic findings. Bile lakes and bile infarcts (Figure 4.7B) are rarely encountered, but when these lesions are present, large-duct biliary obstruction usually can be diagnosed with confidence. Ductal proliferation is a more important feature than ductular proliferation; the latter feature is quite nonspecific (see Chapter 15).

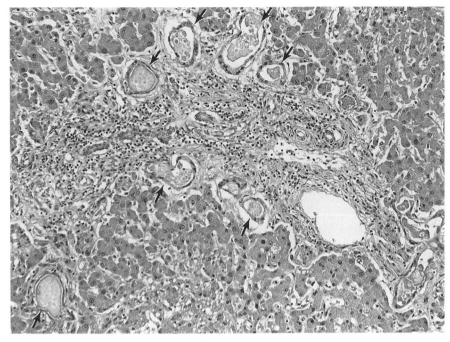

Figure 4.8
Periportal canalicular cholestasis in a patient with septic shock. Canaliculi (arrows) are distended by bile plugs (ductular cholestasis). Mild nonspecific hepatitis is present also.

Inflammatory infiltrates usually are mild and neutrophils often predominate. For neutrophilic or fibrous cholangitis and for periductal fibrosis see Chapter 15. If large-duct biliary obstruction persists, portal fibrosis begins to predominate and ductal proliferation diminishes; even ductopenia may become a feature. In rare instances, obstructive biliary cirrhosis (see Chapter 11) develops within a few months.

Recurrent Intrahepatic Cholestasis

The histologic changes often are indistinguishable from obstruction of large bile ducts (see above). In other instances, portal changes are minimal or absent and pure cholestasis (Chapter 5) appears to prevail. The clinical history is characteristic.[15] An association appears to exist with intrahepatic cholestasis of pregnancy.[16]

Sarcoidosis

In chronic intrahepatic cholestasis of sarcoidosis, biochemical signs of cholestasis are always present, but morphologically cholestasis rarely is a prominent feature. Presence of granulomatous cholangitis (see Chapter 15) is the only diagnostic abnormality.

Sepsis, Hemolysis, and Shock

Cholestasis is common in sepsis and shock, with or without hemolysis. However, the condition is seen more often in autopsy material than in biopsy specimens. In most instances, the cholestasis involves ductules in the periphery of portal tracts (ductular cholestasis), together with reactive nonspecific portal inflammation.[17] Centrilobular and midzonal hepatocanalicular cholestasis may occur also (Figure 4.8).[18] The cholestasis in the hemolytic uremic syndrome and leptospirosis probably is related to the conditions described here.

Wilson's Disease

Steatosis and steatohepatitis are common in Wilson's disease, but this disease usually is not associated with cholestasis. In fulminant Wilson's disease or in late stages of nonfulminant Wilson's disease, cholestasis may be present, but usually without associated fatty change.[19]

Table 4.2 Drugs That May Cause Cholestatic Hepatitis*

Generic or Chemical Name	Product Classification
Acetaminophen	Analgesic and antipyretic
Acetohexamide	Oral hypoglycemic
Allopurinol	Antihyperuricemic
Aminosalicylic acid	Antituberculotic
Amitriptyline hydrochloride	Antidepressant
Amoxicillin-clavulanic acid[20]	Antibiotic
Aprindine	Antiarrhythmic
Atenolol[21]	Antihypertensive: beta-blocking agent
Azathioprine	Immunosuppressant
Captopril[22]	Antihypertensive
Carbamazepine	Anticonvulsant
Carbarsone	Amebicide
Carbimazole	Antithyroid
Carisoprodol	Skeletal muscle relaxant
Cefadroxil monohydrate	Antibiotic
Cefazolin sodium	Antibiotic
Chlorambucil	Antineoplastic
Chlordiazepoxide	Sedative and hypnotic: benzodiazepine
Chlorothiazide	Diuretic
Chlorpromazine	Tranquilizer: phenothiazine

continued on page 44

continued from page 43

Generic or Chemical Name	Product Classification
Chlorpropamide	Oral hypoglycemic
Chlortetracycline	Antibiotic
Chlorthalidone	Diuretic
Cimetidine	H_2 receptor antagonist
Cisplatin	Antineoplastic
Clorazepate dipotassium	Sedative and hypnotic: benzodiazepine
Cyclosporine[23]	Immunosuppressant
Dacarbazine	Antineoplastic
Dantrolene sodium	Skeletal muscle relaxant
Diazepam	Sedative and hypnotic: benzodiazepine
Diclofenac[24]	Anti-inflammatory
Disopyramide phosphate	Antiarrhythmic
Enalapril[25]	Antihypertensive
Erythromycin	Antibiotic
Ethchlorvynol	Hypnotic
Ethionamide	Antituberculotic
Fluoxymesterone	Androgen
Fluphenazine	Tranquilizer: phenothiazine
Flurazepam hydrochloride	Sedative and hypnotic: benzodiazepine
Flutamide[26]	Antiandrogenic
Gold sodium thiomalate	Antarthritic
Griseofulvin	Antifungal antibiotic
Haloperidol	Antipsychotic
Halothane	Inhalation anesthetic
Imipramine	Antidepressant
Indomethacin	Anti-inflammatory
Iodipamide meglumine	Roentgen contrast medium
Isocarboxazid	Antidepressant
Isoniazid	Antituberculotic
Lisinopril (see also Table 9.2)	Antihypertensive
Meprobamate	Tranquilizer
Mercaptopurine	Antineoplastic
Methyldopa	Antihypertensive
Nicotinic acid	Nutrient vitamin
Nifedipine[27]	Calcium channel blocker
Nitrofurantoin	Urinary antibiotic
Oxacillin	Antibiotic
Papaverine hydrochloride	Vasodilator
Penicillamine	Antirheumatic: chelating agent
Penicillin	Antibiotic
Perphenazine	Tranquilizer: phenothiazine
Phenobarbital	Anticonvulsant: barbiturate

continued on page 45

continued from page 44

Generic or Chemical Name	Product Classification
Phenylbutazone	Anti-inflammatory
Phenytoin sodium	Anticonvulsant
Piperazine preparations	Anthelmintic
Piroxicam[28]	Antarthritic
Pizotyline[29]	Tranquilizer: phenothiazine
Polythiazide	Diuretic
Prochlorperazine	Tranquilizer: phenothiazine
Propoxyphene hydrochloride	Analgesic
Quinethazone	Diuretic
Rifampin	Antituberculotic
Sulfamethoxazole[†]	Antibiotic
Sulfasalazine	Antibiotic
Sulfonamide(s), type unspecified	Antibiotic
Sulindac	Anti-inflammatory
Thiabendazole	Anthelmintic
Thiopental sodium	Hypnotic: barbiturate
Thioridazine	Tranquilizer: phenothiazine
Tolazamide	Oral hypoglycemic
Tolbutamide	Oral hypoglycemic
Tranylcypromine sulfate	Antidepressant
Triazolam	Hypnotic: benzodiazepine
Trifluoperazine hydrochloride	Tranquilizer: phenothiazine
Trimethobenzamide hydrochloride	Antinauseant
Trimethoprim[†]	Antibiotic
Tripelennamine	Antihistamine
Troleandomycin[30]	Antibiotic
Valproic acid	Anticonvulsant
Verapamil hydrochloride[31]	Vasodilator

*This list does not include drugs that are unavailable in the United States. For further information, see reference 32.

†Also in combination as trimethoprim-sulfamethoxazole.[33]

References

1. Glover SC, McPhie JL, Brunt PW: Cholestasis in acute alcoholic liver disease. *Lancet* 1:1305-1307, 1977.

2. Sciot R, Van Damme B, Desmet VJ: Cholestatic features in hepatitis A. *J Hepatol* 3:172-181, 1986.

3. Klein S, Nealon WH: Hepatobiliary abnormalities associated with total parenteral nutrition. *Semin Liver Dis* 8:237-246, 1988.

4. Ludwig J: Small-duct primary sclerosing cholangitis. *Semin Liver Dis* 11:11-17, 1991.

5. Dickson ER, Fleming CR, Ludwig J: Primary biliary cirrhosis. *Prog Liver Dis* 6:487-502, 1976.

6. Desmet VJ: Intrahepatic bile ducts under the lens. *J Hepatol* 1:545-559, 1985.

7. Gaskin KJ, Waters DLM, Howman-Giles R, et al: Liver disease and common-bile-duct stenosis in cystic fibrosis. *N Engl J Med* 318:340-346, 1988.

8. Davies SE, Portmann BC, O'Grady JG, et al: Hepatic histological findings after transplantation for chronic hepatitis B virus infection, including a unique pattern of fibrosing cholestatic hepatitis. *Hepatology* 13:150-157, 1991.

9. Shulman HM, Sharma P, Amos D, et al: A coded histologic study of hepatic graft-versus-host disease after human bone marrow transplantation. *Hepatology* 8:463-470, 1988.

10. Demetris AJ, Jaffe R, Starzl TE: A review of adult and pediatric posttransplant liver pathology. *Pathol Annu* 22(II):347-386, 1987.

11. Balistreri WF: Neonatal cholestasis: Lessons from the past, issues for the future. *Semin Liver Dis* 7:1987 (Foreword).

12. Landing BH: Considerations of the pathogenesis of neonatal hepatitis, biliary atresia and choledochal cyst: The concept of infantile obstructive cholangiopathy. *Prog Pediatr Surg* 6:113-139, 1974.

13. Riely CA: Familial intrahepatic cholestatic syndromes. *Semin Liver Dis* 7:119-133, 1987.

14. Nakanuma Y, Ohta G: Histometric and serial section observations of the intrahepatic bile ducts in primary biliary cirrhosis. *Gastroenterology* 76:1326-1332, 1979.

15. Bijleveld CMA, Vonk RJ, Kuipers F, et al: Benign recurrent intrahepatic cholestasis: A long-term follow-up study of two patients. *Hepatology* 9:532-537, 1989.

16. DePagter AGF, van Berge Henegouwen GP, ten Bokkel Huinink JA, et al: Familial benign recurrent intrahepatic cholestasis: Interrelation with intrahepatic cholestasis of pregnancy and from oral contraceptives? *Gastroenterology* 71:202-207, 1976.

17. Lefkowitch JH: Bile ductular cholestasis: An ominous histopathologic sign related to sepsis and "cholangitis lenta." *Hum Pathol* 13:19-24, 1982.

18. Zimmerman HJ, Fang M, Utili R, et al: Jaundice due to bacterial infection. *Gastroenterology* 77:362-365, 1979.

19. Stromeyer FW, Ishak KG: Histology of the liver in Wilson's disease: A study of 34 cases. *Am J Clin Pathol* 73:12-24, 1980.

20. Michielsen PP, van Outryve MJ, van Marck EA, et al: Amoxycillin/clavulanic acid induced cholestasis. *J Hepatol* 11:392, 1990.

21. Schwartz MS, Frank MS, Yanoff A, et al: Atenolol-associated cholestasis. *Am J Gastroenterol* 84:1084-1086, 1989.

22. Rahmat J, Gelfand RL, Gelfand MC, et al: Captopril-associated cholestatic jaundice. *Ann Intern Med* 102:56-58, 1985.

23. Kahan BD, Flechner SM, Lorber MI, et al: Complications of cyclosporin therapy. *World J Surg* 10:348-360, 1986.

24. Iveson TJ, Ryley NG, Kelly PMA, et al: Diclofenac associated hepatitis. *J Hepatol* 10:85-89, 1990.

25. Rosellini SR, Costa PL, Gaudio M, et al: Hepatic injury related to enalapril. *Gastroenterology* 97:810-812, 1989.

26. Møller S, Iverson P, Franzmann M-B: Flutamide-induced liver failure. *J Hepatol* 10:346-349, 1990.

27. Babany G, Uzzan F, Larrey D, et al: Alcoholic-like liver lesions induced by nifedipine. *J Hepatol* 9:252-255, 1989.

28. Hepps K, Maliha G, Estrada R, et al: Severe cholestatic jaundice associated with piroxicam. *Gastroenterology* 101:1737-1740, 1991.

29. Coodley EL, Muro J, Sato RI: Pizotyline-induced cholestatic jaundice. *Arch Intern Med* 144:815-817, 1984.

30. Larrey D, Amouyal G, Danan G, et al: Prolonged cholestasis after troleandomycine-induced acute hepatitis. *J Hepatol* 4:327-329, 1987.

31. Burgunder J-M, Abernethy DR, Lauterburg BH: Liver injury due to verapamil. *Hepatogastroenterology* 35:169-170, 1988.

32. Ludwig J, Axelson R: Drug effects on the liver: An updated tabular compilation of drugs and drug-related hepatic diseases. *Dig Dis Sci* 28:651-666, 1983.

33. Muñoz SJ, Martinez-Hernandez A, Maddrey WC: Intrahepatic cholestasis and phospholipidosis associated with the use of trimethoprim-sulfamethoxazole. *Hepatology* 12:342-347, 1990.

Chapter 5

Pure Cholestasis

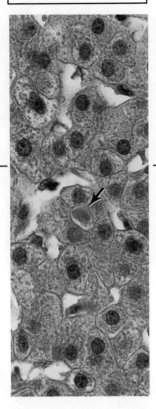

Morphologic Definition

Bile pigment (bilirubin) in hepatic tissue without other morphologic abnormalities or only minimal other changes in portal tracts and lobules is present. The bile pigment usually is found in centrilobular canaliculi. Note: Most conditions with ductular cholestasis are listed in Chapter 4, although the inflammatory changes sometimes are inconspicuous. A clear distinction between cholestatic hepatitis and pure cholestasis is not always possible. For other pigments, see Chapters 13 and 14.

Table 5.1   Clinical Conditions Associated With Pure Cholestasis*

Cholestasis of pregnancy
Drug-induced cholestasis
Uncommon causes:
    Amyloidosis
    Benign postoperative intrahepatic cholestasis
    Cholestasis associated with total parenteral nutrition
    Congenital hepatic fibrosis
    Hepatocellular tumors
    Inspissated bile syndrome
    Lymphoma
    Progressive intrahepatic cholestasis (Byler's disease) and other familial
      intrahepatic cholestatic syndromes
    Recurrent intrahepatic cholestasis
    Sepsis, hemolysis, and shock

*See also Chapter 4.

Clinical Conditions

Amyloidosis

Cholestasis is an uncommon complication of hepatic amyloidosis. The amyloid deposition is the crucial diagnostic finding; it may be more severe in periportal areas, whereas the cholestasis usually is centrilobular. However, centrilobular amyloid and cholestasis may occur together.[1] Exclusive vascular involvement in amyloidosis is not a cause of cholestasis. See also Chapter 14.

Benign Postoperative Intrahepatic Cholestasis

In this condition, transient cholestasis usually occurs within 48 hours after major operations, probably as a result of hepatic bilirubin overload after hemolysis or resorption of hematomas.[2] Centrilobular hepatocanalicular cholestasis is present, with or without evidence of liver cell damage, spotty necrosis, and mild portal inflammation. Kupffer cell erythrophagocytosis and, later, Kupffer cell hemosiderosis are found in some cases.

Cholestasis Associated With Total Parenteral Nutrition

This condition also may occur with cholestatic hepatitis (see Chapter 4) or steatohepatitis (see Chapters 4 and 7).

Cholestasis of Pregnancy

Comments: Cholestasis of pregnancy occurs primarily in the third trimester and disappears postpartum; colicky pain is absent. The condition often is recurrent and may be familial[3]; an association appears to exist with recurrent intrahepatic cholestasis (see below) and with cholestasis after use of oral contraceptives.

Morphologic features: Centrilobular hepatocanalicular cholestasis is the only abnormality in most instances. However, mild portal hepatitis and some Kupffer cell proliferation may be present also.

Congenital Hepatic Fibrosis

The characteristic changes are described and illustrated in Chapter 4.

Drug-Induced Cholestasis

Comments: Although an appropriate clinical history is required for the diagnosis, pure cholestasis should be considered drug-induced unless another diagnosis appears more likely. Information about previous use of steroid-type drugs is not always volunteered. For a list of drugs that may cause pure cholestasis, see Table 5.2.

Morphologic features: Diffuse or centrilobular canalicular cholestasis without appreciable other abnormalities is the most common finding.

Hepatocellular Tumors

Hepatocellular carcinomas and liver cell adenomas may show bile formation. In rare instances, the neoplastic nature of these lesions is not obvious. Of course, tumors also may cause obstructive cholestasis.

Inspissated Bile Syndrome

The pathogenesis of this pediatric condition may resemble that of cholestasis in sepsis, hemolysis, and shock (see Chapter 4) as well as that of benign postoperative intrahepatic cholestasis (see above). The cholestasis is centrilobular and canalicular. Kupffer cell hemosiderosis may be present also.

Lymphoma

Cholestasis may occur as a paraneoplastic syndrome in patients with extrahepatic Hodgkin's lymphoma[4] but also in some instances of non-Hodgkin's lym-

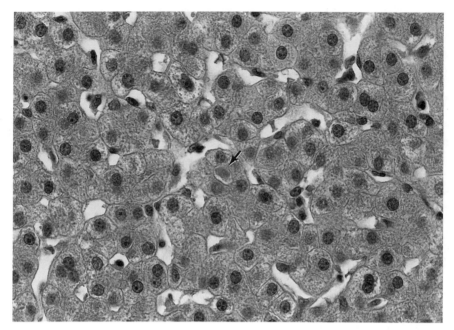

Figure 5.1
Recurrent intrahepatic cholestasis. Note canalicular cholestasis (arrow) in the absence of appreciable hepatocellular changes.

phoma.[5] Obviously, patients with intrahepatic lymphoma or lymphoma in the hepatoduodenal ligament also may develop cholestasis as a result of large-duct biliary obstruction (see Chapter 4). The distinction between these two completely unrelated conditions cannot always be made by histologic study alone. The paraneoplastic cholestasis as well as the obstructive cholestasis in lymphoma tend to be canalicular and centrilobular. However, portal changes usually are minimal or absent in paraneoplastic cholestasis.

Progressive Intrahepatic Cholestasis (Byler's Disease) and Other Familial Intrahepatic Cholestatic Syndromes

Most patients with these syndromes are in the pediatric age group. In addition to Byler's disease, syndromatic (Alagille's syndrome) and nonsyndromatic paucity of intrahepatic bile ducts, Norwegian cholestasis and North American Indian cholestasis must be considered here.[6] Most other familial pediatric liver diseases that may present with cholestasis have additional morphologic features. Examples are alpha-1-antitrypsin deficiency (Chapter 12), cystic fibrosis (Chapter 16), Niemann-Pick lipidosis, galactosemia, and others. However, in Byler's disease[7] and related disorders, centrilobular hepatocanalicular cholestasis may be the leading feature in early stages.

Recurrent Intrahepatic Cholestasis

This condition is described in Chapter 4, because mild inflammatory and ductal changes are often observed. However, pure cholestasis also may be present (Figure 5.1).

Sepsis, Hemolysis, and Shock

The characteristic changes are described and illustrated in Chapter 4.

Table 5.2 Drugs That May Cause Pure Cholestasis*

Generic or Chemical Name	Product Classification
Ethchlorvynol	Hypnotic
Fluoxymesterone	Androgen
Gold sodium thiomalate	Antarthritic
Mestranol	Oral contraceptive
Methandrostenolone	Androgen
Methyltestosterone	Androgen
Norethindrone	Oral contraceptive
Norethynodrel	Oral contraceptive
Norgestrel	Oral contraceptive
Piroxicam[a]	Anti-inflammatory
Prochlorperazine	Tranquilizer: phenothiazine
Warfarin sodium	Anticoagulant

*This list does not include drugs that are unavailable in the United States. For further information, see reference 9.

References

1. Finkelstein SD, Fornasier VL, Pruzanski W: Intrahepatic cholestasis with predominant pericentral deposition in systemic amyloidosis. *Hum Pathol* 12:470-472, 1981.

2. LaMont JT, Isselbacher KJ: Postoperative jaundice. *N Engl J Med* 288:305-307, 1973.

3. Holzbach RT, Sivak DA, Braun WE: Familial recurrent intrahepatic cholestasis of pregnancy: A genetic study providing evidence for transmission of a sex-linked, dominant trait. *Gastroenterology* 85:175-179, 1983.

4. Lieberman DA: Intrahepatic cholestasis due to Hodgkin's disease: An elusive diagnosis. *J Clin Gastroenterol* 8:304-307, 1986.

5. Watterson J, Priest JR: Jaundice as a paraneoplastic phenomenon in a T-cell lymphoma. *Gastroenterology* 97:1319-1322, 1989.

6. Riely CA: Familial intrahepatic cholestatic syndromes. *Semin Liv Dis* 7:119-133, 1987.

7. De Vos R, De Wolf-Peters C, Desmet V, et al: Progressive intrahepatic cholestasis (Byler's disease): Case report. *Gut* 16:943-950, 1975.

8. Caballeria E, Masso RM, Arago JV, et al: Piroxicam hepatotoxicity. *Am J Gastroenterol* 85:898-899, 1990.

9. Ludwig J, Axelson R: Drug effects on the liver: An updated tabular compilation of drugs and drug-related hepatic diseases. *Dig Dis Sci* 28:651-666, 1983.

Chapter 6

Fatty Changes

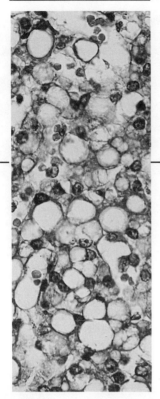

Morphologic Definition

Triglycerides and other lipids in cytoplasmic vacuoles of hepatocytes or lipocytes (Ito cells) are present. If the vacuoles of the hepatocytes are large enough to displace the nuclei, *macrovesicular* fatty changes are present. If the vacuoles are small, leaving the nuclei in their normal position, *microvesicular* fatty changes should be diagnosed. Fatty changes may be diffuse, zonal (in relation to the hepatic lobules), or focal. Frozen sections stained with Sudan IV or another fat stain may be required for the diagnosis, particularly of microvesicular fatty change.

Table 6.1 Clinical Conditions Associated With Fatty Changes

With Macrovesicular or Mixed Microvesicular and Macrovesicular Fatty Changes
   Alcoholic fatty liver
   Focal fatty change (nonalcoholic)
   Nonalcoholic fatty liver (nonalcoholic steatosis of the liver) associated with diabetes
      mellitus, obesity, and many other conditions
With Microvesicular Fatty Changes
   Acute fatty liver of pregnancy
   Alcoholic foamy degeneration (see under "alcoholic fatty liver")
   Drug effects
   Reye's syndrome
   Uncommon causes:
      Heatstroke
      Jamaican vomiting sickness
      Medium-chain and long-chain acyl coenzyme A dehydrogenase deficiency
      Phospholipidoses
      Poisoning by toxic chemicals and bacterial toxins
      Sudden childhood death
      Toxic shock syndrome
      Viral hepatitis D

Clinical Conditions

Acute Fatty Liver of Pregnancy

Comments: Acute fatty liver of pregnancy occurs in the third trimester, usually in a young primigravida, associated with toxemia of pregnancy. Fatalities may occur, but in recent publications survival of most patients was reported.[1]

Morphologic features: Diffuse, uncomplicated microvesicular fatty changes are easy to recognize and near diagnostic in this setting (Figure 6.1). These fatty changes often occur in ballooned hepatocytes, particularly in zones 2 and 3 and early in the course of the disease, together with inflammatory changes, hepatocanalicular cholestasis, and centrilobular endotheliitis (or phlebitis) and necrosis; these features may closely resemble acute viral hepatitis because the fatty changes are often inconspicuous. Therefore, a portion of the specimens should be studied in a frozen section, stained with Sudan IV or another fat stain, whenever this differential diagnosis is under consideration.[2] Extramedullary hematopoiesis and megamitochondria are often present. Electron microscopic studies are particularly useful if frozen sections have not been prepared and if a differential diagnosis with

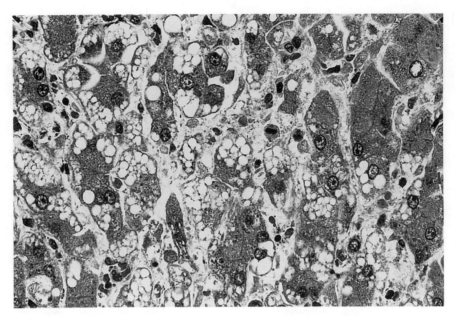

Figure 6.1
Microvesicular fatty changes in patient with acute fatty liver of pregnancy. In this instance, scattered inflammatory changes are present, which would justify the name steatohepatitis, but customarily that term is used only in cases with macrovesicular fatty change, ie, in cases resembling alcoholic hepatitis. Later in the course of fatty liver of pregnancy, the microvesicular fatty changes become inconspicuous.

acute viral hepatitis must be considered. Electron micrographs also allow a morphologic distinction between acute fatty liver of pregnancy and Reye's syndrome[3] (see below).

Alcoholic Fatty Liver

Comments: A history of alcohol abuse or dependence is required for the diagnosis. Most affected patients have hepatomegaly. Acute cholestasis with liver failure,[4] Zieve's syndrome (alcoholic fatty liver with hemolytic anemia, hepatosplenomegaly, and hyperlipidemia), as well as sudden death[5] are possible complications. However, alcoholic fatty liver and alcoholic foamy degeneration (a variant of alcoholic fatty liver)[6] are potentially reversible conditions.

Morphologic features: The macrovesicular fatty change is quite variable but often centrilobular and midzonal (Figure 6.2), or diffuse.[7] Fat cysts and microvesicular fatty changes, lipogranulomas,[7] and cholestasis[4] may be present also. The portal tracts are normal or only minimally inflamed. They sometimes contain lipid. If the inflammatory lesions of alcoholic hepatitis are present (see Chapter 7), the diagnosis "alcoholic fatty liver" is not appropriate. Nevertheless, presence of megamitochondria (see Chapter 12), a few Mallory bodies, or mild sclerosis of ter-

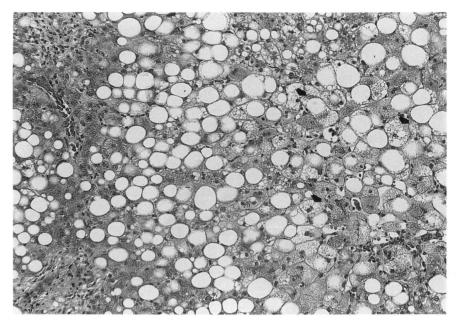

Figure 6.2
Macrovesicular fatty changes in alcoholism. In this instance, fatty changes were primarily in zones 2 and 3. Note that some microvesicular fatty changes (nuclei remain in center of cells) are present also (arrows), a common finding in alcoholic fatty liver.

minal hepatic venules (central veins) is acceptable under this heading. Hepatic vein sclerosis (see Chapter 7) may herald progression of the disease.[8]

A related pattern of alcoholic injury, which has become known under the name "alcoholic foamy degeneration,"[6] consists of microvesicular fatty changes in swollen centrilobular hepatocytes that thus attain a foamy appearance. Bile pigment, megamitochondria, hepatocyte dropout, and perisinusoidal fibrosis are commonly associated features.

Alcoholic Foamy Degeneration

See previous entry.

Drug Effects

An appropriate clinical history is required for the diagnosis. Drugs that may cause macrovesicular or mixed macrovesicular and microvesicular fatty changes (Figure 6.3) are listed in Table 6.2. Drugs that may cause microvesicular fatty changes are listed in Table 6.3. For microvesicular fatty changes in cocaine hepatitis, see Chapter 9.

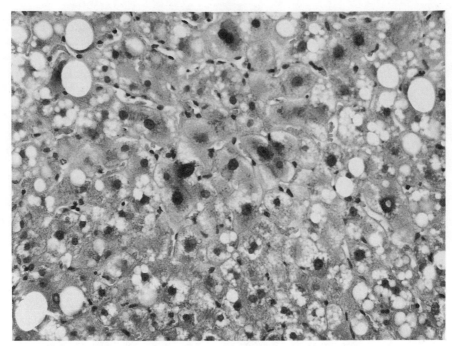

Figure 6.3
Mixed macrovesicular and microvesicular fatty change after methotrexate treatment. Note hyperchroma-
tism and pyknosis of many hepatocellular nuclei; this is a rather characteristic effect of methotrexate.
Kupffer cells are proliferated, and thus some overlap with steatohepatitis is present.

Focal Fatty Change (Nonalcoholic)

Comments: Single or multiple well-defined hepatic lesions are demonstrated
on computed tomographic (CT) scans and sonograms, revealing features that suggest metastatic malignancy. Radionuclide scans may suggest fatty change, and
ultrasound-guided biopsies can confirm the diagnosis.[9] Thus, it is important to
remember that biopsy evidence of fatty change in cases of suspected metastatic
malignancy may reflect the actual lesion, which would obviate further invasive
procedures.

Morphologic features: Macrovesicular fatty changes are found (Figures 6.4A
and 6.4B), sometimes with mild inflammation ("focal steatohepatitis") and an
occasional granuloma. In some instances, the surrounding nonfatty hepatic
parenchyma can be identified.

Heatstroke

Fatty changes occur in fatal exertion heatstroke, together with hemosiderosis

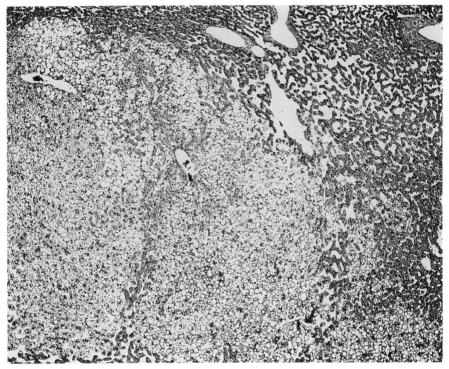

Figure 6.4A
Focal macrovesicular fatty change (nonalcoholic). An overview of the lesion is shown. The surrounding, dark-appearing hepatic parenchyma shows some sinusoidal dilatation but no fatty change.

and congestion, and neutrophilic cholangitis[10] (see Chapter 15), among other lesions. The fatty changes may be microvesicular.[10]

Jamaican Vomiting Sickness

This rare condition occurs in children after consumption of unripe ackee fruits, which contain the toxic agent hypoglycin A.[11] Prominent microvesicular fatty changes occur because hypoglycin A interferes with the mitochondrial oxidation of long-chain fatty acids.

Medium-Chain and Long-Chain Acyl Coenzyme A Dehydrogenase Deficiency

This familial Reye-like syndrome affects infants and young children with an inborn error of intramitochondrial beta-oxidation of fatty acids. The microvesicu-

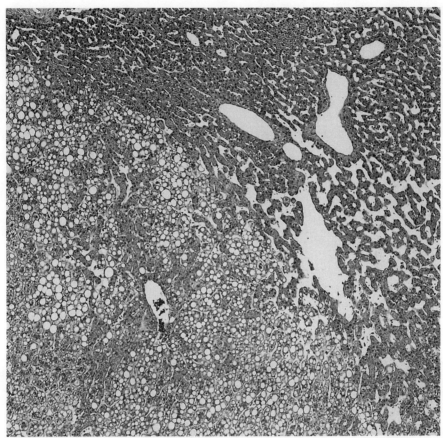

Figure 6.4B
Focal macrovesicular fatty change (nonalcoholic). The macrovesicular fatty changes are clearly identifiable.

lar fatty changes in this condition are not associated with the ultrastructural mitochondrial changes seen in Reye's syndrome.[12]

Nonalcoholic Fatty Liver (Nonalcoholic Steatosis of the Liver)

Comments: A *negative* history of alcohol abuse is required for the diagnosis of nonalcoholic fatty liver (nonalcoholic steatosis of the liver). Hepatomegaly may be present but many other possible complications of alcoholic fatty liver, such as Zieve's syndrome (see above under "Alcoholic Fatty Liver"), are not features of nonalcoholic fatty liver. Clinicopathologic correlations are particularly important for the interpretation of these cases. Possible causes of nonalcoholic fatty liver include the following conditions:

1. Diabetes mellitus (adult-onset)
2. Drug effects (see also Table 6.2)
3. Exposure to occupational and domestic hepatotoxic chemicals; bacterial toxins
4. Gastrointestinal and pancreatic disorders; malabsorption and malnutrition
5. Genetic (familial) liver diseases
6. Hypoxia
7. Obesity
8. Total parenteral nutrition
9. Unknown causes

Obesity and diabetes mellitus undoubtedly are the most common conditions associated with nonalcoholic fatty liver. For further details, see also under "Nonalcoholic Steatohepatitis" (Chapter 7).

Morphologic features: Principally, nonalcoholic fatty changes do not differ from alcoholic fatty liver. As a group, specimens from nonalcoholic patients more often have exclusively or predominantly macrovesicular fatty changes, without any complicating lesions such as microvesicular fatty change or features of foamy degeneration, lipogranulomas, or phlebosclerosis of terminal hepatic venules.

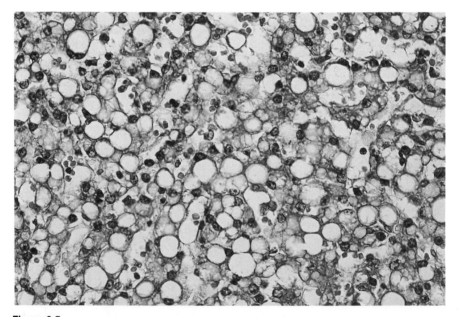

Figure 6.5
Diffuse macrovesicular fatty changes in a newborn with galactosemia. This genetic disease is one of the many causes of nonalcoholic fatty liver. Periportal ductular proliferation is common but not visible in this illustration. Pseudoglandular change with bile plugs within the acini tends to evolve from the fatty change within a few weeks.

Morphologic features associated with specific etiologies—for instance, obesity, gastrointestinal disorders, or drug effect—usually cannot be discerned. Vacuolated hepatocellular nuclei are common in adult-onset diabetes mellitus but also occur in normal specimens. Hypoxia may cause centrilobular fatty change, usually associated with centrilobular necrosis; and certain toxic substances—for instance, phosphorus—cause periportal fatty change or necrosis. In rare instances, sepsis and bacterial toxins can cause severe fatty changes.[13] For fatty changes in hypervitaminosis A, see Chapter 16. In protein deficiency (kwashiorkor), fatty changes also involve periportal regions, at least initially. Severe weight loss and cachectic states in North American patients generally are not associated with steatosis. In patients who had total parenteral nutrition, hepatic fatty changes often are associated with the deposition of pigments (ceroid, lipofuscin, and sometimes hemosiderin and bile); this combination of findings is unusual in other conditions (see Chapter 14). Fatty changes induced by drugs such as steroids have no specific diagnostic features.

In most genetic diseases, clinical and morphologic features often are suggestive of this disease category or even point toward a specific diagnosis, as in glycogen storage disease, type 1.[14] Wilson's disease is described in Chapters 2, 11, and 14. Other conditions in this group include abetalipoproteinemia, galactosemia (Figure 6.5), fructose intolerance, porphyria cutanea tarda, tyrosinemia, cholesteryl ester storage disease, and Wolman's disease, to name some of them. These diseases are quite rare. They may be complicated by cholestasis, hemosiderosis, and cirrhosis. The cholesterol crystals in cholesteryl ester storage disease and in Wolman's disease can be stained in frozen sections or identified as empty clefts in high-power views of paraffin sections. In porphyria cutanea tarda, the fatty changes are usually associated with hemosiderosis (see Chapter 13). Finally, the fatty changes in many specimens are of unknown cause; they often are mild and sometimes focal within the lobules, representing incidental findings of no significance.

Phospholipidoses

The prototype of these conditions is Niemann-Pick disease, in which sphingomyelin is stored in hepatocytes and Kupffer cells. However, most specimens with changes of this type represent drug-induced phospholipidosis—for instance, after amiodarone administration[15]; this condition often is associated with amiodarone-induced steatohepatitis (see Chapter 7).

Poisoning by Toxic Chemicals and Bacterial Toxins

Aflatoxin,[16] margosa oil,[17] and camphor[18] can cause microvesicular fatty changes. Exposure to solvents such as dimethylformamide has caused both microvesicular (acute presentation) and predominantly macrovesicular (chronic presentation) fatty change.[19] Sepsis and bacterial toxins (see above under "Nonalcoholic Fatty Liver") can also cause microvesicular fatty changes, particularly in periportal hepatocytes.[20] For toxic necrosis and related lesions, see Chapter 9.

Reye's Syndrome

Comments: Typically, the disease occurs in pediatric patients, several days after they have a viral-type illness. Intractable vomiting and increasing encephalopathy are observed, leading to coma and often death. Levels of blood ammonia and aminotransferases are elevated. A strong association of the syndrome with aspirin administration is suspected.[21]

Morphologic features: Tissue samples usually represent autopsy specimens. If a biopsy sample is obtained, a small portion should be embedded for electron microscopic study. Whereas light microscopy may only show the microvesicular fatty changes, sometimes with periportal necrosis, ultrastructural studies reveal glycogen depletion, proliferation and dilatation of smooth endoplasmic reticulum, and swelling and distortion of mitochondria.[22] Bile stasis is rare. Features of Reye's syndrome also have been observed after multiple hornet stings.[23]

Sudden Childhood Death

Microvesicular fatty changes of unknown cause have been found in infants and children who died from conditions such as craniocerebral trauma or drowning.[24] The fatty changes usually were diffuse. Thus, this light microscopic finding in the pediatric age group can be quite coincidental.

Toxic Shock Syndrome

Microvesicular fatty change and neutrophilic cholangitis are common findings (see also Chapter 15).

Viral Hepatitis D

Microvesicular fatty changes in viral hepatitis D have been observed in indigent patients in the Amazon River basin (Labrea hepatitis) and other areas in South America, but rarely in North America.[25,26] The described liver biopsy specimens revealed lobular hepatitis (see Chapter 3) in addition to the microvesicular fatty changes.

Table 6.2 Drugs That May Cause Macrovesicular Fatty Changes*

Generic or Chemical Name	Product Classification
Acetaminophen	Analgesic and antipyretic
Asparaginase	Antineoplastic
Azidothymidine (AZT)[†]	For treatment of AIDS
Cisplatin	Antineoplastic

continued on page 65

continued from page 64

Generic or Chemical Name	Product Classification
Clometacin	Analgesic
Corticosteroid(s)	Hormone
Dantrolene sodium	Skeletal muscle relaxant
Etretinate	Antipsoriatic
Floxuridine[‡][27]	Antineoplastic
Flurazepam hydrochloride	Sedative and hypnotic: benzodiazepine
Gold sodium thiomalate	Antarthritic
Halothane	Inhalation anesthetic
Ibuprofen	Anti-inflammatory
Indomethacin	Anti-inflammatory
Isoniazid	Antituberculotic
Methimazole	Antithyroid agent
Methotrexate	Antineoplastic
Methyldopa	Antihypertensive
Nitrofurantoin	Urinary antibiotic
Rifampin	Antituberculotic
Sulindac	Anti-inflammatory
Tamoxifen[28]	Antiestrogen

*This list does not include drugs that are unavailable in the United States. For further information, see reference 32.
†Own observation.
‡By hepatic arterial infusion.

Table 6.3 Drugs That May Cause Microvesicular Fatty Changes*

Generic or Chemical Name	Product Classification
Amiodarone[29]	Antiarrhythmic
Aspirin[†]	Analgesic, anti-inflammatory, and antipyretic
Chlortetracycline	Antibiotic
Didanosine[30]	For the treatment of AIDS
Ketoprofen[31]	Antarthritic
Tetracycline	Antibiotic
Valproic acid	Anticonvulsant

*This list does not include drugs that are unavailable in the United States. For further information, see reference 32.
†May be involved in causation of Reye's syndrome.

References

1. Riely CA, Latham PS, Romero R, et al: Acute fatty liver of pregnancy: A reassessment based on observations in 9 patients. *Ann Intern Med* 106:703-706, 1987.

2. Rolfes DB, Ishak KG: Acute fatty liver of pregnancy: A clinicopathologic study of 35 cases. *Hepatology* 5:1149-1158, 1985.

3. Riely CA: Acute fatty liver of pregnancy. *Semin Liver Dis* 7:47-54, 1987.

4. Morgan MY, Sherlock S, Scheuer P: Acute cholestasis, hepatic failure, and fatty liver in the alcoholic. *Scand J Gastroenterol* 13:299-303, 1978.

5. Randall B: Fatty liver and sudden death. *Hum Pathol* 11:147-154, 1980.

6. Uchida T, Kao H, Quispe-Sjogren M, et al: Alcoholic foamy degeneration: A pattern of acute alcoholic injury of the liver. *Gastroenterology* 84:683-692, 1983.

7. Review by an International Group: Alcoholic liver disease: Morphological manifestations. *Lancet* 1:707-711, 1981.

8. Nakano M, Worner TM, Lieber CS: Perivenular fibrosis in alcoholic liver injury: Ultrastructure and histologic progression. *Gastroenterology* 83:777-785, 1982.

9. Yates CK, Streight RA: Focal fatty infiltration of the liver simulating metastatic disease. *Radiology* 159:83-84, 1986.

10. Rubel LR, Ishak KG: The liver in fatal exertional heatstroke. *Liver* 3:249-260, 1983.

11. Tanaka K: Jamaican vomiting sickness. In Vinken PJ, Bruyn GW (eds): *Handbook of Clinical Neurology, Vol 37*. New York, North-Holland, 1979, pp 511-539.

12. Treem WR, Witzleben CA, Piccoli DA, et al: Medium-chain and long-chain acyl CoA dehydrogenase deficiency: Clinical, pathologic and ultrastructural differentiation from Reye's syndrome. *Hepatology* 6:1270-1278, 1986.

13. Cone LA, Woodard DR, Schlievert PM, et al: Clinical and bacteriologic observations of a toxic shock-like syndrome due to *Streptococcus pyogenes*. *N Engl J Med* 317:146-149, 1987.

14. McAdams AJ, Hug G, Bove KE: Glycogen storage disease, types I to X: Criteria for morphologic diagnosis. *Hum Pathol* 5:463-487, 1974.

15. Poucell S, Ireton J, Valencia-Mayoral P, et al: Amiodarone-associated phospholipidosis and fibrosis of the liver: Light, immunohistochemical and electron microscopic studies. *Gastroenterology* 86:926-936, 1984.

16. Ryan NJ, Hogan GR, Hayes AW, et al: Aflatoxin in B1: Its role in the etiology of Reye's syndrome. *Pediatrics* 64:71-75, 1979.

17. Sinniah D, Baskaran G: Margosa oil poisoning as a cause of Reye's syndrome. *Lancet* 1:487-489, 1981.

18. Jimenez JF, Brown AL, Arnold WC, et al: Chronic camphor ingestion mimicking Reye's syndrome. *Gastroenterology* 84:394-398, 1983.

19. Redlich CA, West AB, Fleming L, et al: Clinical and pathological characteristics of hepatotoxicity associated with occupational exposure to dimethylformamide. *Gastroenterology* 99:748-757, 1990.

20. Ishak KG, Rogers WA: Cryptogenic acute cholangitis—association with toxic shock syndrome. *Am J Clin Pathol* 76:619-626, 1981.

21. Pinsky PF, Hurwitz ES, Schonberger LB, et al: Reye's syndrome and aspirin: Evidence for a dose-response effect. JAMA 260:657-661, 1988.

22. Chang C-H, Uchwat F, Masalskis F, et al: Morphologic grading of hepatic mitochondrial alterations in Reye's syndrome: Potential prognostic implication. Pediatr Pathol 4:265-275, 1985.

23. Weizman Z, Mussafi H, Ishay JS, et al: Multiple hornet stings with features of Reye's syndrome. Gastroenterology 89:1407-1410, 1985.

24. Bonnell HJ, Beckwith B: Fatty liver in sudden childhood death: Implications for Reye's syndrome. Am J Dis Child 140:30-33, 1986.

25. Buitrago B, Popper H, Hadler SC, et al: Specific histologic features of Santa Marta hepatitis: A severe form of hepatitis-virus infection in Northern South America. Hepatology 6:1285-1291, 1986.

26. Lefkowitch JH, Goldstein H, Yatto R, et al: Cytopathic liver injury in acute delta virus hepatitis. Gastroenterology 92:1262-1266, 1987.

27. Zeiss J, Merrick HW, Savolaine ER, et al: Fatty liver change as a result of hepatic artery infusion chemotherapy. Am J Clin Oncol 13:156-160, 1990.

28. Taniya T, Noguchi M, Tajiri K, et al: A case report of hyperlipemia with giant fatty liver during adjuvant endocrine therapy with tamoxifen [in Japanese]. Gan No Rinsho 33:300-304, 1987.

29. Lewis JH, Mullick F, Ishak KG, et al: Histopathologic analysis of suspected amiodarone hepatotoxicity. Hum Pathol 21:59-67, 1990.

30. Lai KK, Gang DL, Zawacki JK, et al: Fulminant hepatic failure associated with 2',3'-dideoxyinosine (ddI). Ann Intern Med 115:283-284, 1991.

31. Dutertre J-P, Bastides F, Jonville A-P, et al: Microvesicular steatosis after ketoprofen administration. Eur J Gastroenterol Hepatol 3:953-954, 1991.

32. Ludwig J, Axelson R: Drug effects on the liver: An updated tabular compilation of drugs and drug-related hepatic diseases. Dig Dis Sci 28:651-666, 1983.

Chapter 7

Steatohepatitis

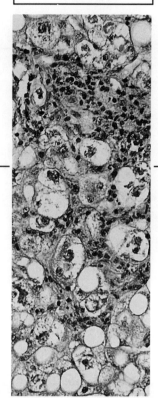

Morphologic Definition

Prominent macrovesicular or mixed macrovesicular and microvesicular fatty changes of hepatocytes with lobular inflammatory infiltrates are present. Portal and periportal inflammation may be found also. However, lobular fatty changes with inflammation only in portal tracts may be the result of two independent causes (for instance, obesity-related fatty changes and nonspecific reactive hepatitis) and thus may not represent the entity "steatohepatitis." Steatohepatitis may be cholestatic (see also Chapter 4). Note: No sharp distinction can be made between mild steatohepatitis and fatty changes with minimal inflammation. Furthermore, inflammatory changes may be patchy and thus not appreciable in each specimen. In some cases, therefore, both Chapters 6 and 7 should be consulted.

Table 7.1 Clinical Conditions Associated With Steatohepatitis

Alcoholic hepatitis (alcoholic steatohepatitis)
Nonalcoholic steatohepatitis (fatty liver hepatitis; steatonecrosis)
    Diabetes mellitus (adult-onset)
    Drug-induced hepatitis or exposure to occupational or domestic hepatotoxic chemicals
    Morbid obesity and effects of weight-reducing surgery or fasting
    Uncomplicated obesity
    Uncommon causes:
        Chronic active hepatitis and related disorders
        Gastrointestinal and pancreatic disorders; malabsorption and malnutrition; extensive
          bowel resection
        Genetic (familial) liver diseases
        Total parenteral nutrition
        Weber-Christian disease and limb lipodystrophy

Clinical Conditions

Alcoholic Hepatitis (Alcoholic Steatohepatitis)

Comments: A history of alcohol abuse or dependence is required for the diagnosis. The condition may be acute and precipitated by particularly heavy drinking, or it may be chronic. Neuropsychiatric disturbances often can be recognized. Biochemical tests show elevated aminotransferase levels, among other abnormalities (see also under "Alcoholic Fatty Liver," Chapter 6).

Morphologic features: Mixed macrovesicular and microvesicular fatty changes with lobular inflammation are characteristic. Portal tracts are also inflamed. Ballooned hepatocytes with Mallory bodies (see Chapter 12), spotty necroses, and mixed inflammatory infiltrates suggest the alcoholic etiology. Clusters of neutrophils often are grouped around foci with Mallory bodies (Figures 7.1A and 7.1B). These inflammatory changes and associated perisinusoidal fibrosis ("sclerosing hyaline necrosis") usually are found in the centrilobular areas, often together with lymphocytic phlebitis, phlebosclerosis or veno-occlusive lesions of central (terminal hepatic) veins.[1] It should be noted that fatty changes are not always prominent in alcoholic hepatitis and that Mallory bodies may be absent.[2] Indeed, severe lobular inflammation in alcoholic hepatitis often is associated with remarkably little fatty change. Centrilobular fibrosis and central-vein changes suggest chronicity. Presence of abundant Mallory bodies usually indicates severe disease (for additional possible histologic features, see also under "Alcoholic Fatty Liver," Chapter 6).

Nonalcoholic Steatohepatitis (Fatty Liver Hepatitis; Steatonecrosis)

Comments: A negative history of alcoholism is required for the diagnosis. Hepatomegaly and complications such as portal hypertension may be present. In rare instances, the disease progresses to cirrhosis and liver failure. Some clinical features are linked to specific causes of nonalcoholic steatohepatitis and therefore are presented separately.

Chronic Active Hepatitis and Related Conditions. Acute or chronic active viral hepatitis B, C, and D can be associated with fatty changes, either because of unrelated causes or unknown reasons (malnutrition? genetic predisposition?), as observed in hepatitis D in South America (see Chapters 3 and 6) or in some Asian patients. Chronic hepatitis, as observed in Mediterranean countries, also has been associated with fatty changes (see below under "Morphologic features"). In idiopathic chronic active hepatitis, fatty changes often are steroid-induced (see Chapter 6).

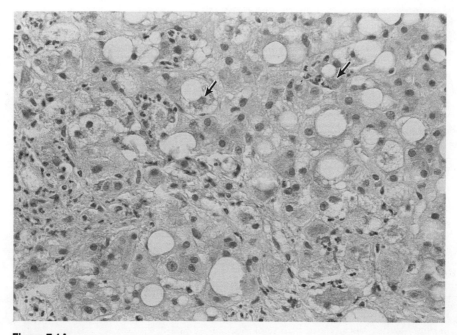

Figure 7.1A
An example of alcoholic steatohepatitis (alcoholic hepatitis). Arrows indicate Mallory bodies.

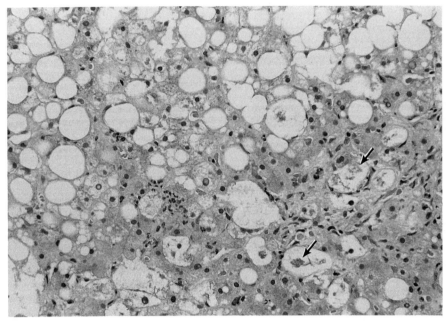

Figure 7.1B
Nonalcoholic steatohepatitis (see also Figures 7.2A and 7.2B). Note the remarkable similarity with Figure 7.1A. Both show macrovesicular fatty changes with fat cysts, spotty necroses, clusters of neutrophils, and Mallory bodies (arrow).

Diabetes Mellitus (Adult-Onset). Most affected patients have adult-onset (type II) diabetes mellitus; they often are also obese. Thus, obesity-related steatohepatitis cannot always be separated from steatohepatitis associated with diabetes mellitus. The steatohepatitis in these patients may be an early manifestation of the diabetes; it has occurred before glucose intolerance was noted.[3] Steatohepatitis associated with juvenile-onset (type I) diabetes mellitus is an uncommon finding.[4]

Drug-Induced Hepatitis or Exposure to Occupational or Domestic Hepatotoxic Chemicals. The diagnosis of drug-induced steatohepatitis can be suggested if an appropriate history has been provided. For a list of drugs that may cause steatohepatitis, see Table 7.2. Hepatotoxic chemicals such as the organic solvent carbon tetrachloride in rare instances have to be considered in this context. For steatohepatitis in the toxic oil syndrome, see Chapters 6 and 15.

Gastrointestinal and Pancreatic Disorders; Malabsorption and Malnutrition; Extensive Bowel Resection. These conditions are discussed together because they can be interrelated. Indeed, the effects of weight-reducing surgery in morbid obesity (see under "Morbid Obesity and Effects of Weight-Reducing Surgery or Fasting") and of total parenteral nutrition (see below) may also belong here. Fatty changes or mild steatohepatitis are common in patients with gastrointestinal and pancreatic disorders, but the clinical situation usually is complex and a clear causative relationship cannot be established. Many intestinal disorders have been implicated, including celiac disease[5] and diverticulosis.[6] Liver abnormalities in malabsorption and malnutrition are equally difficult to interpret.[7] The pathogenetic mechanisms leading to steatohepatitis in these patients may be related to those in patients who have had extensive bowel resection[8] or suffered from bulimia.[9]

Genetic (Familial) Liver Diseases. For histologic changes in Wilson's disease, see Chapters 2, 11, and 14. Abetalipoproteinemia[10] (low-density beta-lipoprotein deficiency) is an example of a hereditary disorder that can be associated with steatohepatitis and cirrhosis (see also Chapter 6).

Morbid Obesity and Effects of Weight-Reducing Surgery or Fasting. The liver abnormalities in these settings undoubtedly are related to the changes observed in uncomplicated obesity. However, they tend to be more severe and indeed may follow a fulminant course leading to hepatic failure. In early reports, most patients had had jejunoileal bypass surgery,[11] but recently, severe steatohepatitis also has been reported following the supposedly safer gastroplasty.[12] The pathogenetic mechanisms appear to be complex. Many patients have preexisting, morbid-obesity related steatohepatitis,[11,13,14] which apparently may be aggravated by precipitous weight loss. Even without surgical procedures, fatal steatohepatitis may occur in morbid obesity if patients fast excessively.[15]

Total Parenteral Nutrition. Patients receiving total parenteral nutrition (TPN) often have been subjected to extensive intestinal resection, and the steatohepatitis therefore may result from both procedures.[16] Malnutrition also may play a role. Although steatohepatitis is not common in patients receiving TPN, it may lead to progressive liver disease if it lasts for more than 4 months.[17] Cirrhosis (see Chapter 11) and hepatic failure may occur.[18]

Uncomplicated Obesity. Nonalcoholic steatohepatitis associated with obesity most commonly occurs in middle-aged women, many of whom also are diabetic.[19,20] The obesity may be mild. Laboratory abnormalities include elevated levels of serum cholesterol and triglycerides.[21] Although the condition often remains stationary, it may progress to cirrhosis.[20] The therapeutic effect of weight loss in such patients has not yet been studied satisfactorily.

Weber-Christian Disease; Limb Lipodystrophy. In a few instances, steatohepatitis has been observed together with extrahepatic diseases of fat tissue. Published examples of Weber-Christian disease[22] and of limb lipodystrophy[23] indicate that a link might exist between such conditions and the steatohepatitis in the affected patients.

Morphologic features: Principally, the morphology of nonalcoholic steatohepatitis does not differ from that of alcoholic hepatitis (Figures 7.1A and 7.1B). As a group, specimens from patients with nonalcoholic conditions have more fat and less hepatocellular damage, inflammation, and fibrosis.[24] Morphologic features usually do not distinguish between the many clinical conditions that may cause or be associated with nonalcoholic steatohepatitis. Nevertheless, some observations merit emphasizing. The steatohepatitis in uncomplicated obesity most often resembles mild alcoholic hepatitis. Weight-reducing surgery or other causes of precipitous weight loss in morbid obesity may result in steatohepatitis with features of severe alcoholic hepatitis (see above and Figures 7.2A and 7.2B). Steatohepatitis in diabetes mellitus resembles mild chronic alcoholic hepatitis, but the correct diagnosis sometimes can be suspected because of the prominent nuclear vacuolation of hepatocytes. Occasionally, the hepatitis in these patients may be predominantly periportal rather than centrilobular.[25] In gastrointestinal and pancreatic disorders, malabsorption and malnutrition, and after extensive bowel resection, steatohepatitis may be found with fatty changes that are zonal or diffuse. Spotty necroses or Mallory bodies, and centrilobular fibrosis and phlebitis are not observed. The same holds true for the steatohepatitis after total parenteral nutrition. Cholestasis and pigment deposition may be diagnostic clues[18] (see Chapters 4 and 14). If chronic active hepatitis or related conditions are associated with fatty changes, diagnostic clues may be provided by the intensity of the periportal inflammation (in steroid-treated idiopathic chronic active hepatitis or in Mediterranean-type chronic hepatitis[26]), the abundance of Councilman bodies, or the presence of microvesicular fatty changes (in some cases of viral hepatitis D; see also Chapter 6). Mallory bodies (see Chapter 12) are not observed in any of these conditions. However, they may occur in Wilson's disease (see above). Some cases of drug-induced hepatitis again closely resemble alcoholic hepatitis. Amiodarone,[27] an

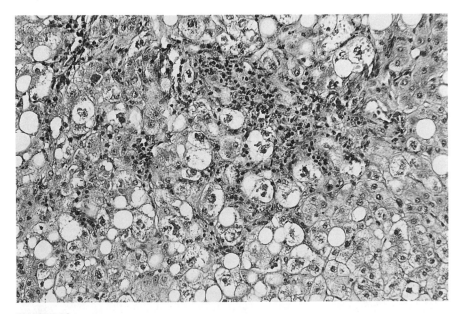

Figure 7.2A
Nonalcoholic steatohepatitis after jejunoileal bypass surgery for morbid obesity. Macrovesicular fatty changes and fat cyst with multiple Mallory bodies are seen, together with mixed inflammatory infiltrates that contain many neutrophils. This is a centrilobular area and also shows some perivenular fibrosis, suggesting that the process had been active for some time (chronic nonalcoholic steatohepatitis).

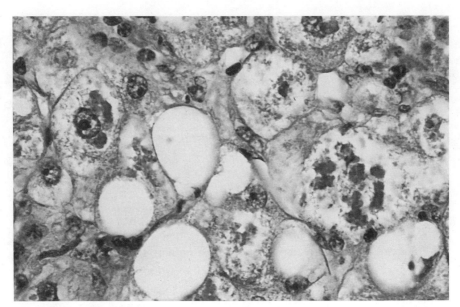

Figure 7.2B
Nonalcoholic steatohepatitis after jejunoileal bypass surgery for morbid obesity. High-power field from some specimens shows classic Mallory bodies.

antiarrhythmic, and the calcium channel blockers nifedipine[28] and perhexiline maleate[29] are the best known examples. If ultrastructural features of phospholipidosis are present or if the Mallory bodies are found in periportal areas, as in some cases of amiodarone hepatitis,[26,30] the drug etiology can be strongly suspected. Hepatotoxic chemicals may cause zonal or diffuse fatty changes and inflammation, but Mallory bodies are not found. However, steatohepatitis with Mallory bodies was found in the liver of a patient with abetalipoproteinemia,[10] and in a case of Weber-Christian disease.[22] In a liver cell adenoma, fatty changes with inflammation and Mallory bodies also have been observed, imparting a picture of alcoholic hepatitis.[31] Steatohepatitis without Mallory bodies but with an occasional noncaseating epithelioid cell or lipoid granuloma may occur in focal fatty change (see Chapter 6).

As stated under the "Morphologic Definition," steatohepatitis can be mimicked by hepatitis of any cause affecting a fatty liver (Figure 7.3).

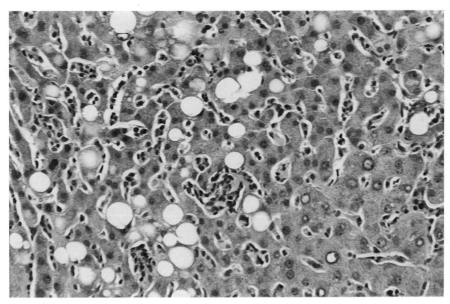

Figure 7.3
Lobular infectious mononucleosis hepatitis in a liver with preexisting fatty change. In this case, steatohepatitis is mimicked by two unrelated processes.

Table 7.2   Drugs That May Cause Steatohepatitis*

Generic or Chemical Name	Product Classification
Amiodarone[†27]	Antiarrhythmic
Diltiazem hydrochloride[†32]	Slow calcium channel blocker: antianginal drug
Methotrexate[33]	Antineoplastic
Naproxen[34]	Anti-inflammatory
Nicardipine[†35]	Calcium channel blocker
Nifedipine[†28]	Calcium channel blocker
Oxacillin[36]	Antibiotic
Perhexiline maleate[†29]	Calcium channel blocker
Spironolactone[37]	Diuretic
Sulfasalazine[38]	Antibiotic

*With the exception of perhexiline maleate, all drugs in this list are available in the United States.
†These drugs may cause steatohepatitis with Mallory bodies, closely resembling alcoholic hepatitis.

References

1. Goodman ZD, Ishak KG: Occlusive venous lesions in alcoholic liver disease: A study of 200 cases. *Gastroenterology* 83:786-796, 1982.

2. Maddrey WC: Alcoholic hepatitis: Clinicopathologic features and therapy. *Semin Liver Dis* 8:91-102, 1988.

3. Batman PA, Scheuer PJ: Diabetic hepatitis preceding the onset of glucose intolerance. *Histopathology* 9:237-243, 1985.

4. Lenaerts J, Verresen L, Van Steenbergen W, et al: Fatty liver hepatitis and type 5 hyperlipoproteinemia in juvenile diabetes mellitus: Case report and review of the literature. *J Clin Gastroenterol* 12:93-97, 1990.

5. Naschitz JE, Yesherun D, Zuckerman E, et al: Massive hepatic steatosis complicating adult celiac disease: Report of a case and review of the literature. *Am J Gastroenterol* 82:1186-1189, 1987.

6. Nazim M, Stamp G, Hodgson HJF: Non-alcoholic steatohepatitis associated with small intestinal diverticulosis and bacterial overgrowth. *Hepatogastroenterology* 36:349-351, 1989.

7. Quigley EMM, Zetterman RK: Hepatobiliary complications of malabsorption and malnutrition. *Semin Liver Dis* 8:218-228, 1988.

8. Peura DA, Stromeyer FW, Johnson LF: Liver injury with alcoholic hyalin after intestinal resection. *Gastroenterology* 79:128-130, 1980.

9. Cuellar RE, Tarter R, Hays A, et al: The possible occurrence of "alcoholic hepatitis" in a patient with bulimia in the absence of diagnosable alcoholism. *Hepatology* 7:878-883, 1987.

10. Partin JS, Partin JC, Schubert WK, et al: Liver ultrastructure in abetalipoproteinemia: Evolution of micronodular cirrhosis. *Gastroenterology* 67:107-118, 1974.

11. Marubbio AT Jr, Buchwald H, Schwartz MZ, et al: Hepatic lesions of central pericellular fibrosis in morbid obesity, and after jejunoileal bypass. *Am J Clin Pathol* 66:684-691, 1976.

12. Hamilton DL, Vest TK, Brown DS, et al: Liver injury with alcoholic-like hyalin after gastroplasty for morbid obesity. *Gastroenterology* 85:722-726, 1983.

13. Fallon WW: Hepatobiliary effects of obesity and weight-reducing surgery. *Semin Liver Dis* 8:229-236, 1988.

14. Klain J, Fraser D, Goldstein J, et al: Liver histology abnormalities in the morbidly obese. *Hepatology* 10:873-876, 1989.

15. Capron J-P, Delamarre J, Dupas J-L, et al: Fasting in obesity: Another cause of liver injury with alcoholic hyaline? *Dig Dis Sci* 27:265-268, 1982.

16. Craig RM, Neumann T, Jeejeebhoy KN, et al: Severe hepatocellular reaction resembling alcoholic hepatitis with cirrhosis after massive small bowel resection and prolonged total parenteral nutrition. *Gastroenterology* 79:131-137, 1980.

17. Klein S, Nealon WH: Hepatobiliary abnormalities associated with total parenteral nutrition. *Semin Liver Dis* 8:237-246, 1988.

18. Bowyer BA, Fleming CR, Ludwig J, et al: Does long-term home parenteral nutrition in adult patients cause chronic liver disease? *JPEN* 9:11-17, 1985.

19. Lee RG: Nonalcoholic steatohepatitis: A study of 49 patients. *Hum Pathol* 20:594-598, 1989.

20. Adler M, Schaffner F: Fatty liver hepatitis and cirrhosis in obese patients. *Am J Med* 67:811-816, 1979.

21. Ludwig J, Viggiano TR, McGill DB: Nonalcoholic steatohepatitis: Mayo Clinic experience with a hitherto unnamed disease. *Mayo Clin Proc* 55:434-438, 1980.

22. Kimura H, Kako M, Yo K, et al: Alcoholic hyalins (Mallory bodies) in a case of Weber-Christian disease: Electron microscopic observations in liver involvement. *Gastroenterology* 78:807-812, 1980.

23. Powell EE, Searle J, Mortimer R: Steatohepatitis associated with limb lipodystrophy. *Gastroenterology* 97:1022-1024, 1989.

24. Diehl AM, Goodman Z, Ishak KG: Alcohollike liver disease in nonalcoholics: A clinical and histologic comparison with alcohol-induced liver injury. *Gastroenterology* 95:1056-1062, 1988.

25. Nagore N, Scheuer PJ: The pathology of diabetic hepatitis. *J Pathol* 156:155-160, 1988.

26. Bruguera M, Zambon D, Ros E, et al: Chronic hepatitis: A possible etiology of fatty liver. *Liver* 5:111-116, 1985.

27. Genève J, Zafrani ES, Dhumeaux D: Amiodarone-induced liver disease. *J Hepatol* 9:130-133, 1989.

28. Babany G, Uzzan F, Larrey D, et al: Alcoholic-like liver lesions induced by nifedipine. *J Hepatol* 9:252-255, 1989.

29. Pessayre D, Bichara M, Feldmann G, et al: Perhexiline maleate-induced cirrhosis. *Gastroenterology* 76:170-177, 1979.

30. Lewis JH, Ranard RC, Caruso A, et al: Amiodarone hepatotoxicity: Prevalence and clinicopathologic correlations among 104 patients. *Hepatology* 9:679-685, 1989.

31. Heffelfinger S, Irani DR, Finegold MJ: "Alcoholic hepatitis" in a hepatic adenoma. *Hum Pathol* 18:751-754, 1987.

32. Beaugrand M, Denis J, Callard P: Tous les inhibiteurs calcique peuvent-ils entraîner des lésions d'hépatite alcoholique (HA)? *Gastroenterol Clin Biol* 1:16(abstract), 1987.

33. Brick JE, Moreland LW, Al-Kawas F, et al: Prospective analysis of liver biopsies before and after methotrexate therapy in rheumatoid patients. *Semin Arthritis Rheum* 19:31-44, 1989.

34. Victorino MM, Silveira JCB, Baptista A, et al: Jaundice associated with naproxen. *Postgrad Med J* 56:368-370, 1980.

35. Isoard B, Daumont M, Pousset G, et al: Hépatite pseudo-alcoholique au cours d'un traitement par la nicardipine. *Presse Med* 17:647-648, 1988.

36. Goldstein LI, Granoff M, Waisman J: Hepatic injury due to oxacillin administration. *Am J Gastroenterol* 70:171-174, 1978.

37. Shuck J, Shen S, Owensby L, et al: Spironolactone hepatitis in primary hyperaldosteronism. *Ann Intern Med* 95:708-710, 1981.

38. Smith MD, Gibson GE, Rowland R: Combined hepatotoxicity and neurotoxicity following sulphasalazine administration. *Aust N Z J Med* 12:76-80, 1982.

Chapter 8

Granulomas and Granulomatous Hepatitis

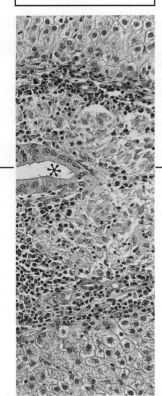

Morphologic Definition

Granulomas are nodules of granulation tissue containing proliferating fibroblasts, capillaries, and modified macrophages resembling epithelial cells, hence the name epithelioid cell granulomas. Many morphologic variations may be present, in particular, giant cells, central necrosis with or without caseation, and peripheral lymphocytic infiltrates. Although the presence of epithelioid cells is the hallmark of granulomas, micronodular inflammatory lesions without well-defined epithelioid cells still can be named granulomas as long as they share the overall appearance. Fungal and mycobacterial infections and immunologic reactions are the most important causes of granuloma formation.

Presence of granulomas in the liver constitutes granulomatous hepatitis. However, if only a few granulomas are found, unaccompanied by an inflammatory response in the remaining tissue, the lesions often are identified without the addition "hepatitis." Because much overlap exists between these presentations, they are discussed here together.

Table 8.1 Clinical Conditions Associated With Granulomas and Granulomatous Hepatitis

Chronic nonsuppurative destructive cholangitis (syndrome of primary biliary cirrhosis)
Drug-induced hepatitis or exposure to occupational or domestic hepatotoxic chemicals
Sarcoidosis
Systemic bacterial and mycobacterial, fungal, parasitic, rickettsial, and viral infections
Uncommon causes:
    Extrahepatic malignant tumors
    Foreign body reactions
    Immune diseases and BCG injection
    Lipogranulomas caused by endogenous fat mobilization
    Lipogranulomas caused by mineral oil
Unknown causes

Clinical Conditions

Chronic Nonsuppurative Destructive Cholangitis (Syndrome of Primary Biliary Cirrhosis)

Comments: Clinical and laboratory findings usually reveal chronic cholestatic liver disease. High titers of antimitochondrial antibodies are characteristic.

Morphologic features: Noncaseating epithelioid cell granulomas often are found in portal tracts and in lobules. The hallmark of the condition is granulomatous cholangitis, that is, destruction of interlobular or septal bile ducts with granuloma formation (for additional descriptions, see the Index); a well-known synonym for this feature is "florid duct lesion" (Figures 8.1A and 8.1B). The granulomas often are poorly defined and thus differ from those in sarcoidosis; they usually consist of clusters of epithelioid cells within accumulations of lymphocytes and other inflammatory cells. A few eosinophils are present in most instances. Langhans' giant cells with asteroid or Schaumann's bodies or with calcium oxalate crystals are quite rare in chronic nonsuppurative destructive cholangitis. Granulomatous cholangitis is found primarily in the early stages of the disease.[1] Presence of granulomas in the syndrome of primary biliary cirrhosis is said to indicate a comparatively good prognosis.[2]

Drug-Induced Hepatitis or Exposure to Occupational or Domestic Hepatotoxic Chemicals

Comments: The diagnosis can be suggested if an appropriate history has been provided. For a list of drugs that may cause granulomas or granulomatous hepatitis, see Table 8.2. Toxic granulomatous hepatitis has become a very rare condition but

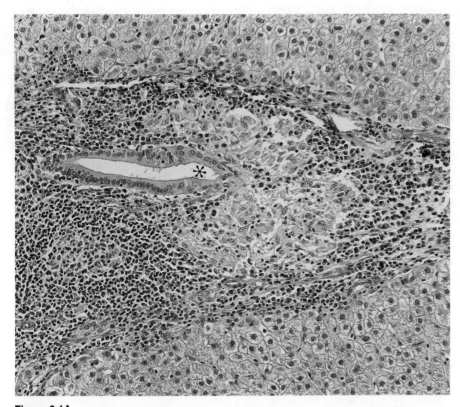

Figure 8.1A
Granulomas in chronic nonsuppurative destructive cholangitis (syndrome of primary biliary cirrhosis). Well-defined noncaseating epithelioid cell granuloma adjacent to a septal bile duct shows swelling of the epithelium within the granuloma (asterisk). Segmental duct destruction is about to occur in this area, a characteristic finding in this condition. This type of granulomatous cholangitis represents a classic florid duct lesion. Note the lymphoid follicle below the left side of the bile duct, which is also common in this condition.

a few cases still can be encountered—for instance, in vineyard workers who used copper sulfate sprays.[3]

Morphologic features: In many instances of drug-induced hepatitis, sarcoid-type granulomas (see below under "Sarcoidosis") are found. However, presence of noncaseating granulomas, with or without eosinophils, does not prove a drug etiology. Associated cholestatic hepatitis may lend support to the diagnosis, but this combination is seen only rarely (see also Table 4.2).

Extrahepatic Malignant Tumors

Noncaseating and even caseating[4] epithelioid cell granulomas, with or without

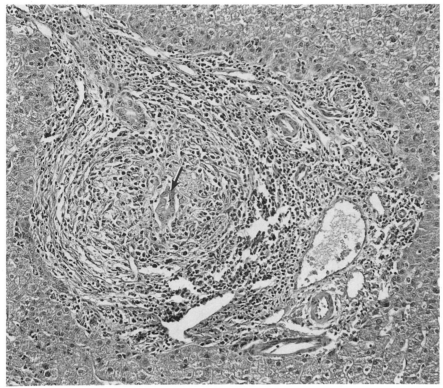

Figure 8.1B
Granulomas in chronic nonsuppurative destructive cholangitis (syndrome of primary biliary cirrhosis). A poorly defined granuloma surrounds the interlobular bile duct (arrow). In this instance, the epithelioid cells have less cytoplasm than those shown in Figure 8.1A, and they are intermingled with more inflammatory cells. This latter type of florid duct lesion is more common but is more difficult to recognize. (See also Figures 1.2, 2.3A, and 2.3B.)

Langhans' giant cells, can be observed in liver biopsy specimens from patients with extrahepatic malignant lymphoma[5] (Figure 8.2) or, in rare instances, extrahepatic carcinoma.[6] The granulomas usually are found in portal tracts.

Foreign Body Reactions

In rare instances, intravenously injected foreign material can be found beyond the pulmonary circulation and thus in the liver—for instance, after use of street preparations of heroin.[7] Use of injectable silicone[8] or intra-arterial embolization of silicone from degenerating, older-model, cardiac ball-valve prostheses may lead to the formation of multiple hepatic foreign body granulomas, primarily in portal tracts. The foreign material is birefringent and thus readily detectable in routine

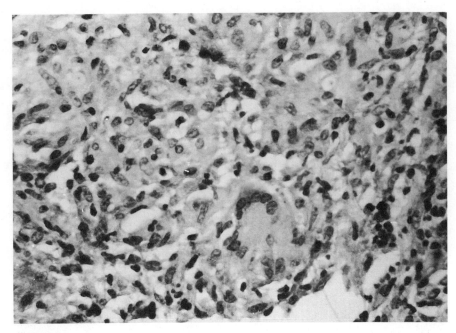

Figure 8.2
Noncaseating epithelioid cell granuloma in a patient with Hodgkin's disease (nodular sclerosing type).
Note Langhans' giant cell at lower edge of granuloma.

slide preparations. Aluminum-containing granulomas may occur in patients who have had long-term hemodialysis.[9] Silicosis[10] and other complications of dust inhalation—for instance, in cement workers[11]—may lead to hepatic foreign body granulomatosis, in addition to the lung involvement (for other foreign material, see Chapter 14).

Immune Diseases and BCG Injection

Sporadic diseases, such as polyarteritis nodosa and familial immune diseases, are possible causes of granulomatous hepatitis.[12] Sarcoidosis or abnormal immunologic reactions to infectious agents[13] or chemicals (eg, in chronic berylliosis) also have been considered in this context.[13] Furthermore, BCG immunotherapy for cancer[14] or for nonmalignant conditions[15] may be accompanied by the development of hepatic noncaseating granulomas.

Lipogranulomas Caused by Endogenous Fat Mobilization

In patients with fatty changes of the liver (see Chapter 6) or steatohepatitis (see Chapter 7), lipogranulomas can be found, particularly in portal tracts and after mobilization of fat.[16] After weight-reducing surgery for morbid obesity, lipogranulomas and noninfectious epithelioid cell granulomas have been observed in the same specimens[17]; the same may occur in focal fatty change.

Lipogranulomas Caused by Mineral Oil

Mineral oil granulomas are a variant of foreign body granulomas (see above under "Foreign Body Reactions"); they are quite common, particularly in elderly patients. Mineral oil granulomas usually are found near portal veins, which they even can occlude[18]; they also are found near central veins (terminal hepatic veins). Vacuolated macrophages surrounded by mixed inflammatory cells and absence of an appreciable epithelioid cell reaction are the main features of mineral oil granulomas.

Sarcoidosis

Comments: This multisystem granulomatous disorder probably represents an abnormal immunologic reaction to many possible agents, including microorganisms. A negative tuberculin test, a positive Kveim test, raised serum angiotensin

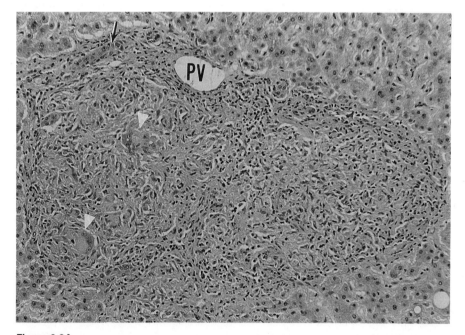

Figure 8.3A
Sarcoid granulomas. There is a portal sarcoid granuloma with Langhans' giant cells (arrowheads). The interlobular bile duct (arrow) and the portal vein (PV) can be seen at the upper edge of the granuloma. Note absence of necrosis. Similarly structured granulomas also may be found in the lobules. At both locations, associated fibrosis may be prominent.

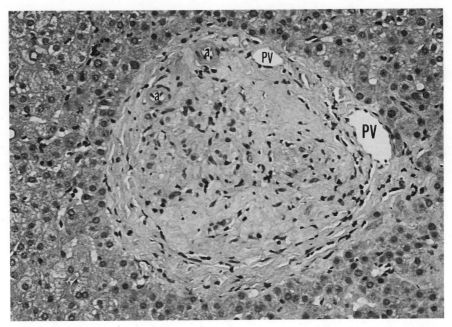

Figure 8.3B
Sarcoid granulomas. Partly hyalinized portal sarcoid granuloma replacing bile duct (a, hepatic artery branches; PV, portal vein branches). Destruction of bile ducts in sarcoidosis is uncommon. Duct destruction in the form of granulomatous cholangitis is the characteristic feature of chronic intrahepatic cholestasis of sarcoidosis; it shares many features with the syndrome of primary biliary cirrhosis.

levels, and radiographic evidence of hilar lymphadenopathy are important clinical features of sarcoidosis. Liver involvement is most common in patients who also have fever or arthralgia or both.[19] Sarcoid liver disease can be a cause of portal hypertension.[20]

Morphologic features: Liver biopsy specimens usually show multiple large noncaseating epithelioid cell granulomas, both in portal tracts and in lobules. These granulomas often contain Langhans' giant cells (Figure 8.3A). In the cytoplasm of these giant cells, Schaumann's bodies, asteroid bodies, or calcium oxalate crystals may be identifiable. Caseation necrosis is not found and special stains for microorganisms are negative. The granulomas may be associated with much scarring (sarcoid fibrosis) or even some evidence of nodular regeneration (sarcoid cirrhosis).

If the sarcoid granulomas appear to destroy entrapped interlobular or septal bile ducts (see Chapter 15), "chronic intrahepatic cholestasis of sarcoidosis" probably is present[21] (Figure 8.3B). The name of this rare clinical condition refers to the laboratory evidence of cholestasis in the affected patients; the biopsy specimens usually show no cholestasis.

Systemic Bacterial and Mycobacterial, Fungal, Parasitic, Rickettsial, and Viral Infections

Comments: Except for some cases of parasitosis, most patients have evidence of systemic infection. If organisms can be cultured from tissue specimens, the results are more reliable than special stains.

Morphologic features: Granulomatous hepatitis in bacterial infections such as brucellosis cannot be subclassified by morphology alone. The granulomas in brucellosis resemble sarcoid granulomas.[22] Granulomas in Whipple's disease often do not contain stainable bacilli,[23] whereas such organisms can be found in Kupffer cells and portal macrophages of these patients.[24] Infection with *Mycobacterium tuberculosis* causes caseating, culture-positive granulomas in most instances,

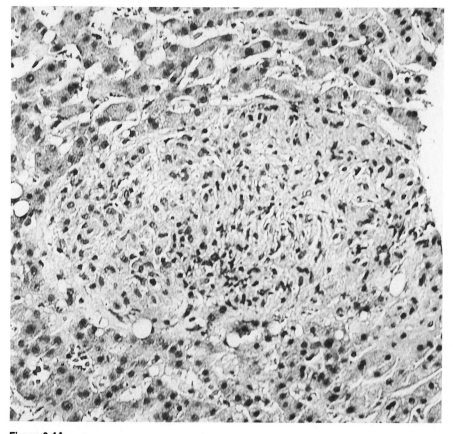

Figure 8.4A
Intralobular granuloma caused by *Mycobacterium avium-intracellulare* in a patient with the acquired immune deficiency syndrome. A sharply outlined granuloma is formed by swollen macrophages; other inflammatory cells are quite sparse. Granulomas of this type are easily overlooked.

although acid-fast stains may be negative. Strongly positive acid-fast stains should be expected after infection with *Mycobacterium avium-intracellulare* in immunocompromised hosts, particularly in patients with the acquired immune deficiency syndrome.[25] In these instances, the granulomas consist of macrophages stuffed with organisms (Figures 8.4A and 8.4B), often in the absence of other inflammatory cells. Organisms also may be seen in Kupffer cells and portal macrophages, unrelated to the granulomas. Even without the use of special stains, identification of these acid-fast intracellular organisms may be possible. Granulomas also may be caused by other atypical mycobacteria, such as *Mycobacterium kansasii* or *Mycobacterium leprae*. In fungal infections such as candidiasis or histoplasmosis, the organisms usually are demonstrable in silver-stained preparations. In viral infections, granulomas

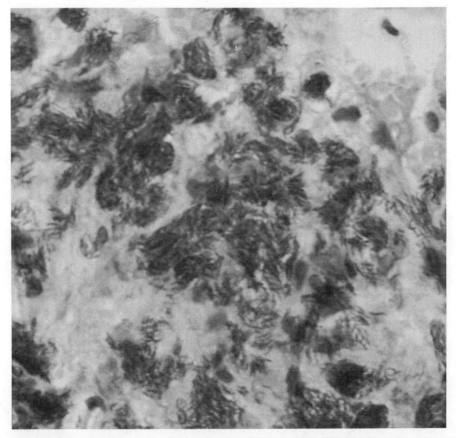

Figure 8.4B
Intralobular granuloma caused by *Mycobacterium avium-intracellulare* in a patient with the acquired immune deficiency syndrome. This high-power view of a Ziehl-Neelsen–stained specimen shows abundant mycobacteria that fill the cytoplasm of the macrophages.

are uncommon but some can be found—for instance, in infectious mononucleosis or cytomegalovirus infection.[26]

In Q fever, a rickettsial infection, granulomas consist of a fibrin ring and a central lipid vacuole.[27] However, it should be noted that similar ring granulomas also have been found in Hodgkin's disease,[28] non-Hodgkin's lymphoma,[29] infectious mononucleosis,[30] cytomegalovirus infection,[31] hepatitis A,[29] visceral leishmaniasis,[32] and allopurinol hepatitis.[33] In parasitic diseases such as schistosomiasis, eggs or remnants of eggs can be found in some granulomas. Necrosis and eosinophils in the center of the granulomas may be caused by parasites such as *Toxocara canis*.[26] Protozoal infections—for instance, toxoplasmosis—, may cause granulomatous hepatitis,[34] occasionally with demonstrable organisms.

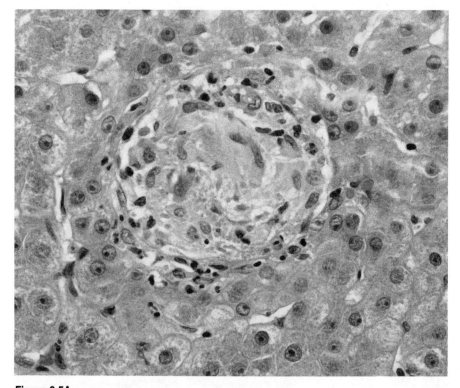

Figure 8.5A
Noncaseating epithelioid cell granulomas of unknown cause. A small intralobular granuloma with a Langhans' giant cell in a patient with chronic hepatitis associated with primary sclerosing cholangitis is shown. Presence of such granulomas may cause confusion with the syndrome of primary biliary cirrhosis because ductopenia may be an associated feature in both conditions. Why some patients with primary sclerosing cholangitis have these granulomas is not clear.

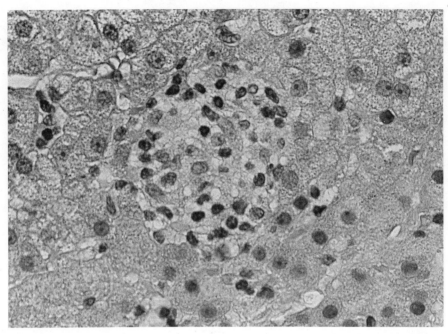

Figure 8.5B
Noncaseating epithelioid cell granulomas of unknown cause. A small granuloma without a giant cell is shown in an otherwise normal liver.

Unknown Causes

Noncaseating epithelioid cell granulomas are common findings in many liver diseases that are not considered granulomatous—for instance, in extrahepatic malignant tumor (see above) and chronic hepatitis associated with primary sclerosing cholangitis (Figure 8.5A). Small granulomas, in particular, appear to develop within hepatic lobules as a response to tissue damage; these microgranulomas are quite nonspecific and of no diagnostic significance. They even may occur in otherwise normal livers (Figure 8.5B). Large hepatic granulomas in the absence of another discernible liver disease are the hallmark of idiopathic granulomatous hepatitis. Some cases of this type might represent hepatic sarcoidosis (see above) without pulmonary involvement or other characteristic features of this disease.

Table 8.2   Drugs That May Cause Granulomas and Granulomatous Hepatitis*

Generic or Chemical Name	Product Classification
Allopurinol	Antihyperuricemic
Aspirin	Analgesic, anti-inflammatory, and antipyretic
Carbamazepine	Anticonvulsant
Cephalexin	Antibiotic
Chlorpromazine	Tranquilizer: phenothiazine
Chlorpropamide	Oral hypoglycemic
Dapsone[3]	Antibacterial: for the treatment of leprosy and dermatitis herpetiformis
Diazepam	Sedative and hypnotic: benzodiazepine
Diltiazem hydrochloride[35]	Slow calcium channel blocker: antianginal drug
Gold sodium thiomalate[3]	Antarthritic
Halothane	Inhalation anesthetic
Hydralazine	Antihypertensive
Isoniazid	Antituberculotic
Mestranol	Oral contraceptive
Methyldopa	Antihypertensive
Metolazone	Diuretic
Nitrofurantoin	Urinary antibiotic
Norethindrone	Oral contraceptive
Norethynodrel	Oral contraceptive
Norgestrel	Oral contraceptive
Oxacillin	Antibiotic
Papaverine hydrochloride	Vasodilator
Penicillin	Antibiotic
Phenylbutazone	Anti-inflammatory
Phenytoin sodium	Anticonvulsant
Procainamide hydrochloride	Antiarrhythmic
Procarbazine hydrochloride	Antineoplastic
Quinidine	Antiarrhythmic
Quinine sulfate[3]	Skeletal muscle relaxant
Ranitidine hydrochloride[3]	H_2 receptor antagonist
Sulfadoxine[3]	Antimalarial agent
Sulfamethoxazole	Antibiotic
Sulfanilamide[3]	Antibiotic
Sulfasalazine	Antibiotic
Sulfathiazole[3]	Antibiotic
Sulfonamide(s), type unspecified	Antibiotic
Tocainide hydrochloride[3]	Antiarrhythmic
Tolbutamide[3]	Oral hypoglycemic
Trichlormethiazide	Diuretic

*This list does not include drugs that are unavailable in the United States. For further information, see reference 36.

References

1. Dickson ER, Fleming CR, Ludwig J: Primary biliary cirrhosis. *Prog Liver Dis* 6:487-502, 1976.

2. Lee RG, Epstein O, Jauregui H, et al: Granulomas in primary biliary cirrhosis: A prognostic feature. *Gastroenterology* 81:983-986, 1981.

3. Ishak KG, Zimmerman HJ: Drug-induced and toxic granulomatous hepatitis. *Baillières Clin Gastroenterol* 2:463-480, 1988.

4. Johnson LN, Iseri O, Knodell RG: Caseating hepatic granulomas in Hodgkin's lymphoma. *Gastroenterology* 99:1837-1840, 1990.

5. Aderka D, Kraus M, Avidor I, et al: Hodgkin's and non-Hodgkin's lymphomas masquerading as "idiopathic" liver granulomas. *Am J Gastroenterol* 79:642-644, 1984.

6. Chagnac A, Kimche D, Zevin D, et al: Liver granulomas: A possible paraneoplastic manifestation of hypernephroma. *Am J Gastroenterol* 80:989-992, 1985.

7. Edland JF: Liver disease in heroin addicts. *Hum Pathol* 3:75-84, 1972.

8. Ellenbogen R, Ellenbogen R, Rubin L: Injectable fluid silicone therapy: Human morbidity and mortality. *JAMA* 234:308-309, 1975.

9. Kurumaya H, Kono N, Nakanuma Y, et al: Hepatic granulomata in long-term hemodialysis patients with hyperaluminumemia. *Arch Pathol Lab Med* 113:1132-1134, 1989.

10. Carmichael GP, Targoff C, Pintar K, et al: Hepatic silicosis. *Am J Clin Pathol* 73:720-722, 1980.

11. Pimental JC, Menezes AP: Pulmonary and hepatic granulomatous disorders due to the inhalation of cement and mica ducts. *Thorax* 33:219-227, 1978.

12. Perks WH, Petheram IS: Familial combined cellular and humoral immune defect with multisystem granulomata. *Thorax* 33:101-105, 1978.

13. Mahida Y, Palmer KR, Lovell D, et al: Familial granulomatous hepatitis: A hitherto unrecognized entity. *Am J Gastroenterol* 83:42-45, 1988.

14. Bodurtha A, Kim YH, Laucius RA, et al: Hepatic granulomas and other hepatic lesions associated with BCG immunotherapy for cancer. *Am J Clin Pathol* 61:747-752, 1974.

15. D'Alessandri RM, Khakoo RA: Granulomatous hepatitis in a healthy adult following BCG injection into a plantar wart. *Am J Gastroenterol* 68:392-395, 1977.

16. Delladetsima JK, Horn T, Poulsen H: Portal tract lipogranulomas in liver biopsies. *Liver* 7:9-17, 1987.

17. Mitros FA, Mason ED: Hepatic granulomas in obesity. *Lab Invest* 44:45(abstract), 1981.

18. Wanless IR, Geddie WR: Mineral oil lipogranulomata in liver and spleen: A study of 465 autopsies. *Arch Pathol Lab Med* 109:283-286, 1985.

19. De Carvalho Hercules H, Bethlem NM: Value of liver biopsy in sarcoidosis. *Arch Pathol Lab Med* 108:831-834, 1984.

20. Tekeste H, Latour F, Levitt RE: Portal hypertension complicating sarcoid liver disease: Case report and review of the literature. *Am J Gastroenterol* 79:389-396, 1984.

21. Bass NM, Burroughes AK, Scheuer PJ, et al: Chronic intrahepatic cholestasis due to sarcoidosis. *Gut* 23:417-421, 1982.

22. Bruguera M, Cervantes F: Hepatic granulomas in brucellosis. *Ann Intern Med* 92:571-572, 1980.

23. Saint Marc Girardin M-F, Zafrani ES, Chaumette M-T, et al: Hepatic granulomas in Whipple's disease. *Gastroenterology* 86:753-756, 1984.

24. Cho C, Linscheer WG, Hirschkorn MA, et al: Sarcoid-like granulomas as an early manifestation of Whipple's disease. *Gastroenterology* 87:941-947, 1984.

25. Klatt EC, Jensen DF, Meyer PR: Pathology of *Mycobacterium avium-intracellulare* infection in acquired immunodeficiency syndrome. *Hum Pathol* 18:709-714, 1987.

26. Ishak KG: Liver granulomas. In Ioachim HL (ed): *Pathology of Granulomas*. New York, Raven Press, 1983, pp 307-369.

27. Hofmann CE, Heaton JW Jr: Q fever hepatitis: Clinical manifestations and pathological findings. *Gastroenterology* 83:474-479, 1982.

28. Voigt JJ, Cassigneul J, Delsol G, et al: Hépatite granulomateuse: A propos de 112 cas chez l'adulte. *Ann Pathol* 4:78-80, 1984.

29. Ponz E, Garcia-Pagan JC, Bruguera M, et al: Hepatic fibrin-ring granulomas in a patient with hepatitis A. *Gastroenterology* 100:268-270, 1991.

30. Nenert M, Mavier P, Dubus N, et al: Epstein-Barr virus infection and hepatic fibrin-ring granulomas. *Hum Pathol* 19:608-610, 1988.

31. Lobdell DH: "Ring" granulomas in cytomegalovirus hepatitis. *Arch Pathol Lab Med* 111:881-882, 1987.

32. Moreno A, Marazuela C, Yebra M, et al: Hepatic fibrin-ring granulomas in visceral leishmaniasis. *Gastroenterology* 95:1123-1126, 1988.

33. Vanderstigel M, Zafrani ES, Lejonc JL, et al: Allopurinol hypersensitivity syndrome as a cause of hepatic fibrin-ring granulomas. *Gastroenterology* 90:188-190, 1986.

34. Weitberg AB, Alper JC, Diamond I, et al: Acute granulomatous hepatitis in the course of acquired toxoplasmosis. *N Engl J Med* 300:1093-1096, 1979.

35. Sarachek NS, London RL, Matulewicz TJ: Diltiazem and granulomatous hepatitis. *Gastroenterology* 88:1260-1262, 1985.

36. Ludwig J, Axelson R: Drug effects on the liver: An updated tabular compilation of drugs and drug-related hepatic diseases. *Dig Dis Sci* 28:651-666, 1983.

Chapter 9

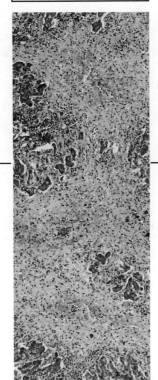

Necrosis and Postnecrotic States

Morphologic Definition

Hepatic necrosis is characterized by death of hepatocytes involving the entire liver (massive hepatic necrosis), major portions of the liver (submassive hepatic necrosis), the same parts of all or most hepatic lobules (zonal necrosis), or circumscribed areas in random distribution throughout the liver (focal or spotty necrosis, and infarcts). With the exception of infarcts, necrotic hepatocytes rarely are visible in biopsy specimens from patients with these conditions because these cells are very quickly removed from the tissue. Therefore, hepatic necrosis usually is diagnosed by the presence of mesenchymal liver tissue in which the hepatic cell plates have been replaced by blood or blood components and inflammatory cells, or by the collapsed mesenchyme. Large areas of necrosis present as postnecrotic collapse with condensation of reticulum fibers and, eventually, collagen deposition. Small areas of necrosis usually present as tissue defects with accumulation of Kupffer cells, other inflammatory cells, and pigmented, PAS-D–positive macrophages. Thus, by convention, use of the term "necrosis" in liver biopsy interpretation often refers to a postnecrotic state, with or without regenerative changes (ductular prolif-eration, formation of hepatocellular rosettes) and fibrosis. Because of this peculiari-ty, necroses and postnecrotic states are considered here together, as also shown in the following definitions for special types of hepatic necrosis.

Piecemeal Necrosis

Lymphocytic
Death or disappearance of periportal or paraseptal hepatocytes or of hepato-cytes in the periphery of regenerative nodules occurs, caused by or associated with infiltrates consisting of lymphocytes and other inflammatory cells. Before cell death, the affected hepatocytes often show hydropic degeneration and rosette for-mation. This is the "classic" piecemeal necrosis, most commonly observed in chronic active hepatitis.

Biliary
Feathery degeneration and death or disappearance of periportal or paraseptal hepatocytes or of hepatocytes in the periphery of regenerative nodules occur, pro-ducing a "halo" that probably is a result of cholate stasis. The affected hepatocytes often contain copper and copper-protein; they also may contain bile pigment and Mallory bodies. In biliary piecemeal necrosis, vacuolated or foamy macrophages are found also, sometimes with bile pigment in their cytoplasm. Lymphocytes, neu-trophils, other inflammatory cells, and bile plugs in canaliculi may be present.

Fibrous
Degeneration and death or disappearance of periportal or paraseptal hepato-cytes or of hepatocytes in the periphery of regenerative nodules occur, caused by proliferated connective tissue that has entrapped groups of hepatocytes, with little evidence of cellular inflammation. Around portal tracts, the condition may lead to formation of new limiting plates that border the seemingly enlarged portal tracts; evidence of continuing inflammation or necrosis may be absent. Fibrous piecemeal necrosis is a common finding in the syndrome of primary sclerosing cholangitis; it may be a late-stage biliary piecemeal necrosis.

Ductular
Death or disappearance of periportal or paraseptal hepatocytes or of hepato-cytes in the periphery of regenerative nodules occurs, associated with prominent ductular proliferation. Mixed inflammatory infiltrates with predominance of neu-trophils often are present between the proliferated ductules. This type of piecemeal necrosis is not common; it is found in the syndrome of primary biliary cirrhosis (often together with lymphocytic piecemeal necrosis), in primary sclerosing cholangitis, and (rarely) in other chronic liver diseases.

Bridging Necrosis

Death or disappearance of a large group of hepatocytes occurs in zones that bridge portal tracts or central veins (terminal hepatic veins) or portal tracts with central veins, in any combination. If bridging necrosis is severe or widespread, it may represent submassive hepatic necrosis.

Multilobular (Confluent) Necrosis

Death or disappearance of hepatocytes involving several adjacent hepatic lob-ules occurs. Multilobular necrosis is the typical histologic manifestation of massive or submassive (nonzonal) hepatic necrosis. As stated above, the terms "massive" or "submassive" hepatic necrosis refer to changes in the entire liver.

Zonal Necrosis

Centrilobular
Death or disappearance of hepatocytes occurs in the centrilobular regions of the liver.

Midzonal
Death or disappearance of hepatocytes occurs in the midzonal regions of the liver. Midzonal and centrilobular necrosis often occur together; if zonal necrosis is widespread, it may represent submassive (zonal) hepatic necrosis.

Periportal
Death or disappearance of hepatocytes occurs in the periportal (peripheral lobular) regions of the liver.

Focal Necrosis

Death or disappearance of hepatocytes occurs involving small groups of liver cells at any site, usually associated with lobular hepatitis. Recently, the term *focal necrosis* has been used to describe rare nonzonal lesions of the size of a lobule or at least a major part of a lobule, whereas the term *spotty necrosis* is used for the minute lesions, as defined below.

Spotty Necrosis

Death or disappearance of hepatocytes occurs involving small groups of liver cells at any site, usually associated with lobular hepatitis or periportal hepatitis (see Chapters 2 and 3).

Table 9.1 Clinical Conditions Associated With Necrosis or Postnecrotic States

With Spotty Necrosis
   See conditions listed under "Periportal Hepatitis" (see also Table 2.1) and
      "Lobular Hepatitis" (see also Table 3.1) below
   Systemic bacterial, fungal, protozoal, and viral infections
      (see also under "Cytomegalovirus Hepatitis" below)
With Focal Necrosis
   Systemic bacterial, fungal, protozoal, and viral infections (see also under "Herpes Simplex
      Hepatitis" below)
With Piecemeal and Bridging Necrosis
   See conditions listed under "Periportal Hepatitis" (see also Table 2.1)
      and "Lobular Hepatitis" (see also Table 3.1) below
With Multilobular (Confluent) Necrosis
   Acute hepatic allograft failure
   Acute or unresolved viral hepatitis
   Chronic active hepatitis
   Drug-induced hepatitis
   Eclampsia (toxemia of pregnancy)
   Idiopathic neonatal hemochromatosis
   Massive or submassive hepatic necrosis of unknown cause
   Systemic viral infections (see under "Systemic Bacterial, Fungal, Protozoal,
      and Viral Infections" below)
With Centrilobular and Midzonal Necrosis
   Circulatory failure: heart disease and shock
   Cocaine hepatitis
   Drug-induced hepatitis
   Hepatic allograft rejection
   Nongestational disseminated intravascular coagulation
   Toxic hepatitis (toxic necrosis)
With Midzonal Necrosis
   Yellow fever hepatitis
With Periportal (Nonpiecemeal) Necrosis
   Cocaine hepatitis
   Eclampsia (toxemia of pregnancy)
   Halothane hepatitis
   Labetalol hepatitis
   Phosphorus and ferrous sulfate poisoning
With Focal Nonzonal (Multilobular) Necrosis
   Anemic infarcts
   Oral contraceptive–induced hemorrhagic necrosis and infarcts
   Systemic bacterial, fungal, protozoal, and viral infections (see also under
      "Herpes Simplex Hepatitis" below)
   Tumor necrosis

Clinical Conditions

Acute Hepatic Allograft Failure

The necrosis occurs within days after orthotopic liver transplantation and may be caused by primary graft damage. Although the necrosis is multilobular, it is not as severe as in an anemic infarction (Figures 9.1A and 9.1B).

Acute or Unresolved Viral Hepatitis

Acute viral hepatitis B and non-A, non-B are the prototypes of lobular hepatitis (see Chapter 3), and unresolved viral hepatitis may feature lobular or periportal (see Chapter 2) hepatitis. The necrosis in these conditions is spotty, of bridging type (Figure 9.2), or multilobular (confluent), reflecting the severity of the condition. Multilobular necrosis is a feature of fulminant or subfulminant viral hepatitis. In hepatitis A, necrosis is an uncommon finding but may occur in zone 1; fulminant hepatitis A infection with multilobular necrosis is particularly rare.[1] Zone 3 necrosis occurs in some cases of acute hepatitis B.

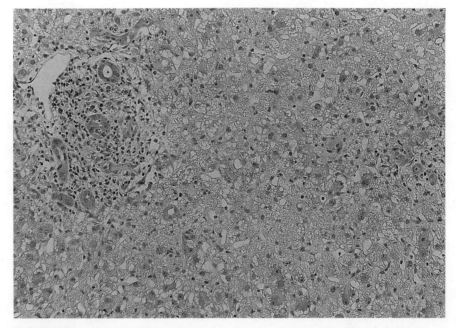

Figure 9.1A
Necrosis in allograft. Multilobular (confluent) necrosis in acute hepatic allograft failure is shown 2 days after orthotopic liver transplantation. Note ductular proliferation and granulocytes in portal tract on the left. Most hepatocytes appear pale and show a vesicular cytoplasm with loss of nuclei. A few darker regenerating hepatocytes are interspersed.

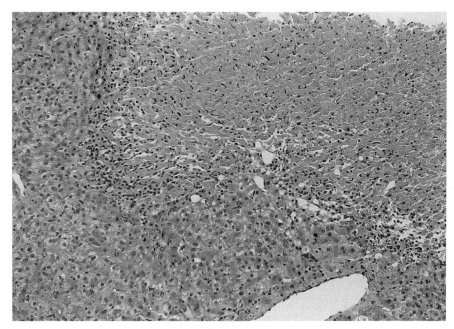

Figure 9.1B
Necrosis in allograft. Anemic infarct in a biopsy specimen from a hepatic allograft 1 month after ortho-topic liver transplantation is shown.

Anemic Infarcts

Anemic hepatic infarcts are rare, and most appear to be caused by vascular occlusions associated with the growth of malignant tumors. Hepatic allografts may show subcapsular infarcts (Figure 9.1B), particularly in the first weeks after implan-tation.[2] Undoubtedly, hypoperfusion plays a role here also. For ischemic lesions associated with nongestational disseminated intravascular coagulation or eclamp-sia, see below. Finally, inadvertent surgical ligation, and thrombosis or embolic occlusion of the hepatic artery must be considered as causes of hepatic infarcts. For another association, see below under "Oral Contraceptive–Induced Hemorrhagic Necrosis and Infarcts." Histologically, a faint outline of the necrotic hepatic tissue is noted. The infarct usually is surrounded by granulation tissue with dilated capil-laries and inflammatory infiltrates. Cavitation or abscess formation is observed pri-marily in very large infarcts.

Chronic Active Hepatitis

Lymphocytic piecemeal necrosis (Figure 9.3) is the hallmark of chronic active hepatitis, and bridging necrosis or multilobular (confluent) necrosis may occur as added features in severe cases. For the clinical findings in chronic active hepatitis and for additional histologic features, see Chapter 2.

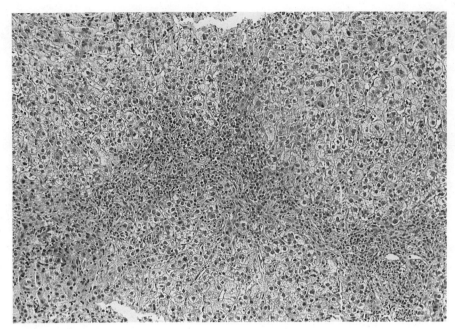

Figure 9.2
Bridging necrosis in unresolved viral hepatitis. The "bridge" runs from left to right in the midsection of the illustration (it probably represents portal to central bridging).

Circulatory Failure: Heart Disease and Shock

Hepatic dysfunction in left ventricular failure with low cardiac output sometimes leads to biopsy because the condition is misinterpreted as primary liver disease. The clinical findings of right ventricular failure may or may not be present.[3] In noncardiogenic hypotension and shock, similar hepatic abnormalities may be noted. Biopsy specimens show centrilobular and midzonal necrosis. Particularly in shock-like states, these changes may be associated with periportal ductular cholestasis as well as hepatocanalicular cholestasis in midzonal areas (see also Chapter 4). If sinusoidal dilatation is a prominent feature, right ventricular failure probably is involved.

Cocaine Hepatitis

Cocaine is hepatotoxic and may cause centrilobular and midzonal necrosis.[4] Massive zonal necrosis with involvement of periportal hepatocytes also may occur. Inflammatory changes are mild. Microvesicular fat droplets are found in the preserved hepatocytes.[4] Isolated periportal necrosis in a cocaine user also has been described.[5]

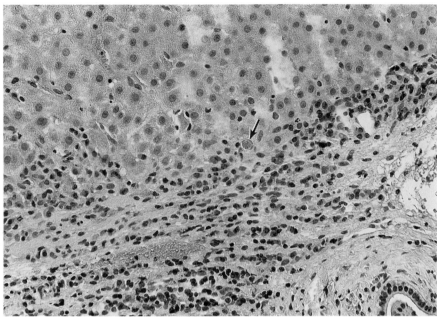

Figure 9.3
Lymphocytic piecemeal necrosis in chronic active hepatitis. Note accumulation of lymphocytes and of other inflammatory cells invading the hepatic parenchyma at the limiting plate surrounding this large portal tract. Actual cell necrosis often cannot be appreciated; one Councilman body is present (arrow).

Cytomegalovirus Hepatitis

Currently, the condition is observed most commonly in hepatic allografts[6] but it also is seen in livers from other immunosuppressed patients, particularly in association with the acquired immunodeficiency syndrome.[7] The inclusion bodies can be found in both epithelial and mesenchymal cells; they are not always associated with necrosis or an inflammatory response. However, in many cases, spotty necrosis can be found in the hepatic parenchyma, with clusters of neutrophils that impart the features of microabscesses. In some of these lesions, hepatocytes or other cells with inclusion bodies can be identified (Figure 9.4). If such cells are not present, nonspecific-reactive hepatitis (see Chapter 3) must be ruled out. Immunostains with monoclonal and polyclonal antibodies, in situ DNA hybridization,[8] and the polymerase chain reaction[9] can be used to detect the antigen.

Drug-Induced Hepatitis

The diagnosis can be suggested if an appropriate history has been provided. For a list of drugs that may cause centrilobular and midzonal hepatic necrosis, see

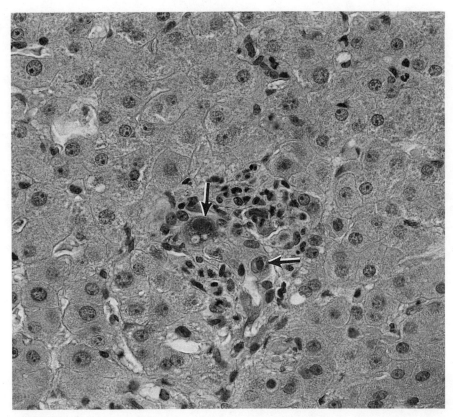

Figure 9.4
Spotty necrosis in cytomegalovirus hepatitis. Note hepatocytes with nuclear inclusions (arrows) surrounded by inflammatory cells, mostly neutrophils.

Table 9.2. For a list of drugs that may cause multilobular (confluent) necrosis, see
Table 9.3. Drug-induced centrilobular damage also may lead to centrilobular
hepatitis. For other manifestations of drug-induced hepatitis, see also under
"Cocaine Hepatitis," "Halothane Hepatitis," "Labetalol Hepatitis" and "Oral Contraceptive–Induced Hemorrhagic Necrosis and Infarcts."

Eclampsia (Toxemia of Pregnancy)

Biopsy evidence of periportal hemorrhage with patchy hepatocellular necrosis
can be found in both eclampsia and preeclampsia. The most characteristic findings
are fibrin thrombi in dilated periportal sinusoids (Figure 9.5) and sometimes also in
portal vein branches or portal arterioles and arteries. Later in the course of the disease, an inflammatory response can be seen. Severe subcapsular and intrahepatic

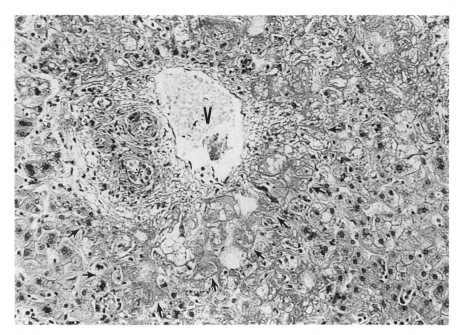

Figure 9.5
Periportal necrosis in eclampsia. A zone of necrotic hepatocytes and fibrin deposition (arrows) border an intact parenchyma. The portal vein (V), artery, and bile duct (asterisk) can be identified.

---

hemorrhages, focal or diffuse necrosis and infarction, and capsular rupture also may occur[10] (see also Chapter 16).

Halothane Hepatitis

Among the many forms of halothane-induced hepatic injury (see Tables 2.2, 4.2, 8.2, 9.2, and 9.3), periportal necrosis also has been described.[11] In Figure 9.6, an example of severe centrilobular and midzonal necrosis associated with halothane hepatitis is shown.

Hepatic Allograft Rejection

For centrilobular necrosis and related findings in hepatic allografts, see Chapter 15.

Herpes Simplex Hepatitis (Herpes Simplex Necrosis)

Most patients with herpes simplex hepatitis have been immunosuppressed. Large nonzonal coagulative hepatic necroses are found in most instances. In fatal

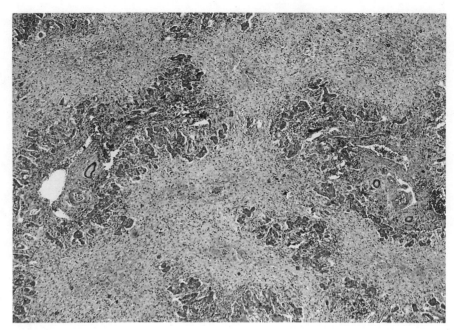

Figure 9.6
Centrilobular and midzonal hepatic necrosis associated with halothane hepatitis. The necrosis was widespread and thus fatal (massive hepatic necrosis, zonal type). In patients with severe shock, livers also
may show zonal necrosis as shown here. Note that massive or submassive hepatic necrosis in viral
hepatitis is of the nonzonal type.

---

herpes simplex hepatitis, these necroses may be confluent. The diagnostic changes
are at the margins of the lesions where eosinophilic inclusions can be found in the
nuclei of many hepatocytes; these inclusion bodies may be surrounded by a halo
(Cowdry type A inclusion bodies). The diagnosis of herpes simplex hepatitis can
be confirmed with immunoperoxidase stains.[12] Most infections are caused by herpes simplex virus type 1. Hepatitis after herpes simplex virus type 2 (genital herpes
simplex) infection is extremely rare in adults.[13]

Idiopathic Neonatal Hemochromatosis

See Chapter 13.

Labetalol Hepatitis

Massive and submassive zonal necrosis has occurred in this condition but also
periportal (zone 1) necrosis (see also Tables 9.2 and 9.3).

Lobular Hepatitis

Acute viral hepatitis is the prototype of this condition. For other causes of lobular hepatitis, see Chapter 3. Spotty necrosis, lymphocytic piecemeal necrosis, bridging necrosis, and multilobular (confluent) necrosis can be found in these conditions. Bridging and multilobular necrosis, in particular, are features of severe and progressive disease.

Massive or Submassive Hepatic Necrosis of Unknown Cause

Patients may present with symptoms of fulminant hepatic failure without any evidence of hepatitis virus infection or of exposure to a drug or hepatotoxic substance. Histologic study usually cannot solve this dilemma. In young patients, copper stains and chemical copper studies should be done to rule out fulminant Wilson's disease.[14,15] If nonzonal coagulative necrosis is present, a careful search should be made for viral inclusion bodies (see also above under "Herpes Simplex Hepatitis"). If zonal (centrilobular and midzonal) coagulation necrosis is present, viral hepatitis can be ruled out and conditions such as circulatory failure or cocaine hepatitis (see above) should be considered. Information on drug exposure may not be volunteered, even if the drug can be obtained legally—for instance, if acetaminophen was used in a suicide attempt. Severe zonal necrosis also can be caused by inhalable hepatotoxic substances such as carbon tetrachloride or after mushroom poisoning (usually by *Amanita phalloides*). Presence of associated fatty changes may be a diagnostic clue. Liver transplantation is a therapeutic option in some of these cases.[15,16]

Nongestational Disseminated Intravascular Coagulation

In disseminated intravascular coagulation (DIC), centrilobular coagulation necrosis can be observed, either as a result of the shock that led to DIC or due to the occlusion of portal vessels by fibrin thrombi.[17] Damage of centrilobular hepatocytes without necrosis occurs if fibrin thrombi develop in the sinusoids of these areas. Changes related to DIC usually are found only at autopsy.[17] Patchy periportal necrosis also may be found.

Oral Contraceptive–Induced Hemorrhagic Necrosis and Infarcts

Multilobular hemorrhagic necrosis and infarcts have been observed after use of oral contraceptives.[18,19] Narrowing of hepatic arterioles due to drug-related medial hyperplasia and intimal swelling, as well as obstruction of small hepatic veins, may have accounted for the hemorrhagic necroses.[18] In the patient who developed actual infarcts, occlusion (presumably thrombotic) of the proper hepatic artery was found.[19]

Periportal Hepatitis

Chronic active hepatitis is the prototype of this condition. For other causes of periportal hepatitis, see Chapter 2. Spotty necrosis, lymphocytic and sometimes fibrous, biliary, or ductular piecemeal necrosis (see also Figures 11.6A and 11.6B), bridging necrosis, and multilobular (confluent) necrosis can be found in these conditions.

Phosphorus and Ferrous Sulfate Poisoning

These toxic substances can cause periportal necrosis.[20] In the case of phosphorus poisoning, portal inflammation, periportal fatty change, and periportal cholestasis also have been observed.

Systemic Bacterial, Fungal, Protozoal, and Viral Infections

In listeriosis, melioidosis, salmonellosis, and other bacterial infections with septicemia and pyema, necroses with neutrophilic infiltrates as well as microabscesses may be found. Infections with *Cryptococcus*, *Candida*, and *Aspergillus* species may cause similar lesions. Spotty necroses are found in toxoplasmic mononucleosis and in several viral infections, including cytomegalovirus hepatitis (see above), infectious mononucleosis, and rubella hepatitis.[21] Small coagulative necroses may result from Coxsackie virus infection, and large necroses are typical of herpes simplex hepatitis (see above). In systemic varicella-zoster infection, focal hepatic necroses develop, with Cowdry type A inclusion bodies in adjacent hepatocytes. For pertinent publications, see reference 21. For necrosis in adenovirus hepatitis, see Chapter 12. Multilobular necrosis may be found in Coxsackie or ECHO virus infection, infectious mononucleosis, and yellow fever.[21]

Toxic Hepatitis (Toxic Necrosis)

Many toxic substances may cause massive necrosis—for instance, chlorinated benzenes, or zonal necrosis, either in zone 1 (allyl compounds, ferrous sulfate) or in zones 3, or 2 and 3 (aflatoxin, carbon tetrachloride, ethylene dichloride, and many others). Most of the organic compounds that cause centrilobular necrosis also cause fatty changes (see Table 6.1). For a synopsis of hepatotoxic substances, see reference 22. Recently, some herbal and "health food" products have proved to be toxic. For instance, a herbal compound called Chaparral Leaf has caused extensive centrilobular hepatic necrosis (herbal hepatitis).[23]

Tumor Necrosis

Necrotic tissue in needle biopsy specimens may represent tumor tissue. The necrosis is coagulative, and therefore faint outlines of the tissue often can be iden-

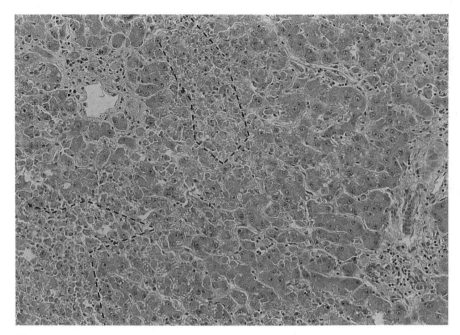

Figure 9.7
Midzonal necrosis in yellow fever hepatitis (outlined by broken line). Inflammatory infiltrates and fatty changes are quite mild in this instance.

tified. Superinfection of necrotic tissue may result in abscess formation. For changes that may occur in the vicinity of tumors, see Chapter 16.

Yellow Fever Hepatitis

In fatal cases of this tropical group B arbovirus infection, extensive midzonal (zone 2) necroses can be found (Figure 9.7). Councilman bodies abound. A few hepatocellular nuclei may contain eosinophilic inclusions (Torres bodies). Hepatocellular fatty changes, lipochrome pigmentation, and Kupffer cell hemosiderosis often are present also.

Table 9.2   Drugs That May Cause Centrilobular and Midzonal Necrosis*

Generic or Chemical Name	Product Classification
Acetaminophen	Analgesic and antipyretic
Allopurinol	Antihyperuricemic
Chlortetracycline	Antibiotic
Daunorubicin hydrochloride	Antineoplastic
Desipramine hydrochloride	Antidepressant
Diazepam	Sedative and hypnotic: benzodiazepine
Disulfiram[24]	For treatment of chronic alcoholism
Enflurane	Inhalation anesthetic
Ethionamide	Antituberculotic
Halothane	Inhalation anesthetic
Imipramine	Antidepressant
Indomethacin	Anti-inflammatory
Iodipamide meglumine	Roentgen contrast medium
Isoniazid	Antituberculotic
Labetalol hydrochloride[25]	Antihypertensive
Lisinopril[26]	Antihypertensive
Mercaptopurine	Antineoplastic
Methoxyflurane	Inhalation anesthetic
Methyldopa	Antihypertensive
Norfloxacin	Antibacterial agent
Pirprofen	Anti-inflammatory
Propranolol[27]	Antihypertensive
Quinidine	Antiarrhythmic
Rifampin	Antituberculotic
Sulfasalazine	Antibiotic
Sulindac	Anti-inflammatory
Tolazamide	Oral hypoglycemic
Valproic acid	Anticonvulsant

*This list does not include drugs that are unavailable in the United States. For further information, see reference 36.

Table 9.3 Drugs That May Cause Multilobular Necrosis*

Generic or Chemical Name	Product Classification
Allopurinol	Antihyperuricemic
Amitriptyline hydrochloride	Antidepressant
Captopril[28]	Antihypertensive
Carbamazepine	Anticonvulsant
Chlordiazepoxide	Sedative and hypnotic: benzodiazepine
Cimetidine	H_2 receptor antagonist
Dacarbazine	Antineoplastic
Dantrolene sodium	Skeletal muscle relaxant
Dapsone[29]	Antibacterial: For the treatment of leprosy and dermatitis herpetiformis
Diclofenac[30]	Anti-inflammatory
Disulfiram[31]	For treatment of chronic alcoholism
Erythromycin[32]	Antibiotic
Ethacrynic acid	Diuretic
Halothane	Inhalation anesthetic
Hydralazine	Antihypertensive
Indomethacin	Anti-inflammatory
Isoflurane[33]	Inhalation anesthetic
Isoniazid	Antituberculotic
Ketoconazole	Antifungal agent
Labetalol hydrochloride[25]	Antihypertensive
Mephobarbital	Anticonvulsant: barbiturate
Methoxyflurane	Inhalation anesthetic
Methyldopa	Antihypertensive
Mitomycin	Antineoplastic
Nicotinic acid[34]	Antihypercholesterolemic
Nitrofurantoin	Urinary antibiotic
Pemoline	Central nervous system stimulant
Phenelzine sulfate	Antidepressant
Phenobarbital	Anticonvulsant: barbiturate
Phenylbutazone	Anti-inflammatory
Phenytoin	Anticonvulsant
Piroxicam[35]	Anti-inflammatory
Probenecid	Uricosuric agent
Prochlorperazine	Tranquilizer: phenothiazine
Propylthiouracil	Antithyroid agent
Sulfamethoxazole	Antibiotic
Sulfonamide(s), type unspecified	Antibiotic
Valproic acid	Anticonvulsant

*This list does not include drugs that are unavailable in the United States. For further information, see reference 36.

References

1. Akriviadis EA, Redeker AG: Fulminant hepatitis A in intravenous drug users with chronic liver disease. *Ann Intern Med* 110:838-839, 1989.

2. Russo PA, Yunis EJ: Subcapsular hepatic necrosis in orthotopic liver allografts. *Hepatology* 6:708-713, 1986.

3. Ross RM: Hepatic dysfunction secondary to heart failure. *Am J Gastroenterol* 76:511-518, 1981.

4. Kanel GC, Cassidy W, Shuster L, et al: Cocaine-induced liver cell injury: Comparison of morphologic features in man and in experimental models. *Hepatology* 11:646-651, 1990.

5. Perino LE, Warren GH, Levine JS: Cocaine-induced hepatotoxicity in humans. *Gastroenterology* 93:176-180, 1987.

6. Snover DC, Hutton S, Balfour HH Jr, et al: Cytomegalovirus infection of the liver in transplant recipients. *J Clin Gastroenterol* 9:659-665, 1987.

7. Klatt EC, Shibata D: Cytomegalovirus infection in the acquired immunodeficiency syndrome: Clinical and autopsy findings. *Arch Pathol Lab Med* 112:540-544, 1988.

8. Naoumov NV, Alexander GJM, O'Grady JG, et al: Rapid diagnosis of cytomegalovirus infection by in-situ hybridisation in liver grafts. *Lancet* 1:1361-1363, 1988.

9. Chehab FF, Xiao X, Kan YW, et al: Detection of cytomegalovirus infection in paraffin-embedded tissue specimens with the polymerase chain reaction. *Mod Pathol* 2:75-78, 1989.

10. Alexander J, Cuellar RE, van Thiel DH: Toxemia of pregnancy and the liver. *Semin Liv Dis* 7:55-58, 1987.

11. Benjamin SB, Goodman ZD, Ishak KG, et al: The morphologic spectrum of halothane-induced hepatic injury: Analysis of 77 cases. *Hepatology* 5:1163-1171, 1985.

12. Marrie TJ, McDonald ATJ, Conen PE, et al: Herpes simplex hepatitis: Use of immunoperoxidase to demonstrate the viral antigen in hepatocytes. *Gastroenterology* 82:71-76, 1982.

13. Rubin MH, Ward DM, Painter CJ: Fulminant hepatic failure caused by genital herpes in a healthy person. *JAMA* 253:1299-1301, 1985.

14. McCullough AJ, Fleming CR, Thistle JL, et al: Antemortem diagnosis and short-term survival of a patient with Wilson's disease presenting as fulminant hepatic failure. *Dig Dis Sci* 29:862-864, 1984.

15. Rakela J, Kurtz SB, McCarty JT, et al: Fulminant Wilson's disease treated with postdilution hemofiltration and orthotopic liver transplantation. *Gastroenterology* 90:2004-2007, 1986.

16. Klein AS, Hart J, Brems JJ, et al: Amanita poisoning: Treatment and the role of liver transplantation. *Am J Med* 86:187-193, 1989.

17. Esaki Y, Hirokawa K, Fukazawa T, et al: Immunohistochemical study on the liver in autopsy cases with disseminated intravascular coagulation (DIC) with reference to clinicopathologic analysis. *Virchows Arch [A]* 404:229-241, 1984.

18. Zafrani ES, Pinaudeau Y, Le Cudonnec B, et al: Focal hemorrhagic necrosis of the liver: A clinicopathologic entity possibly related to oral contraceptives. *Gastroenterology* 79:1295-1299, 1980.

19. Jacobs MB: Hepatic infarction related to oral contraceptive use. *Arch Intern Med* 144:642-643, 1984.

20. Kent G, Orfei E: Hepatic manifestations of toxic and therapeutic agents. In Sunderman FW Jr (ed): *Laboratory Diagnosis of Diseases Caused by Toxic Agents*. St Louis, Warren H. Green Inc, 1970, pp 460-469.

21. Ishak KG: New developments in diagnostic liver pathology. In Farber E, Phillips MJ, Kaufman N (eds): *Pathogenesis of Liver Diseases*. Baltimore, Williams & Wilkins, 1987, pp 223-373.

22. Zimmerman HJ: *Hepatotoxicity: The Adverse Effects of Drugs and Other Chemicals on the Liver*. New York, Appleton Century Crofts, 1978.

23. Katz M, Saibil F: Herbal hepatitis: Subacute hepatic necrosis secondary to Chaparral Leaf. *J Clin Gastroenterol* 12:203-206, 1990.

24. Cereda J-M, Bernuau J, Degott C, et al: Fatal liver failure due to disulfiram. *J Clin Gastroenterol* 11:98-100, 1989.

25. Clark JA, Zimmerman HJ, Tanner LA: Labetalol hepatotoxicity. *Ann Intern Med* 113:210-213, 1990.

26. Larrey D, Babany G, Bernuau J, et al: Fulminant hepatitis after lisinopril administration. *Gastroenterology* 99:1832-1833, 1990.

27. Roschlau G, Baumgarten R, Binus R: Arzneimittelhepatitis durch Propranolol (Obsidan®): Ein Bericht über 3 Fälle. *Z Klin Med* 42:1985-1988, 1987.

28. Bellary SV, Isaacs PET, Scott AWM: Captopril and the liver. *Lancet* 2:514, 1989.

29. Jayalakshmi P, Ting HC: Dapsone-induced liver necrosis. *Histopathology* 17:89-91, 1990.

30. Helfgott SM, Sandberg-Cook J, Zakimd D, et al: Diclofenac-associated hepatotoxicity. *JAMA* 264:2660-2662, 1990.

31. Bartle WR, Fisher MM, Kerenyi N: Disulfiram-induced hepatitis: Report of two cases and review of the literature. *Dig Dis Sci* 30:834-837, 1985.

32. Gholson CF, Warren GH: Fulminant hepatic failure associated with intravenous erythromycin lactobionate. *Arch Intern Med* 150:215-216, 1990.

33. Brunt EM, White H, Marsh JW, et al: Fulminant hepatic failure after repeated exposure to isoflurane anesthesia: A case report. *Hepatology* 13:1017-1021, 1991.

34. Mullin GE, Greenson JK, Mitchell MC: Fulminant hepatic failure after ingestion of sustained-release nicotinic acid. *Ann Intern Med* 111:253-255, 1989.

35. Planas R, De Léon R, Quer JC, et al: Fatal submassive necrosis of the liver associated with piroxicam. *Am J Gastroenterol* 85:468-470, 1990.

36. Ludwig J, Axelson R: Drug effects on the liver: An updated tabular compilation of drugs and drug-related hepatic diseases. *Dig Dis Sci* 28:651-666, 1983.

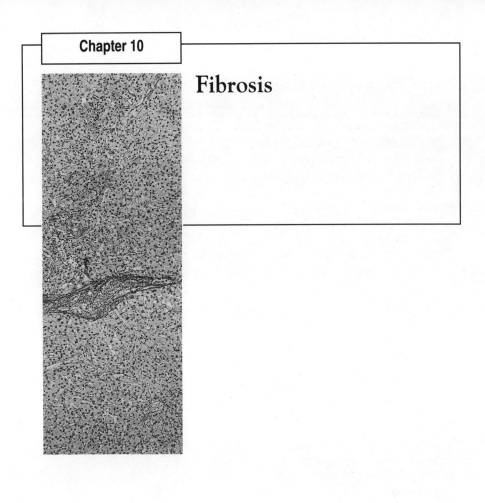

Chapter 10

Fibrosis

Morphologic Definition

Excessive fibrous tissue is present in any location. In the liver, fibrosis may be portal, periportal, septal, centrilobular, or unrelated to specific anatomic structures, as in old infarcts or areas of previous postnecrotic collapse. Deposition of fibrous tissue also can be confined to perivascular areas—for instance, in perisinusoidal fibrosis—or to periductal tissue (periductal fibrosis). Appearance of the coarse, doubly refractile bundles of type I collagen is generally considered irreversible, whereas presence of newly formed type III collagen (reticulin) is a potentially reversible feature.

Table 10.1 Clinical Conditions Associated With Fibrosis

With Periductal Fibrosis
    Nonsuppurative cholangitis, all types
    Obstruction of large (extrahepatic or perihilar intrahepatic) bile ducts
    Primary sclerosing cholangitis
    Unknown causes
With Portal Fibrosis
    Alcoholic liver disease
    Congenital hepatic fibrosis
    Idiopathic portal hypertension (hepatoportal sclerosis)
    Obstruction of large (extrahepatic or perihilar intrahepatic) bile ducts
    Primary sclerosing cholangitis
    Schistosomiasis
    Toxic fibrosis
    Unknown causes
With Periportal Fibrosis
    Conditions listed above under "With Portal Fibrosis"
    Chronic active hepatitis and other conditions listed under "Periportal Hepatitis"
       (see Table 2.1) and under "Piecemeal Necrosis" (see Table 9.1)
    Unresolved viral hepatitis
With Septal Fibrosis
    Conditions listed under "Cirrhosis" (see Table 11.1)
    Genetic (familial) liver diseases
With Centrilobular and Perisinusoidal Fibrosis
    Chronic alcoholic hepatitis (active or healed)
    Chronic congestion
    Chronic nonalcoholic steatohepatitis (active or healed)
    Healed centrilobular necroses in hepatic allografts
    Hypervitaminosis A
    Syphilis (neonatal syphilitic hepatitis)
Fibrosis Unrelated to Specific Anatomic Structures
    Conditions listed under "Nonzonal (Multilobular) Necrosis" (see Table 9.1).
    Healed infarcts
    Treated neoplasms or postinfectious states

Clinical Conditions

Chronic Active or Unresolved Viral Hepatitis

Comments: The duration of chronic active hepatitis is 6 months or longer. Unresolved viral hepatitis is diagnosed 2 to 5 months after onset. Chronic active hepatitis is either idiopathic or caused by hepatitis viruses B or non-A, non-B (hepatitis C, D, and possibly other hitherto undescribed viruses). See also Chapters 2 and 3.

Morphologic features: Lymphocytic piecemeal necrosis (see Chapter 9), the hallmark of chronic active hepatitis, may be associated with periportal proliferation of immature fibroblasts and, eventually, periportal fibrosis. Tongue-shaped proliferations may lead to "active septa," that is, bridging (or septal) fibrosis. Portal-to-central bridging may set the stage for the development of cirrhosis. Fibroplastic proliferation of this type in acute or unresolved viral hepatitis often heralds progressive disease and chronicity, particularly in older patients.[1] Other types of periportal hepatitis (see Chapter 2) also may lead to periportal and septal fibrosis.

Chronic Alcoholic Hepatitis

Comments: A history of alcohol abuse or dependence is required for the diagnosis (see also Chapters 6 and 7).

Morphologic features: The features of chronicity in alcoholic hepatitis are

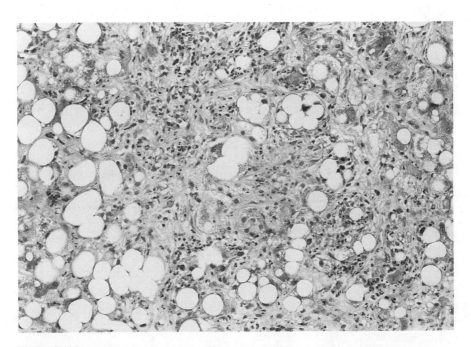

Figure 10.1A
Fibrosis in chronic alcoholic hepatitis. Centrilobular fibrosis is associated with fatty changes, spotty necroses with neutrophils, and Mallory bodies (not clearly visible at this magnification). The scarring in the center of the field suggests chronicity; a vein cannot be identified. The inflammatory changes are the features of ongoing acute alcoholic hepatitis.

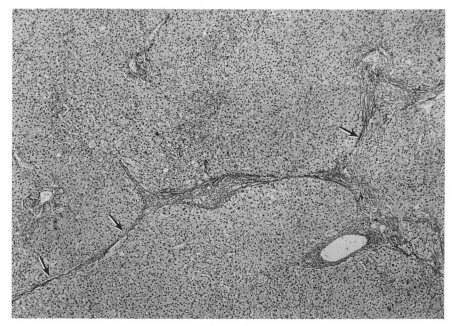

Figure 10.1B
Fibrosis in chronic alcoholic hepatitis. Slender fibrous septa (arrows) are the only remnants of previous chronic alcoholic hepatitis in a patient who stopped drinking. The fibrous septa replace central veins or are found in their vicinity.

perisinusoidal fibrosis, particularly in centrilobular areas ("sclerosing hyaline necrosis"), and lymphocytic phlebitis, phlebosclerosis, or veno-occlusive lesions of central (terminal hepatic) veins (Figure 10.1A). These centrilobular changes are accompanied by portal and periportal fibroplasia, which eventually leads to portal-to-central bridging and cirrhosis (for other features of alcoholic hepatitis, see Chapter 7). If a patient with chronic alcoholic hepatitis stops drinking, the biopsy evidence of alcoholic liver disease disappears within a few months, except for the telltale centrilobular scars (Figure 10.1B).

Chronic Congestion

Chronic congestive heart failure is the most common cause of this condition. Biopsy specimens may show centrilobular fibrosis, central-to-central bridging (septal fibrosis) and, very rarely, true congestive cirrhosis. The combination of centrilobular sinusoidal dilatation, centrilobular scarring, and presence of normal portal tracts surrounded by normal hepatic parenchyma provides the most important diagnostic clue. (For further details and references, see Chapter 16).

Chronic Nonalcoholic Steatohepatitis

Comments: A negative history of alcoholism is required for the diagnosis. Hepatomegaly and complications such as portal hypertension may be present. The most common underlying disorders appear to be uncomplicated or morbid obesity and adult-onset diabetes mellitus. (See also Chapter 7.)

Morphologic features: The morphologic changes are indistinguishable from the changes in chronic alcoholic hepatitis (see above). Although nonalcoholic steatohepatitis usually is milder than alcoholic hepatitis, chronicity may be associated with centrilobular scarring, septal fibrosis, and, eventually, cirrhosis.

Congenital Hepatic Fibrosis

Comments: This hereditary hamartomatous disorder of the liver may be entirely asymptomatic or may be associated with symptoms of portal hypertension or complications of associated fibrocystic diseases of the liver or biliary tract, such as choledochal cyst or focal dilatation of intrahepatic bile ducts (Caroli's disease).

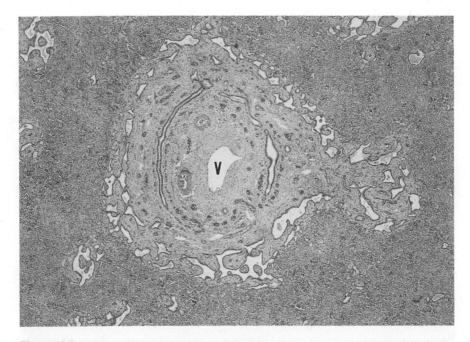

Figure 10.2
Congenital hepatic fibrosis. Note enlarged and fibrosed portal tract with proliferated hamartomatous bile ducts, forming microcysts near the limiting plates. Portal vein (V) hypoplasia is not evident in this illustration.

Morphologic features: Dilated and proliferated bile ducts are embedded in excess portal and periportal connective tissue (Figure 10.2), resulting in enlargement of portal tracts and septal fibrosis. Bile plugs may be present in the ducts. Hypoplasia of portal vein branches may be a prominent finding. Evidence of biliary infection with neutrophilic cholangitis is not a feature of uncomplicated congenital hepatic fibrosis. However, infective cholangitis can be found if congenital hepatic fibrosis is associated with focal dilatation of intrahepatic bile ducts (segmental Caroli's disease).

Genetic (Familial) Liver Diseases

In hereditary metabolic disorders such as mucopolysaccharidoses, slender fibrous septa may connect the portal tracts and thus appear to encircle the lobules.[2] Periportal and septal fibrosis also occur in argininosuccinic aciduria, atransferrinemia, glycogenosis types I, III, VI, IX, and X, as well as in cholesteryl ester storage disease and many other conditions in this category. (Also included here are all hereditary disorders listed under "Cirrhosis and Hepatocellular Nodules Without Cirrhosis" in Chapter 11.)

Healed Centrilobular Necroses in Hepatic Allografts

Centrilobular necroses in hepatic allografts most often appear to be related to persistent rejection. In some instances, the necroses persist until the graft is lost, but if the graft recovers they seem to disappear or heal by centrilobular scarring.[3]

Healed Infarcts

Anemic hepatic infarcts are rare, particularly in biopsy specimens. Although massive hepatic infarction is not survivable, small infarcts may heal and form irregular scars, particularly in the subcapsular regions. Tumor in the liver is a common cause of infarcts. Subcapsular infarcts are also found in many allografts.[4] Nongestational disseminated intravascular coagulation and eclampsia are other possible causes of infarcts (see Chapter 16). Infarcts of Zahn (see Chapter 16) are not associated with tissue necrosis or scarring.

Hypervitaminosis A

Even moderate amounts of vitamin A can cause liver damage if the intake occurred over a long period.[5] The resulting fibrosis is panlobular and primarily perisinusoidal; it may be associated with periportal sinusoidal dilatation (see Chapter 16). Central veins also may become sclerosed and adjacent hepatocytes atrophied. Characteristic is the swelling of the perisinusoidal lipocytes (Ito cells). If frozen sections can be prepared, these lipocytes show a characteristic, quickly fading green fluorescence, which confirms the diagnosis. However, if a patient with an appropriate history and elevated levels of serum retinol has swollen, vacuolated lipocytes, the diagnosis of hypervitaminosis A is reasonably certain, even without the study of fluorescence.

Idiopathic Portal Hypertension

Biopsy specimens may appear normal, but large wedge specimens typically show subendothelial thickening of portal vein branches. In advanced cases, most specimens show portal fibrosis with obliteration or loss of small portal vein branches (see Figure 16.6). Organized portal vein thrombi may be present also. The hepatic lobules usually are normal.[6] These histologic features are incorporated in the synonyms for idiopathic (or primary) portal hypertension, "noncirrhotic portal fibrosis" and "hepatoportal sclerosis." It should be noted that similar histologic changes can be found in extrahepatic portal vein obstruction. Idiopathic portal hypertension probably can have many causes, which appear to differ geographically. The observed histologic changes might represent either the cause of the portal hypertension—for instance, after portal vein microembolism—or they

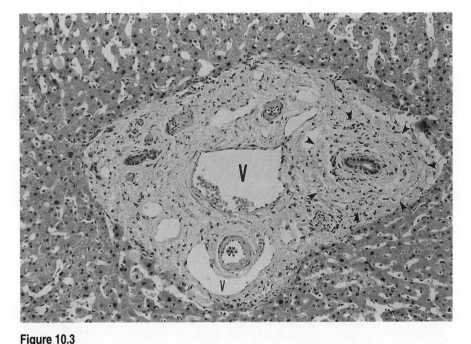

Figure 10.3
Portal fibrosis and fibrous cholangitis in a patient with persistent choledocholithiasis. The interlobular bile duct is surrounded by a fibrous collar with interspersed chronic inflammatory cells (arrowheads). It should be noted that the periductal inflammation is not an obligatory feature. Several hepatic artery (asterisks) and portal vein branches (V) can be seen in this slightly fibrosed portal tract. The expected ductal proliferation cannot be appreciated in this portal tract.

might be the result of the condition as one would expect if truly functional primary portal hypertension does indeed exist. For the characteristic vascular changes, see Chapter 16.

Nonsuppurative Cholangitis, All Types

Periductal fibrosis may represent the healing stage of all types of nonsuppurative cholangitis that have been listed in Table 15.1. It appears that lymphocytic, pleomorphic (mixed cell), fibrous, and granulomatous cholangitis may lose their inflammatory features, which then are replaced by a fibrous collar.

Obstruction of Large (Extrahepatic or Perihilar Intrahepatic) Bile Ducts

Comments: Biopsy often is done because of negative cholangiographic or ultrasound studies. In many instances, parenchymal liver disease is suspected.

Morphologic features: The typical biopsy findings have been described in Chapter 2. Periductal fibrosis is a prominent feature in a few cases; it may represent late-stage fibrous cholangitis. Characteristically, a collar of concentrically arranged collagen fibers surrounds interlobular or septal bile ducts. Persistence of biliary obstruction often leads to increased density of the portal connective tissue (portal fibrosis; Figure 10.3) and to periportal collagen deposition in the form of fibrous piecemeal necrosis (see Chapter 9). Intermittently, new limiting plates are formed. In these instances, the periportal fibrosis may be misinterpreted as being part of unusually large portal tracts. Eventually, portal-to-portal bridging (septal fibrosis) can be observed. This pattern of hepatic fibrosis is rather characteristic of many chronic biliary diseases and therefore has been named "biliary fibrosis." Cases designated as biliary cirrhosis because of the presence of garland-shaped regenerative nodules often have a preserved lobular and vascular architecture and therefore represent biliary fibrosis, which is a potentially reversible condition.

Primary Sclerosing Cholangitis

Comments: Clinical and laboratory findings usually reveal chronic cholestatic liver disease. Typical cholangiographic findings confirm the diagnosis. Most patients have chronic ulcerative colitis.

Morphologic features: All types of biliary fibrosis described above under "Obstruction of Large (Extrahepatic or Perihilar Intrahepatic) Bile Ducts" may also occur in primary sclerosing cholangitis. Indeed, the presence of enlarged portal tracts after periportal collagen deposition and the formation of portal-to-portal bridges (septal fibrosis) have been used as the criteria for the disease stages 2 and 3, respectively.[7,8] Fibrosis and other changes confined to the portal tracts characterize stage-1 disease, and presence of diffuse fibrosis with true regenerative nodules is the hallmark of stage-4 disease. These features can be found in both small-duct and large-duct primary sclerosing cholangitis.

Schistosomiasis

Hepatosplenic schistosomiasis can be caused by *Schistosoma mansoni*, *Schistosoma japonicum*, and *Schistosoma mekongi*. The last two are restricted to parts of the Far East.[9] In chronic cases, characteristic patterns of portal and septal fibrosis can be observed ("pipestem fibrosis"), consisting of serpiginous septa connecting fibrotic portal tracts. Granulomas with ova are diagnostic but they are not always present. Portal veins often are tortuous and show intimal proliferation; thrombi or adult worms sometimes can be found in their lumina. After infection with *S mansoni*, intrahepatic bile duct changes have been described, consisting of periductal fibrosis, hyperplasia and degeneration of bile duct epithelium, and ductular proliferation.[10]

Syphilis

Neonatal syphilitic hepatitis (congenital syphilis) leads to diffuse pericellular (perisinusoidal) hepatic fibrosis, together with portal fibrosis and diffuse chronic inflammatory infiltrates. The diagnosis can be confirmed with silver stains, which will reveal *Treponema pallidum* throughout the lobules and in blood vessels.

Toxic Fibrosis

Exposure to arsenic or copper solutions and industrial poisons such as vinyl chloride may cause hepatic fibrosis (see also Chapters 11 and 16).

Treated Neoplasms or Postinfectious States

Irregular scars resembling old infarcts may be observed after successful irradiation or chemotherapy of tumors,[11] or after healing of abscesses or of granulomatous inflammation. Calcification in such lesions suggests an infectious etiology.[12] Calcification in tumors is an uncommon finding.

Unknown Causes

Prominent periductal fibrosis can be an incidental finding in many liver diseases and in otherwise normal livers. It is not clear whether this feature always represents a healing stage of previous cholangitis or whether it may be a variant of normal. Periductal fibrosis is not a reliable sign of primary sclerosing cholangitis! Other types of hepatic fibrosis—in particular, portal and septal fibrosis—may be found in specimens from patients who have no history of liver disease and who are asymptomatic. The fibrotic lesions in these cases probably represent healing stages after asymptomatic infections. Only descriptive diagnoses can be provided.

References

1. Bianchi L: Histopathology of viral hepatitis. *Proc Clin Biol Res* 143:66-76, 1983.

2. Parfrey NA, Hutchins GM: Hepatic fibrosis in mucopolysaccharidoses. *Am J Med* 81:825-829, 1986.

3. Ludwig J, Gross JR Jr, Perkins JD, et al: Persistent centrilobular necroses in hepatic allografts. *Hum Pathol* 21:656-661, 1990.

4. Russo PA, Yunis EJ: Subcapsular hepatic necrosis in orthotopic liver allografts. *Hepatology* 6:708-713, 1986.

5. Minuk GY, Kelly JK, Hwang W-S: Vitamin A hepatotoxicity in multiple family members. *Hepatology* 8:272-275, 1988.

6. Sarin SK: Non-cirrhotic portal fibrosis (progress report). *Gut* 30:406-415, 1989.

7. Ludwig J, LaRusso NF, Wiesner RH: Primary sclerosing cholangitis. In Peters RL, Craig JR (eds): *Liver Pathology*. New York, Churchill Livingstone, 1986, pp 193-213.

8. Ludwig J: Surgical pathology of the syndrome of primary sclerosing cholangitis. *Am J Surg Pathol* 13:43-49, 1989.

9. De Cock KM: Hepatosplenic schistosomiasis: A clinical review. *Gut* 27:734-745, 1986.

10. Vianna MR, Gayotto LCCC, Telma R, et al: Intrahepatic bile duct changes in human hepatosplenic schistosomiasis mansoni. *Liver* 9:100-109, 1989.

11. Quizlbash A, Kontozoglou T, Sianos J, et al: Hepar lobatum associated with chemotherapy and metastatic breast cancer. *Arch Pathol Lab Med* 111:58-61, 1987.

12. Okuda K, Kimura K, Takara K, et al: Resolution of diffuse granulomatous fibrosis of the liver with antituberculous chemotherapy. *Gastroenterology* 91:456-460, 1986.

Chapter 11

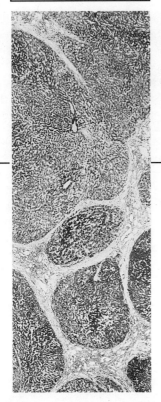

Cirrhosis and Hepatocellular Nodules Without Cirrhosis

Morphologic Definition

Cirrhosis is an endstage of many liver diseases, characterized by fibrosis, nodular regeneration, and disturbed vascular architecture throughout the liver. The fibrosis is septal or multilobular, and the regenerative changes are micronodular, macronodular, or mixed. The disturbance of the vascular architecture has been demonstrated in many studies but is not apparent in routine tissue preparations. For all practical purposes, cirrhosis is considered irreversible. In some conditions—in particular, biliary and congestive fibrosis—the histologic appearance may be that of cirrhosis, although parenchymal regeneration and altered vascular architecture still have not reached the level of true cirrhosis and therefore may be potentially reversible. Other conditions that do not meet the criteria for cirrhosis as defined here include macroregenerative nodules in submassive or massive hepatic necrosis, congenital hepatic fibrosis[1] (see Chapter 10), focal nodular hyperplasia,[2] liver cell adenoma or adenomatosis,[3] nodular regenerative hyperplasia,[4] partial nodular transformation,[5] and subcapsular fibrosis with nodular regeneration in atrophic livers. Note: Because the term "cirrhosis" implies irreversibility, the histopathologic diagnosis should be based on convincing changes, identified in a specimen of adequate size. If only minute fragments are available for study, a reticulum stain should be prepared; presence of cirrhosis can be suspected if condensed reticulin fibers are found in the periphery of the fragments. This feature is considered evidence of nodular regeneration and hence is suggestive of cirrhosis.

Table 11.1 Clinical Conditions Associated With Cirrhosis and Hepatocellular Nodules Without Cirrhosis*

Cirrhosis With Prominent Fatty Changes
  Alcoholic cirrhosis
  Cirrhosis caused by nonalcoholic steatohepatitis (nonalcoholic steatohepatitic cirrhosis)
  Cirrhosis of any type with superimposed fatty change—for instance,
    after prednisone treatment (not listed in this chapter)
  Uncommon causes:
    Cirrhosis associated with total parenteral nutrition
    Cirrhosis caused by genetic (familial) liver diseases (galactosemia, hereditary
      fructose intolerance, porphyria cutanea tarda, tyrosinemia, Wilson's disease)
    Congestive cirrhosis
    Drug-induced cirrhosis
    Toxic cirrhosis
Cirrhosis With Much Hemosiderosis, With or Without Fatty Changes
  Pigment cirrhosis in primary hemochromatosis or associated with alcoholism,
    erythropoietic disorders, or venovenous shunts
Cirrhosis With Much Cholestasis
  Biliary cirrhosis in infantile obstructive cholangiopathy (see under
    "Obstructive Biliary Cirrhosis")
  Biliary cirrhosis associated with primary sclerosing cholangitis (see under
    "Small-Duct Biliary Cirrhosis Other Than Primary Biliary Cirrhosis")
  Obstructive biliary cirrhosis (large-duct biliary cirrhosis; secondary biliary cirrhosis)
  Primary biliary cirrhosis
  Uncommon causes: (see under "Small-Duct Biliary Cirrhosis Other Than
    Primary Biliary Cirrhosis")
      Chronic intrahepatic cholestasis of sarcoidosis
      Drug-induced cholangitis
      Ductopenic (chronic) hepatic allograft rejection
      Graft-versus-host disease
      Idiopathic adulthood ductopenia
      Infantile obstructive cholangiopathy
Cirrhosis With Other Special Histologic Features
  Cirrhosis associated with alpha-1-antitrypsin deficiency

continued on page 123

continued from 122
Uncommon causes:
Cirrhosis associated with hereditary hemorrhagic telangiectasia (Rendu-Weber-Osler disease)
Cirrhosis caused by other genetic (familial) liver diseases (cystic fibrosis [mucoviscidosis]; erythropoietic protoporphyria; galactosemia; glycogen storage disease, type IV; hereditary fructose intolerance; mucopolysaccharidosis; porphyria cutanea tarda; tyrosinemia; Wolman's disease)
Congestive cirrhosis
Indian childhood cirrhosis
Sarcoid cirrhosis
Cirrhosis Without Fatty Changes, Hemosiderosis, Cholestasis, or Other Special Features
Cryptogenic cirrhosis
Drug-induced cirrhosis
Posthepatitic cirrhosis
Conditions Associated With Hepatocellular Nodules in the Absence of Cirrhosis
Focal nodular hyperplasia
Liver cell adenoma
Macroregenerative nodules (in massive or submassive hepatic necrosis)
Mixed hamartoma
Nodular regenerative hyperplasia
Partial nodular transformation

*Because of their special microscopic features, some types of cirrhosis or conditions leading to cirrhosis have been listed here under more than one subheading.

Clinical Conditions

Alcoholic Cirrhosis

Comments: A history of alcohol abuse or dependence is required for the diagnosis. Neuropsychiatric disturbances often can be recognized. Biochemical tests show elevated aminotransferase levels, among other abnormalities. Alcoholic cirrhosis may be associated with symptoms of acute alcoholic hepatitis. After a patient has stopped drinking, alcoholic cirrhosis gradually assumes the clinical and morphologic features of cryptogenic cirrhosis (see below).

Morphologic features: Alcoholic cirrhosis in an active drinker shows all the histologic changes described under "Alcoholic Hepatitis" (see Chapter 7), with the added feature of nodular regeneration (Figure 11.1A). If cholestasis is present, a distinction must be made between alcoholic cirrhosis with cholestasis, and biliary or other types of cirrhosis with cholestasis-induced Mallory bodies (see Chapter 12). In biliary cirrhosis, Mallory bodies are found in the periphery of the regenerative nodules, and fatty changes, if present, tend to be mild. In alcoholic

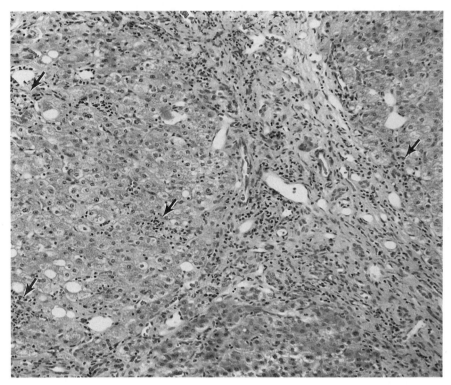

Figure 11.1A
Alcoholic cirrhosis. This cirrhosis can be considered active because of the inflammatory changes and spotty necroses (arrows) within the lobules. In active posthepatitic cirrhosis, the nodules would be surrounded by lymphocytic piecemeal necrosis.

cirrhosis, Mallory bodies often are found in a more random distribution and the fatty changes usually are prominent.

As stated above, alcoholic cirrhosis loses the features of alcoholic hepatitis after the patient has stopped drinking; this usually happens within a few months and certainly in less than 1 year (Figure 11.1B). If sclerosis or obliteration of hepatic vein branches can be identified, the cause of the cirrhosis can be tentatively diagnosed even after that time.

Cirrhosis Associated With Alpha-1-Antitrypsin Deficiency

Alpha-1-antitrypsin deficiency is a hereditary disorder of protein metabolism that may lead to cirrhosis, usually in the 6th to 8th decade of life. Chronic obstructive pulmonary disease is another important complication. Clinical onset of the liver disease is earlier in homozygotes (ZZ) than in heterozygotes (MZ and SZ) and thus, cirrhosis is found more commonly in homozygotes.[6] The livers resemble

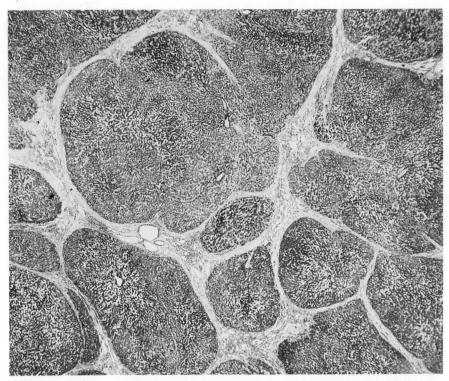

Figure 11.1B
Alcoholic cirrhosis. Inactive alcoholic cirrhosis is shown in a patient who had stopped drinking several years earlier. This specimen was obtained at the time of orthotopic liver transplantation. Note the sharp outline of the regenerative nodules, characteristic of cirrhosis without inflammatory activity.

---

posthepatitic or cryptogenic cirrhosis. The diagnostic findings are PAS-positive, diastase-resistant granules and globules in the cytoplasm of hepatocytes (see Figures 12.2A and 12.2B). Immunostains for alpha-1-antitrypsin show staining of the cytoplasm rather than staining of the inclusions. The largest globules can be found in the periphery of the regenerative nodules. A rough correlation appears to exist between the number of globules and the phenotype—that is, globules are most prominent in homozygotes. For additional descriptions, see the Index.

Cirrhosis Associated With Hereditary Hemorrhagic Telangiectasia (Rendu-Osler-Weber Disease)

Whether cirrhosis can actually be caused by hereditary hemorrhagic telangiectasia is controversial. Some authors claim to have documented such an association,[7] but others have pointed out that many of these patients do not have true cirrhosis[8]; artery-to-portal vein shunts and other vascular abnormalities seem to cause nodular transformation akin to focal nodular hyperplasia or nodular regenerative hyperplasia, and this may imitate cirrhosis. In any event, in specimens from affected patients the typical telangiectasias can be found, and that establishes the presence of this familial angiomatosis. The cause of the cirrhosis must be determined on a case-by-case basis.

Cirrhosis Associated With Total Parenteral Nutrition

The condition probably is caused by multiple hepatotoxic factors related to parenteral nutrition. Biopsy specimens may show features of chronic hepatitis with cholestasis, or of steatohepatitic cirrhosis, often with ceroid, lipochrome, and other pigments. For further details and for references, see Chapters 7 and 14.

Cirrhosis Caused by Genetic (Familial) Liver Diseases

Most of these conditions are quite rare, and the liver disease in many instances is only one of many manifestations. The following list comprises the majority of genetic liver diseases that have led to cirrhosis.

Alpha-1-Antitrypsin Deficiency
This has been discussed above.

Cystic Fibrosis (Mucoviscidosis)
Most livers of patients with this hereditary disorder of unknown pathogenesis have only fatty changes and portal fibrosis, but in a few cases, inspissated mucus can be found in small bile ducts, with or without biliary cirrhosis (focal or multilobular biliary cirrhosis).[9] After infancy, cholestasis is quite rare in this condition. Deformities of large bile ducts with hepatolithiasis,[10] carcinoma of extrahepatic bile ducts,[11] and amyloidosis[12] also have been described in cystic fibrosis. (See also Chapter 15.)

Erythropoietic Protoporphyria
In this rare hereditary disorder of heme biosynthesis, the congenital deficiency of ferrochelatase can cause cirrhosis, and liver failure may develop. The histologic diagnosis can be based on the presence of abundant and characteristic pigment deposits in epithelial cells as well as mesenchymal liver cells; they represent protoporphyrin.[13,14] In frozen sections under polarized light, the pigment appears bright red with a centrally located black Maltese cross in each granule. Electron microscopically, the pigment shows a characteristic "star-burst" pattern. (See also Chapter 14.)

Galactosemia
In this rare hereditary disorder of carbohydrate metabolism, a congenital deficiency of galactose-1-phosphate uridyl transferase (galactosemia, type 1) or

galactokinase (galactosemia, type 2), the cirrhosis is associated with pseudoglandular transformation of the hepatic parenchyma with canalicular cholestasis, and fatty changes. (For the resemblance with changes in hereditary fructose intolerance, see below.) Giant cell transformation and liver cell adenomas also have been observed. The cirrhosis develops in infancy. (See also Chapter 6.)

Glycogen Storage Disease

More than 10 subtypes exist of this rare hereditary disorder of carbohydrate metabolism,[15] all characterized by congenital deficiency of different enzymes. Only glycogenosis, type IV (amylopectinosis; congenital deficiency of alpha-1,4-glucan-6-glycosyl transferase) has led to well-documented cirrhosis.[16] The diagnostic features in this condition are spherical or rhombohedral inclusions in the cytoplasm of hepatocytes; they are stainable with PAS (partially resistant to diastase), Hale's iron, and alcian blue. Thus, these inclusions are indistinguishable from Lafora bodies (see Chapter 12).

Hemochromatosis

Primary hemochromatosis is a hereditary disorder of unknown pathogenesis affecting iron deposition. Many cases of hemochromatosis associated with alcoholism probably also belong in this category. The morphologic features are discussed below.

Hereditary Fructose Intolerance

In this rare hereditary disorder of carbohydrate metabolism, the cirrhosis is caused by a congenital deficiency of fructose-1-phosphate aldolase or fructose-1,6-diphosphatase. Giant cell transformation, pseudoglandular rearrangement of hepatocytes, and fatty change in the earlier stages (closely resembling the above-mentioned changes in galactosemia), and fibrosis and cirrhosis in the late stages are the expected findings. The cirrhosis in this condition may be reversible, and thus these cases may not meet all the criteria for true cirrhosis.

Hereditary Hemorrhagic Telangiectasia (Rendu-Osler-Weber Disease)

This has been discussed above.

Mucopolysaccharidosis

At least 7 subtypes exist of this rare hereditary disorder of glycoprotein metabolism (lysosomal storage disorder), all characterized by congenital deficiency of different enzymes. Whether true cirrhosis develops in mucopolysaccharidosis (MPS) is not quite clear but prominent hepatic fibrosis has been documented in Hurler's syndrome (MPS, type 1), Hunter's syndrome (MPS, type 2), and Sanfilippo's syndrome (MPS, types 3A and 3B).[17] Swelling of hepatocytes (particularly in periportal or paraseptal areas) and of Kupffer cells can be appreciated in all areas. The histochemical demonstration of the mucopolysaccharides requires preparation of frozen sections and alcian blue staining. Because of the solubility of this material, even this staining procedure may not be successful.

Niemann-Pick Disease

See Chapter 12.

Porphyria Cutanea Tarda

The accumulation of uroporphyrins in this condition results from a reduced activity of uroporphyrinogen decarboxylase. Alcoholism, certain drugs, and possibly other factors appear to trigger the full expression of this disease. Porphyria cutanea tarda may not always be a hereditary disorder. The cirrhosis in some of these cases may be alcoholic or of some other type. Typically, the histologic sections show fatty changes and small intralobular aggregates of inflammatory cells with Kupffer cells containing iron and ceroid.[18] With the ferric ferricyanide reduction reaction and sometimes with van Gieson stains, needle-shaped cytoplasmic inclusions can be identified in paraffin sections; they appear to be specific for this condition.[19] Hemosiderosis in hepatocytes in the periphery of the nodules can be found also. (See also Chapter 14.)

Progressive Intrahepatic Cholestasis (Byler's Disease)

This hereditary disorder is characterized by an abnormal secretion of bilirubin and bile acids. The condition leads to biliary-type cirrhosis, liver failure, and death in infancy or childhood. For other familial conditions resembling progressive intrahepatic cholestasis, see Chapter 4.

Tyrosinemia

In this rare hereditary disorder of amino acid metabolism, the cause of the liver disease is unclear; liver abnormalities precede the appearance of increased concentrations of tyrosine and methionine. The cirrhosis in tyrosinosis, type 1 (chronic form) develops in infancy and may be associated with hepatocellular carcinoma.[20] Some regenerative nodules may contain diffuse fatty changes and ballooning whereas adjacent nodules lack these features. Hepatocellular rosettes and dysplastic changes of hepatocytes also may be present.[21]

Wilson's Disease

The histologic changes in this hereditary disorder of copper metabolism are described in Chapters 2, 12, and 14. In the cirrhotic stage of this disease, presence of high copper levels may be the only feature with which Wilson's disease can be distinguished from posthepatitic cirrhosis. For methods of demonstrating the copper, see Chapter 14.

Wolman's Disease

This rare hereditary disorder of lipid metabolism leads to cirrhosis and death in infancy; it is caused by a deficiency of lysosomal acid lipase. Hepatocytes and Kupffer cells are stuffed with cholesteryl esters and triglycerides so that these two cell types become difficult to distinguish. In a related condition, cholesteryl ester storage disease, the manifestations are milder but hepatic fibrosis still may develop. (See also Chapter 12.)

Cirrhosis Caused by Nonalcoholic Steatohepatitis (Nonalcoholic Steatohepatitic Cirrhosis)

Comments: A negative history of alcoholism is required for the diagnosis. For possible causes of steatohepatitic cirrhosis, see under "Nonalcoholic Steatohepatitis"

(Chapter 7). Nonalcoholic steatohepatitis of any etiology is a much less common cause of cirrhosis than alcoholic steatohepatitis (alcoholic hepatitis).

Morphologic features: Principally, nonalcoholic steatohepatitic cirrhosis cannot be distinguished from alcoholic cirrhosis. As described under "Nonalcoholic Steatohepatitis" (see Chapter 7), the morphologic features of the two conditions are the same, but as a group histologic features of nonalcoholic steatohepatitis tend to be milder. Nonalcoholic steatohepatitic cirrhosis most often resembles alcoholic cirrhosis in a patient who has not been drinking for several weeks.

Congestive Cirrhosis

This condition is extremely rare. It is caused by prolonged hepatic venous outflow impairment in congestive heart failure or in hepatic vein thrombosis and other conditions that are considered causes of the Budd-Chiari syndrome (including occlusion of the hepatic or suprahepatic inferior vena cava) and hepatic veno-occlusive disease. Sinusoidal dilatation, fibrous bridging—particularly between central veins (terminal hepatic veins)—and nodular regeneration, with or without fatty change, are the diagnostic features. In most instances, the islands of parenchyma have portal tracts in their centers and thus represent pseudonodules rather than true regenerative nodules. In these cases, the diagnosis "congestive fibrosis" should be used. (See also Chapter 16.)

Cryptogenic Cirrhosis

Comments: If clinical history, biochemistry, histology, and other pertinent studies fail to reveal the cause of the condition, the term *cryptogenic cirrhosis* is applicable. If no attempts were made to determine the cause of the cirrhosis or if the data are unavailable, the correct designation is "cirrhosis, type undetermined." Most patients with cryptogenic cirrhosis probably have posthepatitic cirrhosis following asymptomatic chronic active hepatitis non-A, non-B, or inactive alcoholic or nonalcoholic steatohepatitic cirrhosis. If a history of alcoholism is volunteered, the tentative diagnosis of alcoholic cirrhosis still can be made (see above).

Morphologic features: Typically, fibrosis, nodular regeneration, and mild inflammatory changes are the only histologic findings. If fatty changes are prominent, they are either unrelated to the cirrhosis or they are a sign of antecedent steatohepatitis. Iron stains are negative or at least not in the range of pigment cirrhosis (see below). Staining with PAS-D fails to reveal the globules of alpha-1-antitrypsin deficiency (see Chapter 12). Stains for copper or copper-associated protein are negative or only weakly positive. Cholestasis generally is not a feature of cryptogenic cirrhosis either.

Drug-Induced Cirrhosis

The diagnosis can be suggested if an appropriate history has been provided. For a list of drugs that may cause cirrhosis, see Table 11.2. It should be noted that drug-induced cirrhosis is quite rare and that exposure to a drug listed on Table 11.2 still does not prove an etiologic association.

Focal Nodular Hyperplasia

In this circumscribed lesion, hepatocellular nodules surround a central fibrous scar (Figure 11.2). Bile ductules usually can be identified, but normal portal tracts are not present. The lesions are thought to develop in response to an arterial anomaly.[22] Focal nodular hyperplasia is not related to cirrhosis.

Indian Childhood Cirrhosis

This condition might represent a genetic disease but also could be the result of exogenous copper overload; cases with similar features have been observed in the United States[23] and Germany.[24] The patients in both studies disclosed no Indian heritage or parental consanguinity. In the German family with two affected siblings,[24] chronic copper contamination of the drinking water was demonstrated

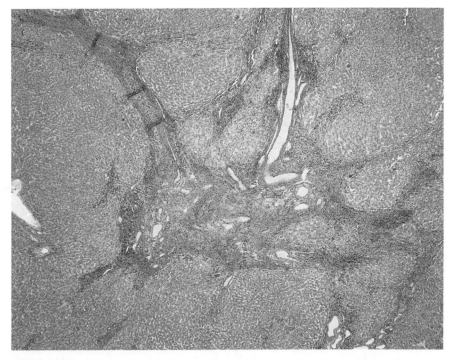

Figure 11.2
Focal nodular hyperplasia. Note central scar with fibrous septa imparting a star-like configuration. This is a focal lesion but microscopic specimens may be interpreted as representing cirrhosis.

(see Chapter 14). All cases with this condition show micronodular cirrhosis in which the nodules are indeed minuscule, having the size of a lobule or less. The hepatocytes are ballooned and Mallory bodies are abundant. Spotty inflammatory infiltrates with neutrophils are a characteristic feature. Stains for copper and copper-associated protein are strongly positive. The fibrous septa show chronic inflammation, ductular proliferation, and edema. Pericellular fibrosis and fibrosis of hepatic vein branches have been noted. Fatty change is not a feature of this condition.

Liver Cell Adenoma

This tumor rarely occurs spontaneously but is fairly common in women taking oral contraceptives or in patients taking anabolic steroids. Adenomas also occur in patients with glycogen storage disease, type I, or with tyrosinosis. The hepatocytes in the adenomas often are enlarged and may be hydropic. Vascular changes and hemorrhages are found in many of these tumors, as described in Chapter 16. In some adenomas, hepatocellular rosettes with bile plugs, or hepatocytes with Mallory bodies and fatty changes are present; hepatocellular giant cells also may be found.[22] If foci of fibrodegenerative change are present, the distinction from focal nodular hyperplasia comes into consideration. Liver cell adenomas are not related to cirrhosis.

Macroregenerative Nodules

These nodules occur not only in cirrhosis but also in massive or submassive hepatic necrosis (see Chapter 9). Although these conditions often are fatal, they are potentially reversible and therefore not cirrhosis.

Mixed Hamartoma

This is a rare solitary tumor of hepatocytes, bile ductules, and dense fibrous tissue. Mixed hamartomas lack the central scars that are found in focal nodular hyperplasia.[22] Also, in mixed hamartomas bile ductules are only present at the interface between fibrous and hepatocellular tissue, not among the hepatic cell plates. This tumor is not related to cirrhosis.

Nodular Regenerative Hyperplasia

In this condition, multiple hepatocellular nodules are distributed throughout the liver (Figure 11.3), usually in response to obliteration of small portal veins.[25] The condition has been observed in a large number of systemic diseases. It may be associated with portal hypertension. The nodules rarely measure more than a few millimeters in diameter. In biopsy specimens, nodular regenerative hyperplasia is best recognized after use of a reticulum stain. Fibrosis is absent in this condition, and therefore it is not related to cirrhosis.

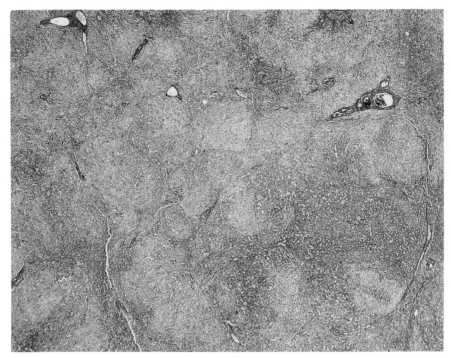

Figure 11.3
Nodular regenerative hyperplasia in a patient with multiple myeloma and amyloidosis. Note multiple light hepatocellular nodules and dark, partly compressed hepatic parenchyma, without fibrosis. Although this is a diffuse lesion, it does not represent cirrhosis since fibrosis is absent.

Obstructive Biliary Cirrhosis (Large-Duct Biliary Cirrhosis; Secondary Biliary Cirrhosis)

Comments: This type of biliary cirrhosis can be diagnosed after prolonged obstruction of extrahepatic or large perihilar intrahepatic bile ducts. The cirrhosis can develop within a few months after the biliary obstruction has become manifest. Biliary cirrhosis complicating small-duct biliary disease is either primary biliary cirrhosis or it should be identified by its specific etiology—for instance, biliary cirrhosis associated with graft-versus-host disease. (See also below under "Small-Duct Biliary Cirrhosis Other Than Primary Biliary Cirrhosis.")

Morphologic features: Septal fibrosis and edema, nodular regeneration, proliferation of ducts and ductules, and cholestasis with bile lakes and bile infarcts are typical findings. Neutrophilic and fibrous cholangitis are common additional features. Cholangitic abscesses may complicate the condition. In some instances, prolonged large-duct biliary obstruction leads to loss of interlobular bile ducts. Because of the resulting ductopenia, obstructive biliary cirrhosis may bear a close resemblance to primary biliary cirrhosis.

Partial Nodular Transformation

In this rare condition, large regenerative nodules (up to 4 cm) are found in the perihilar area, probably in response to thrombosis of portal vein branches. The patients have portal hypertension.[25,26] Pericellular fibrosis and fibrosis of hepatic vein branches have been noted. Fatty change is not a feature of this condition.

Pigment Cirrhosis in Primary Hemochromatosis or Associated With Alcoholism, Erythropoietic Disorders, or Venovenous Shunts

Comments: The clinical presentations of hemochromatosis (used here as a name for a group of clinical conditions) and the suspected relationships between hemochromatosis and alcoholism, erythropoietic disorders, or venovenous (portacaval) shunts are presented in Chapter 13. In any of these conditions, hepatic iron concentration should be measured. Paraffin-embedded tissue can be used to obtain dried specimens for flameless atomic absorption spectrophotometry. Formalin fixation and paraffin embedding have no effect on the results of these studies.[27]

Morphologic features: Pigment cirrhosis in untreated primary (genetic) hemochromatosis shows fibrosis, nodular regeneration, severe hemosiderosis of hepatocytes, epithelial cells of bile ducts and ductules, and mesenchymal cells including Kupffer cells and portal fibroblasts. (Note: The term "hemosiderosis" connotes a histologic finding, not "mild hemochromatosis.") The hepatocellular hemosiderosis is most severe in the periphery of the regenerative nodules. Patches of ferritin (see Chapter 13) may be found in some nodules. Typically, pigment cirrhosis is quite inactive, that is, inflammatory changes are minimal (Figure 11.4). After a prolonged phlebotomy program, most or all of the stainable iron may have left the liver. Bile duct epithelial cells store hemosiderin the longest. Exclusive iron staining of these cells is diagnostic for treated hemochromatosis. In the rare neonatal or perinatal hemochromatosis,[28] true cirrhosis appears to be uncommon.

Pigment cirrhosis in alcoholic patients may show both hemosiderosis, as in primary hemochromatosis, and the features of alcoholic cirrhosis (see above). Thus, fatty changes and inflammation are the most common added features. Often the hemosiderosis is considerably milder than in primary hemochromatosis without alcoholism; the alcohol abuse undoubtedly precipitates the development of cirrhosis in these conditions.

In erythropoietic disorders, the pigment cirrhosis may be indistinguishable from that in primary hemochromatosis. If inflammation and piecemeal necrosis are prominent added features, chronic viral hepatitis may have complicated the condition.

The presence of postshunt hemochromatosis can be proved by the absence of stainable iron in a cirrhotic liver at the time of shunt surgery (portacaval shunt or comparable procedures) and the subsequent accumulation of iron, imparting the features of typical pigment cirrhosis.[29] The causes of this complication are poorly understood; increased iron absorption may play a role. The histologic changes— apart from the hemosiderosis—depend on the type of preexisting cirrhosis.

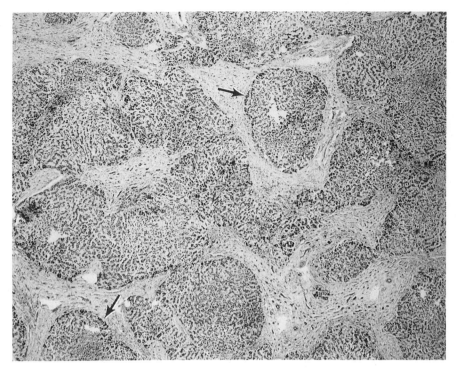

Figure 11.4
Pigment cirrhosis in primary hemochromatosis. Even in this low-power illustration, hemosiderin can be identified as a dark pigment in the periphery of the regenerative nodules (arrows). Note the absence of inflammatory infiltrates, a rather characteristic finding in this disorder. Most regenerative nodules are not complete (compare with Figure 11.5).

Posthepatitic Cirrhosis

Comments: Patients with posthepatitic cirrhosis had unresolved viral or chronic active hepatitis, as described in Chapters 2 and 3, respectively. Biochemical features of ongoing viral hepatitis may or may not be present, depending on the activity of the underlying disease.

Morphologic features: Fibrosis and nodular regeneration are the only constant features. If fatty changes are prominent, they usually are unrelated to the cirrhosis; they may be the result of steroid treatment. Iron stains are negative or at least not in the range of pigment cirrhosis (see also above under "Hemochromatosis"). Staining with PAS-D fails to reveal the globules of alpha-1-antitrypsin deficiency (see Chapters 2 and 12). Stains for copper and copper-associated protein are negative or only weakly positive. Cholestasis rarely is a prominent feature of posthepatitic cirrhosis. Thus, posthepatitic cirrhosis and cryptogenic cirrhosis may be morphologically indistinguishable. One important exception is cases of chronic active hepatitis B with posthepatitic cirrhosis,

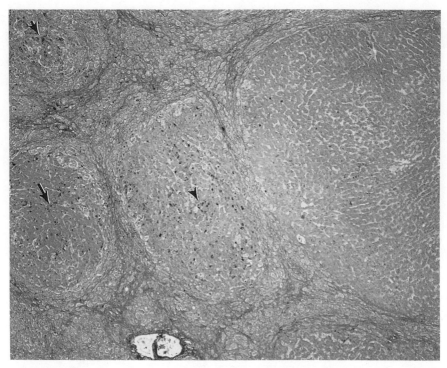

Figure 11.5
Posthepatitic cirrhosis. Advanced nodular regeneration and much fibrosis are present. This cirrhosis is of mixed micronodular and macronodular type. Inflammatory changes are minimal. This is an orcein stain (Shikata's stain), which shows elastic fibers but also hepatitis B surface antigen in hepatocytes. Note the irregular distribution of the stained hepatocytes; they are visible even at this low power (arrows).

because the viral antigens usually are stainable in these instances (Figure 11.5). In all cases of posthepatitic cirrhosis, the activity of the underlying disease (viral or autoimmune) can be estimated by the degree of lymphocytic piecemeal necrosis in the periphery of the regenerative nodules. However, the inflammatory activity often varies considerably from nodule to nodule, and therefore judgment of overall disease activity in posthepatitic cirrhosis is less reliable than in chronic active hepatitis without cirrhosis.[30]

Primary Biliary Cirrhosis

Comments: The clinical manifestations are the same as those in the early stages (see Chapters 1 and 2). Portal hypertension and hepatic failure are common complications of primary biliary cirrhosis.

Morphologic features: Septal fibrosis connotes the presence of stage 3 disease, and true cirrhosis is classified as chronic nonsuppurative destructive cholangitis, stage 4 (see also Chapter 2). Typically, specimens show septal fibrosis and garland-shaped regenerative nodules (see below), often surrounded by ductular, fibrous, or biliary piecemeal necrosis (see Chapter 9). Cholestasis, cholate stasis, and Mallory bodies are common findings at the interface between regenerative nodules and fibrous septa (Figures 11.6A and 11.6B). Rhodanine stains for copper are strongly positive.

Sarcoid Cirrhosis

Hepatic involvement in sarcoidosis is common; it is characterized by the presence of many noncaseating epithelioid cell granulomas, often with prominent fibrosis in the vicinity. In a few instances, cirrhosis and portal hypertension have been reported in this condition.[31] It is still not clear whether the cirrhosis in these cases was caused by the sarcoidosis or whether it was coincidental. For the biliary cirrhosis complicating chronic cholestasis of sarcoidosis, see next entry; the pathogenesis of that condition is quite different.

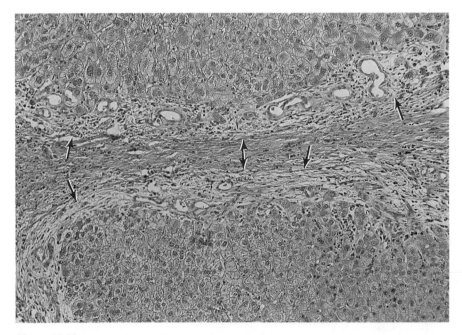

Figure 11.6A
Primary biliary cirrhosis. Periphery of two regenerative nodules with fibrous and ductular piecemeal necrosis is shown. Note the light "halo" (arrows) that surrounds the regenerative nodules; this is caused by edema associated with this type of piecemeal necrosis. These features are common in biliary cirrhosis of any type.

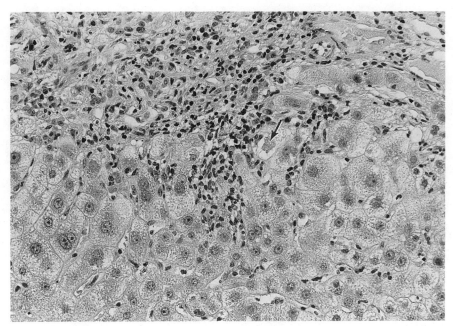

Figure 11.6B
Primary biliary cirrhosis. Focus of primarily lymphocytic piecemeal necrosis in primary biliary cirrhosis. Many hepatocytes in this area appear swollen and pale (cholate stasis); one contains a Mallory body (arrow).

Small-Duct Biliary Cirrhosis Other Than Primary Biliary Cirrhosis

Biliary cirrhosis due to loss of small bile ducts (ductopenia) occurs not only in primary biliary cirrhosis but also in several other conditions with quite different etiologies (see also Chapter 15)[32]; they are chronic intrahepatic cholestasis of sarcoidosis, drug-induced cholangitis, ductopenic (chronic) hepatic allograft rejection, graft-versus-host disease, infantile obstructive cholangiopathy, and the syndrome of primary sclerosing cholangitis (Figure 11.7), including small-duct primary sclerosing cholangitis ("pericholangitis").[33] Finally, in a few adult patients with this type of biliary cirrhosis, the cause of the underlying ductopenia is not apparent, hence the name "idiopathic adulthood ductopenia."[34]

Toxic Cirrhosis

Cirrhosis due to exposure to occupational or domestic and dietary hepatotoxic chemicals is extremely rare, particularly in North America and Europe. Fatty changes may be present. Almost all convincing cases of toxic cirrhosis in the Western world represent drug-induced cirrhosis after prolonged consumption of

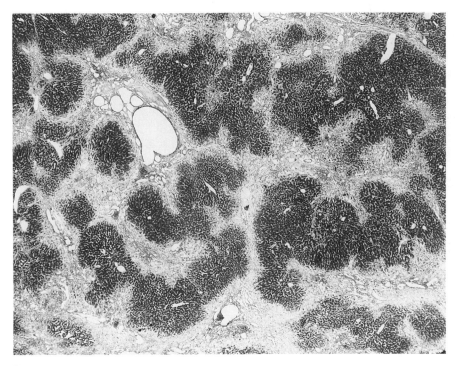

Figure 11.7
Biliary cirrhosis with typical garland-shaped regenerative nodules in a patient with primary sclerosing cholangitis involving both large ducts and small ducts. Note that many of the darkly stained regenerative nodules still display central veins. Therefore, this condition might not represent true cirrhosis at this stage but rather biliary fibrosis. However, since the underlying diseases tend to be irreversible, this condition by convention is called biliary cirrhosis.

hepatotoxic drugs such as methotrexate (see also Table 7.2). Arsenic also can cause cirrhosis—for instance, after intake of Fowler's solution for psoriasis.[35] It should be noted that Indian childhood cirrhosis (see above) might be a toxic cirrhosis.

Table 11.2   Drugs That May Cause Cirrhosis*

Generic or Chemical Name	Product Classification
Acetaminophen	Analgesic and antipyretic
Acetohexamide	Oral hypoglycemic
Amiodarone[36]	Antiarrhythmic
Chlorothiazide	Diuretic
Chlorpromazine	Tranquilizer: phenothiazine
Dantrolene sodium	Skeletal muscle relaxant
Ferrous fumarate (or other salts of iron)	Nutrient mineral
Halothane	Inhalation anesthetic
Isoniazid	Antituberculotic
Mercaptopurine	Antineoplastic
Methotrexate	Antineoplastic
Methyldopa	Antihypertensive
Methyltestosterone	Androgen
Nitrofurantoin	Urinary antibiotic
Papaverine hydrochloride[37]	Vasodilator
Perhexiline maleate	Calcium channel blocker
Phenylbutazone	Anti-inflammatory
Thiabendazole[38]	Anthelmintic
Valproic acid	Anticonvulsant

*This list does not include drugs that are unavailable in the United States. For further information, see reference 39.

References

1. Hodgson HJF, Davies DR, Thompson RPH: Congenital hepatic fibrosis. *J Clin Pathol* 29:11-16, 1976.

2. Wanless IR, Mawdsley C, Adams R: On the pathogenesis of focal nodular hyperplasia of the liver. *Hepatology* 5:1194-1200, 1985.

3. Brophy CM, Bock JF, West AB, et al: Liver cell adenomatosis: Diagnosis and treatment of a rare hepatic neoplastic process. *Am J Gastroenterol* 84:429-432, 1989.

4. Colina F, Alberti N, Solis JA, et al: Diffuse nodular regenerative hyperplasia of the liver (DNRH): A clinicopathologic study of 24 cases. *Liver* 9:253-265, 1989.

5. Wanless IR, Lentz JS, Roberts EA: Partial nodular transformation of liver in an adult with persistent ductus venosus: Review with hypothesis on pathogenesis. *Arch Pathol Lab Med* 109:427-432, 1985.

6. Rakela J, Goldschmiedt M, Ludwig J: Late manifestations of chronic liver disease in adults with alpha-1-antitrypsin deficiency. *Dig Dis Sci* 32:1358-1362, 1987.

7. Deviere J, Brohee D, Hiden M, et al: Hepatic telangiectasia and cirrhosis. *J Clin Gastroenterol* 10:111-114, 1988.

8. Wanless IR, Gryfe A: Nodular transformation of the liver in hereditary hemorrhagic telangiectasis. *Arch Pathol Lab Med* 110:331-335, 1986.

9. Park RW, Grand RJ: Gastrointestinal manifestations of cystic fibrosis: A review. *Gastroenterology* 81:1143-1161, 1981.

10. Bass S, Connon JJ, Ho CS: Biliary tree in cystic fibrosis: Biliary tract abnormalities in cystic fibrosis demonstrated by endoscopic retrograde cholangiography. *Gastroenterology* 84:1592-1596, 1983.

11. Abdul-Karim FW, King TA, Dahms BB, et al: Carcinoma of extrahepatic biliary system in an adult with cystic fibrosis. *Gastroenterology* 82:758-762, 1982.

12. Biberstein M, Wolf P, Pettross B, et al: Amyloidosis complicating cystic fibrosis. *Am J Clin Pathol* 80:752-754, 1983.

13. Bloomer JR, Enriquez R: Evidence that hepatic crystalline deposits in a patient with protoporphyria are composed of protoporphyrin. *Gastroenterology* 82:569-572, 1982.

14. Bloomer JR, Weimer MK, Bossenmaier IC, et al: Liver transplantation in a patient with protoporphyria. *Gastroenterology* 97:188-194, 1989.

15. McAdams AJ, Hug G, Bove KE: Glycogen storage disease, types I to X: Criteria for morphologic diagnosis. *Hum Pathol* 5:463-487, 1974.

16. Schochet SS Jr, McCormick WF, Zellweger H: Type IV glycogenosis (amylopectinosis): Light and electron microscopic observations. *Arch Pathol* 90:354-363, 1970.

17. Parfrey WA, Hutchins GM: Hepatic fibrosis in mucopolysaccharidoses. *Am J Med* 81:825-829, 1986.

18. Lefkowitch JH, Grossman ME: Hepatic pathology in porphyria cutanea tarda. *Liver* 3:19-29, 1983.

19. Fakan F, Chlumska A: Demonstration of needle-shaped hepatic inclusions in porphyria cutanea tarda using the ferric ferricyanide reduction test. *Virchows Arch [Pathol Anat]* 411:365-368, 1987.

20. Mielas LA, Esquivel CO, van Thiel DH, et al: Liver transplantation for tyrosinemia: A review of 10 cases from the University of Pittsburgh. *Dig Dis Sci* 35:153-157, 1990.

21. Dehner LP, Snover DC, Sharp HL, et al: Hereditary tyrosinemia type 1 (chronic form): Pathologic findings in the liver. *Hum Pathol* 20:149-158, 1989.

22. Craig J, Peters RL, Edmondson HA: Tumors of the liver and intrahepatic bile ducts. *Atlas of Tumor Pathology*, 2nd series, fascicle 26. Washington, DC: Armed Forces Institute of Pathology, 1989.

23. Lefkowitch JH, Honig CL, King ME, et al: Hepatic copper overload and features of Indian childhood cirrhosis in an American sibship. *N Engl J Med* 307:271-277, 1982.

24. Müller-Höcker J, Meyer U, Wiebecke B, et al: Copper storage disease of the liver and chronic dietary copper intoxication in two further German infants mimicking Indian childhood cirrhosis. *Pathol Res Pract* 183:39-45, 1988.

25. Wanless IR: Micronodular transformation (nodular regenerative hyperplasia) of the liver: A report of 64 cases among 2,500 autopsies and a new classification of benign hepatocellular nodules. *Hepatology* 11:787-797, 1990.

26. Wanless IR, Lentz JS, Roberts EA: Partial nodular transformation of liver in an adult with persistent ductus venosus: Review with hypothesis on pathogenesis. *Arch Pathol Lab Med* 109:427-432, 1985.

27. LeSage GD, Baldus WP, Fairbanks VF, et al: Hemochromatosis: Genetic or alcohol-induced? *Gastroenterology* 84:1471-1477, 1983.

28. Adams PC, Searle J: Neonatal hemochromatosis: A case and review of the literature. *Am J Gastroenterol* 83:422-425, 1988.

29. Lombard CM, Strauchen JA: Postshunt hemochromatosis with cardiomyopathy. *Hum Pathol* 12:1149-1151, 1981.

30. Ludwig J, Czaja AJ: The role of liver biopsy interpretation in the management of chronic active hepatitis. In Cohen S, Soloway RD (eds): *Contemporary Issues in Gastroenterology*. New York, Churchill Livingstone, 1983, vol 2, pp 171-187.

31. Tekeste H, Latour F, Levitt RE: Portal hypertension complicating sarcoid liver disease: Case report and review of the literature. *Am J Gastroenterol* 79:389-396, 1984.

32. Ludwig J: New concepts in biliary cirrhosis. *Semin Liver Dis* 7:293-301, 1987.

33. Ludwig J: Small-duct primary sclerosing cholangitis. *Semin Liver Dis* 11:11-17, 1991.

34. Ludwig J, Wiesner RH, LaRusso NF: Idiopathic adulthood ductopenia: A cause of chronic cholestatic liver disease and biliary cirrhosis. *J Hepatol* 7:193-199, 1988.

35. Nevens F, Fevery J, Van Steenbergen W, et al: Arsenic and non-cirrhotic portal hypertension: A report of eight cases. *J Hepatol* 11:80-85, 1990.

36. Lewis JH, Mullick F, Ishak KG, et al: Histopathologic analysis of suspected amiodarone hepatotoxicity. *Hum Pathol* 21:59-67, 1990.

37. Poncin E, Silvain C, Touchard G, et al: Papaverin-induced chronic liver disease. *Gastroenterology* 90:1051-1053, 1986.

38. Roy MA, Nugen FW, Aretz HT: Micronodular cirrhosis after thiabendazole. *Dig Dis Sci* 34:938-941, 1989.

39. Ludwig J, Axelson R: Drug effects on the liver: An updated tabular compilation of drugs and drug-related hepatic diseases. *Dig Dis Sci* 28:651-666, 1983.

Chapter 12

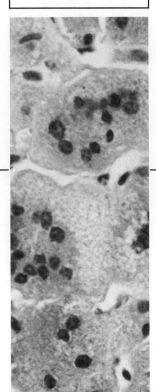

Abnormal Hepatocytes

Morphologic Definition

An enormous variety of hepatocellular abnormalities can be observed. With the exception of the degenerative changes, they are grouped here on the basis of morphologic resemblances. The categories are groundglass hepatocytes, hepatocellular storage cells, intracytoplasmic inclusions, intranuclear inclusions, and multinucleated giant hepatocytes. For hepatocytes with fatty changes, see Chapters 6 and 7. For hepatocytes with abnormal pigments, see Chapters 13 and 14.

Degenerative Changes

The main degenerative hepatocellular changes can be defined as follows:

Acidophilic Bodies

Rounded necrotic hepatocytes are present, with pyknotic nuclei or without nuclei; the cytoplasm is strongly eosinophilic and often hyalin-like. Acidophilic bodies with tiny fat droplets and ceroid pigment were first described in cases of yellow fever hepatitis (some of these cases actually may have been hepatitis D) and since then have been named Councilman bodies.[1] Currently, the terms acidophilic body and Councilman body can be considered synonyms. These degenerative cell bodies occur most commonly in periportal hepatitis (Chapter 2), lobular hepatitis (Chapter 3), and most other conditions associated with necrosis (Chapter 9).

Apoptotic Bodies

Fragments of hepatocellular cytoplasm are present, particularly in areas of piecemeal necrosis (see Chapter 9), but also at other sites in inflamed lobules. Apoptotic bodies are much smaller than acidophilic bodies, but otherwise they are very similar; apoptotic bodies do not contain nuclear material. The shedding of cytoplasm leading to the formation of apoptotic bodies is called apoptosis.

Ballooning Degeneration

Swelling of hepatocytes is present, resulting in paleness of the cytoplasm (hepatocellular edema). This type of cell damage most often occurs in lobular hepatitis (see also Chapter 3). Ballooning degeneration associated with cholestasis has been named feathery degeneration (see below).

Calcification

This is an uncommon finding in the liver. Calcium usually is easy to identify in routine sections but its presence can be confirmed with von Kossa's stain. See also below under "Hepatic Allografts" and "Hyperparathyroidism."

Councilman Bodies

See above under "Acidophilic Bodies."

Dysplasia

Enlarged hepatocytes with prominent pleomorphic hyperchromatic nuclei are commonly found in advanced cirrhosis, particularly in patients with chronic hepatitis B infection. Liver cell dysplasia indicates an increased likelihood that a hepatocellular carcinoma is present or will develop.

Feathery Degeneration

Swelling of hepatocytes is present, resulting in paleness and a foamy appearance of the cytoplasm. The condition is a feature of cholestasis and thus most commonly found in cholestatic hepatitis (Chapter 4). Feathery degeneration in periportal or paraseptal hepatocytes or in the periphery of regenerative nodules occurs most commonly in primary biliary cirrhosis (see Chapter 11) and has been named cholate stasis; this phenomenon probably is caused by toxic bile acids.

Clusters of hepatocytes with feathery degeneration are described as "pseudo-xanthomatous change," in contradistinction to "xanthomatous change," which refers to similar features in macrophages. With routine preparations, the distinction is not always possible.

Groundglass Hepatocytes

Cells with this feature are often swollen; the cytoplasm is opaque and usually granular and eosinophilic. The groundglass cytoplasm may appear to fill out the entire cell but more often resembles a large inclusion, which is separated from the cell wall by a space or halo. Groundglass hepatocytes must be distinguished from hepatic oncocytes as described below under "Alcoholic Liver Disease" and from induction cells as described below under "Drug-Induced Hepatitis or Hepatopathy."

Hepatocellular Storage Cells

Storage cells are defined here as hepatocytes with accumulated metabolites in the cytoplasm, leading to cytomegaly. These metabolites include cholesterol, fibrinogen, glycolipids, glycoprotein, mucolipids, mucopolysaccharides, phospholipids, and sphingomyelin. For clinical conditions in which these metabolites are stored, see below.

Intracytoplasmic Inclusions

Proteinaceous globules or irregularly shaped bodies are present, identifiable in paraffin sections. The affected hepatocytes often appear swollen. Several types of inclusions can be identified and defined as follows:

Acidophilic Bodies After Bone Marrow Transplantation

Hepatocellular intracytoplasmic inclusions of proteinaceous material (probably plasma) are present, linked to bone marrow transplantation. The pathogenesis of the finding is unknown. For morphologic features and staining characteristics, see below.

Acidophilic Bodies After Thermal Injury

Hepatocellular intracytoplasmic inclusions of proteinaceous material (probably plasma) are present, linked to thermal injury. The pathogenesis of the finding is unknown. For morphologic features and further clinical information, see below.

Alpha-1-Antitrypsin Globules

Affected hepatocytes have round granules or globules in the cytoplasm; they are strongly PAS-positive and diastase-resistant. The surface of the globules and the cytoplasm of the affected hepatocytes can be shown immunohistochemically to contain alpha-1-antitrypsin.[2] The granules and globules vary considerably in size, measuring between 1 and 40 μm in diameter. The smaller the inclusions, the larger is their number in each hepatocyte.

Giant Lysosomes

When lysosomes become active in breakdown processes, they can be identified in paraffin section as PAS-positive, diastase-resistant granules or globules. Ultrastructurally, they are membrane-bound, electron-dense bodies (secondary lysosomes). Enlarged lysosomes often contain lipid (lipolysosomes).

Hyaline Globules in Congestion

Hepatocellular intracytoplasmic inclusions of proteinaceous material (probably plasma) are present, linked to passive congestion of the liver. The pathogenesis of this finding is unknown. For morphologic features and staining characteristics, see below.

Mallory Bodies

Hepatocellular intracytoplasmic inclusions of deranged cytokeratin intermediate filaments are present,[3] linked to alcoholic liver disease but also to many nonalcoholic hepatic abnormalities. Irregular clumps of proteinaceous material are present in the cytoplasm. The material often forms sausage-shaped or antler-shaped rods that wrap themselves around the nuclei in a semicircular configuration. The affected hepatocytes often appear swollen. Mallory bodies are PAS-negative; their presence can be confirmed by immunoperoxidase staining with a monoclonal antibody.[4]

Megamitochondria

These organelles can be found in the cytoplasm of hepatocytes. For morphologic features and staining characteristics, see below.

Phagocytized Erythrocytes

They may resemble round megamitochondria (see above). Comparison with extracellular hepatocytes is helpful.

Viral Inclusion Bodies

Viral inclusion bodies rarely occur in the cytoplasm of hepatocytes, but they can be found after cytomegalovirus infection. However, even in that condition most inclusions are in the nuclei (see also below under "Intranuclear Inclusions").

Intranuclear Inclusions

Glycogen Inclusions

These PAS-positive, diastase-digestible inclusions present as vacuolated nuclei in routine preparations. This may be a normal finding, particularly in childhood, but glycogen inclusions are also common in conditions such as adult-onset diabetes mellitus.

Lead Inclusion Bodies

Hepatocellular intranuclear inclusions are present, linked to lead poisoning. For the putative chemical composition of these inclusions, see below.

Lipid Inclusions

Hepatocellular intranuclear inclusions of lipid are present, without a consistent link to specific liver diseases.

Pseudoinclusions

Invaginations of nuclear membranes are a common finding; they contain cytoplasm. Unless the mouth of the invagination in the nuclear membrane is in the plane of sectioning, the finding resembles a true nuclear inclusion.

Sanded Nuclei

Hepatocellular intranuclear inclusions of viral antigen are linked to viral hepatitis B and D. The appearance of affected nuclei differs from that of other viral inclusion bodies (see below).

Viral Inclusions

Hepatocellular intranuclear inclusions of viral antigen are present, as observed in adenovirus hepatitis, cytomegalovirus hepatitis, and herpes simplex hepatitis. For morphologic features of these conditions, see below.

Multinucleated Giant Hepatocytes

Hepatocellular giant cells with many nuclei are found primarily in pediatric liver diseases, but they also occur in adults. The pathogenesis of this finding is poorly understood. The presence of multinucleated giant hepatocytes is not linked to any specific etiology.

Table 12.1   Clinical Conditions Associated With Abnormal Hepatocytes*

Degenerative Changes (degeneration products in parentheses)
    Conditions listed under "Periportal Hepatitis" (Chapter 2), "Lobular Hepatitis" (Chapter 3),
        "Cholestatic Hepatitis" (Chapter 4), and most conditions listed under "Necrosis"
        (Chapter 9). See also above under "Morphologic Definitions."
    Hepatic allografts (calcification)
    Hyperparathyroidism (calcification)
Groundglass Hepatocytes (type of cell or stored material in parentheses)
    Cirrhosis: Alcoholic, posthepatitic, and other types (oncocytes)
    Drug-induced hepatitis or hepatopathy (induction cells)
    Fibrinogen storage disease (fibrinogen)
    Glycogen storage disease, type IV (amylopectin)
    Hepatocellular carcinoma (fibrinogen)
    Progressive familial myoclonic epilepsy (Lafora bodies)
    Viral hepatitis B, with or without cirrhosis (hepatitis B surface antigen; oncocytes)
Hepatocellular Storage Cells (type of stored material in parentheses)[†]
    Cholesteryl ester storage disease (cholesterol)
    Drug-induced hepatitis or hepatopathy (hydroxyethyl starch; phospholipids)

continued on page 148

continued from page 147
    Fabry's disease (glycosphingolipid)
    Fibrinogen storage disease (fibrinogen)
    Fucosidosis (glycolipid, glycoproteins, and other metabolites)
    Glycogen storage disease (glycogen or related carbohydrates in most types; see below in text)
    Hepatocellular carcinoma (fibrinogen)
    I-cell disease (mucolipid)
    Mannosidosis (alpha-D-mannose)
    Mauriac's syndrome (glycogen)
    Mucolipidosis (mucolipid)
    Mucopolysaccharidosis (mucopolysaccharide)
    Niemann-Pick disease (sphingomyelin)
    Wolman's disease (cholesterol)
Intracytoplasmic Inclusions
    Mallory bodies
        Alcoholic liver disease
        Autoimmune chronic active hepatitis
        Biliary obstruction and other causes of cholestasis
        Chronic nonsuppurative destructive cholangitis (primary biliary cirrhosis)
        Diabetes mellitus
        Drug-induced hepatitis or hepatopathy
        Glycogen storage disease, type Ia
        Hepatocellular carcinoma
        Indian childhood cirrhosis
        Nonalcoholic fatty changes or nonalcoholic steatohepatitis
        Primary sclerosing cholangitis
        Wilson's disease
    Inclusions other than Mallory bodies (type of inclusion in parentheses)
        Acute fatty liver of pregnancy (megamitochondria)
        Alcoholic liver disease (alpha-1-antitrypsin; megamitochondria)
        Alpha-1-antichymotrypsin deficiency (alpha-1-antichymotrypsin)
        Alpha-1-antitrypsin deficiency (alpha-1-antitrypsin)
        Bone marrow transplantation (acidophilic bodies)
        Congestion (hyaline globules)
        Cytomegalovirus hepatitis (viral inclusion bodies)
        Hypoxia (acidophilic bodies)
        Thermal injury (acidophilic bodies)
Intranuclear Inclusions (type of inclusion in parentheses)
    Adenovirus hepatitis (viral inclusion bodies)
    Cytomegalovirus hepatitis (viral inclusion bodies)
    Diabetes mellitus (glycogen)
    Glycogen storage disease (glycogen)
    Herpes simplex hepatitis (viral inclusion bodies)

continued on page 149

continued from page 148
    Lead poisoning (lead-protein)
    Viral hepatitis B (core antigen)
    Viral hepatitis D (delta antigen)
Multinucleated Hepatocytes
    Autoimmune chronic active hepatitis
    Acute or unresolved viral hepatitis non-A, non-B
    Chronic active hepatitis non-A, non-B
    Drug-induced hepatitis or hepatopathy
    Hepatic allografts
    Hepatocellular carcinoma
    Neonatal liver disease
    Syncytial giant cell hepatitis
    Toxic hepatitis
    Wilson's disease

*Morphologic classification—for instance, groundglass hepatocytes vs storage cells—is somewhat arbitrary. All appropriate categories should be considered if a diagnostic problem exists.
†Conditions such as Gaucher's disease are not included here because the abnormal metabolites are stored in mesenchymal cells. However, these cells may swell to such an extent that they resemble hepatocellular storage cells.

Clinical Conditions

Acute and Unresolved Viral Hepatitis (Hepatitis Virus Hepatitis)

See below under "Viral Hepatitis B and Non-A, Non-B (C, D)."

Acute Fatty Liver of Pregnancy

See Chapter 6.

Adenovirus Hepatitis

Comments: This is a rare type of viral hepatitis that occurs in immuno-compromised hosts. Currently, most patients are pediatric liver transplant recipients; serotypes 1 and 2 appear to predominate.[5]

Morphologic features: Nonzonal necroses and collections of mononuclear-histiocytic cells and neutrophils are found. Some hepatocytes in these areas are slightly enlarged and contain intranuclear viral inclusion bodies. Immunostains with monoclonal antibodies on frozen sections reveal viral antigen in nuclei and cytoplasm of affected hepatocytes.

Alcoholic Liver Disease

Comments: A history of alcohol abuse or dependence is required for the diagnosis. For other clinical findings, see Chapters 6, 7, and 11.

Morphologic features: In alcoholic fatty liver or alcoholic hepatitis, Mallory bodies are found primarily in ballooned centrilobular hepatocytes. In alcoholic cirrhosis, cells with Mallory bodies are found in a more random distribution, including the periphery of the regenerative nodules. Clusters of neutrophils often are noticed in the vicinity of hepatocytes with Mallory bodies (Figures 12.1A and 12.1B). For staining characteristics of these inclusions, see above under "Morphologic Definitions." Other intracytoplasmic hepatocellular inclusions, found in approximately 25% of the cases, are megamitochondria (giant mitochondria).[6] Megamitochondria most often occur in centrilobular areas, just as Mallory bodies do; they are highly suggestive features of alcoholic liver disease.[7] They are PAS-negative and appear bright red with the Masson trichrome stain. These organelles must be distinguished from phagocytized erythrocytes, giant lysosomes, alpha-1-antitrypsin globules (see below), and round Mallory bodies (see also Table 12.1). Finally, in alcoholic cirrhosis, hepatic oncocytes[8] can be found; they present as groundglass hepatocytes (see below). Their cytoplasm is opaque-

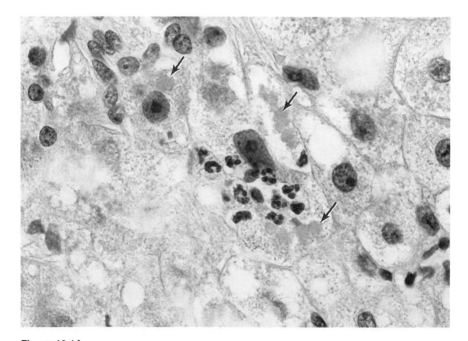

Figure 12.1A
Mallory bodies in steatohepatitis. Alcoholic hepatitis is shown with a cluster of neutrophils in the vicinity of some Mallory bodies (arrows). This is a common finding in such cases.

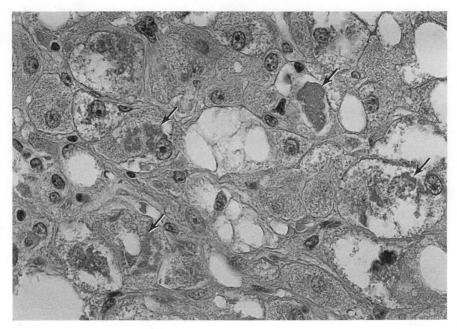

Figure 12.1B
Mallory bodies in steatohepatitis. Obesity-related steatohepatitis is shown with ballooned hepatocytes containing Mallory bodies of many sizes and shapes (arrows).

---

granular and strongly eosinophilic. This change is caused by the accumulation of densely packed mitochondria; they can be demonstrated as blue granules with the phosphotungstic acid–hematoxylin stain. Hepatic oncocytes are not specific for any particular etiology. For alpha-1-antitrypsin globules in alcoholic liver disease, see under "Alpha-1-Antitrypsin Deficiency."

Alpha-1-Antichymotrypsin Deficiency

A patient with intermediate deficiency of alpha-1-antichymotrypsin (A1ACT), a rare endoplasmic reticulum storage disease,[9,10] showed chronic hepatitis and cirrhosis with granules of A1ACT, primarily in periportal and paraseptal hepatocytes. Some were slightly PAS-positive.

Alpha-1-Antitrypsin Deficiency

Comments: This hereditary disorder affects secretion of alpha-1-antitrypsin (alpha-1-proteinase inhibitor) from the liver. It is associated with chronic active hepatitis (see Chapter 2), cirrhosis, and hepatocellular carcinoma (in cirrhosis) in adulthood, and with infantile obstructive cholangiopathy (in particular, neonatal hepatitis and nonsyndromatic paucity of intrahepatic bile ducts; see Chapters 3 and 15, respectively). Adult patients with the ZZ phenotype appear to develop cirrhosis earlier than patients with the SZ and MZ phenotype.[11] Presence of a defective M variant allele such as M malton may be responsible for typical inclusions in patients who apparently have a normal phenotype; the proteins have similar mobilities with isoelectric focusing techniques.[12] However, a small number of alpha-1-antitrypsin globules can be found in some patients with cryptogenic or alcoholic cirrhosis or in elderly patients with high disease activity who had no evidence of alpha-1-antitrypsin deficiency.[12] In these instances, hepatocytes appear to have produced more alpha-1-antitrypsin than they can secrete. As shown below, the size of the globules may allow a distinction.

Morphologic features: The intracytoplasmic globules of alpha-1-antitrypsin, which characterize this disease, are found primarily in periportal hepatocytes and in the periphery of regenerative nodules (Figures 12.2A and 12.2B). Inclusions greater than 3 μm are highly specific for carriers of the PiZ allele.[13] For staining characteristics and other features, see above under "Morphologic Definitions." In rare instances, alpha-1-antitrypsin globules may be found in epithelial cells of bile ducts and ductules.[14] In the first months of life, immunostains or electron microscopy are needed to identify alpha-1-antitrypsin.

Autoimmune Chronic Active Hepatitis

Comments: For clinical features, see Chapter 2.

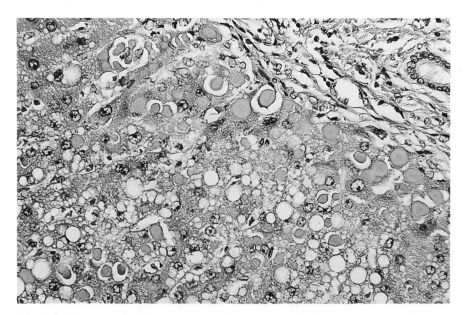

Figure 12.2A
Liver in alpha-1-antitrypsin deficiency with cirrhosis. Note pale inclusion in hepatocytes; they are weakly eosinophilic in the hematoxylin-eosin stain.

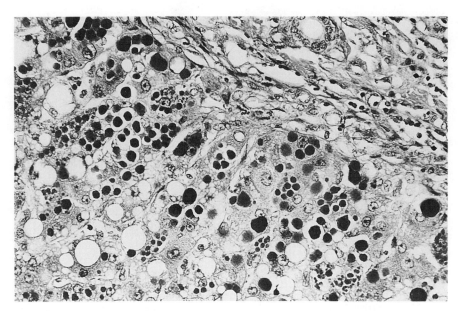

Figure 12.2B
Liver in alpha-1-antitrypsin deficiency with cirrhosis. In a PAS stain with diastase digestion the globules appear bright red. Note that the largest globules are found in the most peripheral hepatocytes.

Morphologic features: Multinucleated giant hepatocytes appear to form in some of these cases.[15] However, in the majority of instances, the patients have evidence of chronic non-A, non-B infection (see below under "Viral Hepatitis"). In rare cases of autoimmune chronic active hepatitis, a few Mallory bodies can be found in periportal hepatocytes or in the periphery of regenerative nodules, possibly related to ultrastructural bile accumulation (see next entry).

Biliary Obstruction and Other Causes of Cholestasis

Comments: For clinical features of cholestatic hepatitis and of pure cholestasis, see Chapters 4 and 5.

Morphologic features: In chronic nonsuppurative destructive cholangitis (syndrome of primary biliary cirrhosis) and in primary sclerosing cholangitis, cholestasis-induced Mallory bodies often are found in periportal and paraseptal hepatocytes (see below); the affected cells show features of feathery degeneration (see Chapter 11) because of cholate stasis. If cirrhosis is present, the changes are found in the periphery of regenerative nodules, sometimes together with ductular and biliary piecemeal necrosis (see also Chapter 11). Copper is almost always present (see also Chapter 14). In prolonged large-duct biliary obstruction, similar changes may occur. In pure cholestasis, Mallory bodies are not common. In contradistinction to alcoholic liver disease (see above), fatty changes usually are absent in the above-mentioned cholestatic syndromes. For additional morphologic features, see Chapters 4 and 5.

Bone Marrow Transplantation

Comments: In three patients who had bone marrow transplantation for acute leukemia, hepatocellular cytoplasmic inclusions were found.[16]

Morphologic features: Large eosinophilic bodies were found in the cytoplasm, usually near the nuclei. Some hepatocytes contained multiple inclusions, and in others most of the cytoplasm was replaced by one eosinophilic body. The material was PAS-negative, and histochemical or immunohistochemical stains for alpha-1-antitrypsin, alpha-fetoprotein, glycogen, and lipid were negative also. Electron microscopically, the inclusions were membrane-bound and appeared granular, sometimes with small vesicles.

Cholesteryl Ester Storage Disease

This condition is related to Wolman's disease (see below) but may remain asymptomatic until adulthood.[17]

Chronic Active Hepatitis, Autoimmune or Viral

See under "Autoimmune Chronic Active Hepatitis" and under "Viral Hepatitis B and Non-A, Non-B (C, D)."

Chronic Nonsuppurative Destructive Cholangitis

See under "Biliary Obstruction and Other Causes of Cholestasis."

Cirrhosis

For alpha-1-antitrypsin globules in cryptogenic cirrhosis, see under "Alpha-1-Antitrypsin Deficiency." For oncocytes in alcoholic cirrhosis, see under "Alcoholic Liver Disease." Oncocytes also occur in posthepatitic and other types of cirrhosis. For an illustration of oncocytes in biliary cirrhosis see Figure 12.6B.

Congestion

Comments: Evidence of chronic right ventricular failure usually is present. (See also Chapter 16.) Some patients had prolonged extracorporeal circulation.

Morphologic features: Hyaline globules have been found in the cytoplasm of hepatocytes in or near zones of centrilobular passive congestion.[18] The globules usually were invisible in hematoxylin-stained sections but they were strongly positive in PAS stains after diastase digestion. Immunohistochemical staining for alpha-1-antitrypsin and fibrinogen was positive in most instances. In electron microscopic preparations, fibrillar material was seen in these globules, unassociated with endoplasmic reticulum. The material sometimes contained rod-shaped inclusions. The globules measured between 3 and 20 μm in diameter and differed from alpha-1-antitrypsin granules in several staining properties, their preferred location, and the clinical setting.[18] These globules probably represent phagosomes with imbibed serum proteins; the process appears to be triggered in some way by passive congestion.

Cytomegalovirus Hepatitis

Comments: Cytomegalovirus (CMV) infection is the most common systemic viral disease in transplant recipients. In contradistinction to adenovirus infection (see above), CMV can be found in all age groups. Other immunocompromised hosts also may be affected.

Morphologic features: The inclusion bodies can be found in hepatocytes, bile duct epithelial cells, and endothelial cells. If hepatocytes are involved, viral inclusion bodies may be found in the cytoplasm. However, the most characteristic

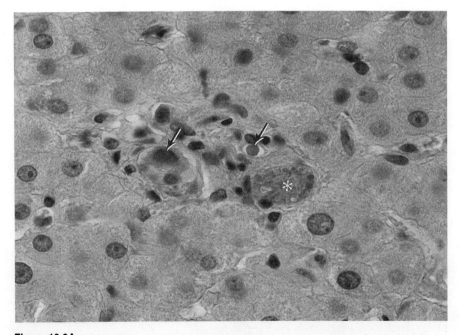

Figure 12.3A
Viral inclusions. Cytomegalovirus inclusions in nuclei (arrows) and cytoplasm (asterisk) are shown. The arrow to the right shows a nuclear inclusion with a halo (owl's eye).

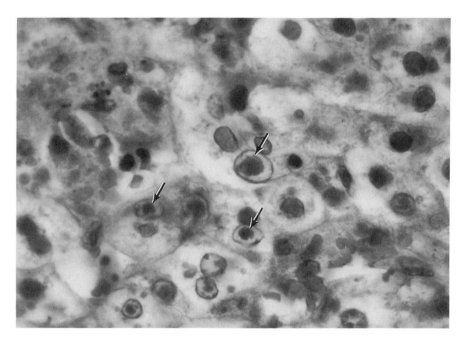

Figure 12.3B
Viral inclusions. Nuclear inclusions (arrows) in herpes simplex hepatitis are shown.

inclusions are in the nuclei (Figures 12.3A and, for comparison, 12.3B); they are amphophilic or basophilic and are separated from the nuclear membrane by a halo. This halo imparts the "owl's eye" appearance. The inclusions are Feulgen-positive and bright red in Masson's trichrome stain; they are PAS-negative. Multiple methods to demonstrate CMV antigen are available,[19-21] but routine histology probably is the best diagnostic approach overall.

Diabetes Mellitus

For changes in adult-onset diabetes mellitus, see below under "Nonalcoholic Fatty Changes or Nonalcoholic Steatohepatitis." For changes in juvenile-onset diabetes mellitus, see below under "Mauriac's Syndrome."

Drug-Induced Hepatitis or Hepatopathy

Comments: The diagnosis can be suggested if an appropriate history has been provided. For a list of drugs that may be associated with the formation of Mallory bodies, see Table 7.2.

Morphologic features: Drug-induced Mallory bodies generally are found together with the features of steatohepatitis (see Chapter 7). However, in some instances, the fatty changes may be inconspicuous or absent and the Mallory bodies may be most prominent in periportal hepatocytes. Amiodarone (an antiarrhythmic) hepatitis may show these features,[22] together with phospholipidosis affecting macrophages and hepatocytes of these livers. Because of the appearance of phospholipid storage cells, the histologic changes in these patients may resemble those in Niemann-Pick disease (see below). Similar drug-induced changes have occurred after use of trimethoprim-sulfamethoxazole (see Table 4.2) and in Great Britain after the use of the antianginal agent perhexiline maleate.[23] Another storage phenomenon has been observed in patients with renal failure who had received infusions with hydroxyethyl starch, a colloidal plasma substitute; they accumulated that substance in liver cells, causing portal hypertension. The hepatocytes resembled storage cells.[24] A common drug-induced abnormality of hepatocytes is the formation of induction cells. Drugs such as azathioprine, chlorpromazine, or barbiturates may cause the smooth endoplasmic reticulum of some hepatocytes to proliferate.[25,26] The affected cells attain a groundglass appearance and are found primarily in a periportal and centrilobular distribution; their cytoplasm becomes stainable with PAS-D, whereas special stains for hepatitis B surface antigen (see below) are negative. After administration of disulfiram[27] or cyanamide[28] (both for the treatment of chronic alcoholism; cyanamide is not available in the United States), groundglass hepatocytes with features of Lafora bodies (see below under "Progressive Familial Myoclonic Epilepsy") may appear, either in the periportal zone or in a random distribution. Finally, drug-induced multinucleated hepatocytes have been observed after the use of methotrexate,[29] para-aminosalicylic acid,[30] 6-mercaptopurin,[31] and clometacin (not used in the United States).[32] In toxic hepatopathy after exposure to vinyl chloride, this feature also has been observed.[33]

Fabry's Disease (Angiokeratoma Corporis Diffusum)

Comments: This is a hereditary x-linked disorder of lipid metabolism, characterized by a congenital deficiency of lysosomal ceramide trihexoside alpha-galactosidase.

Morphologic features: Lipid (glycolipid, glycosphingolipid) is stored in the cytoplasm of hepatocytes, Kupffer cells, and portal macrophages, and in blood vessels.

Fibrinogen Storage Disease

Comments: This very rare condition is linked to alpha-1-antitrypsin deficiency by the collective disease designation, "endoplasmic storage disease."

Morphologic features: The fibrinogen accumulation in the cytoplasm produces a groundglass appearance of the affected hepatocytes.[34] The material is weakly eosinophilic and separated from the cell membrane by a space or halo. The fibrinogen stains bright red with Masson's trichrome stain. PAS-D stains and special stains for hepatitis B surface antigen (see below under "Viral Hepatitis") are negative. For positive identification of the fibrinogen, immunoperoxidase staining is required. Electron microscopic studies also give characteristic results.[34]

Fucosidosis

Comments: This is a hereditary disorder of glycoprotein metabolism, characterized by a congenital deficiency of alpha-L-fucosidase. This is a childhood disease; one type is fatal between 4 and 6 years of age, the other has a much slower course.

Morphologic features: Hepatocytes and Kupffer cells show cytoplasmic vacuolation; the cells store fucose-containing glycolipids, glycoproteins, and polysaccharides or oligosaccharides.

Glycogen Storage Disease

Comments: A group of hereditary disorders of carbohydrate metabolism is

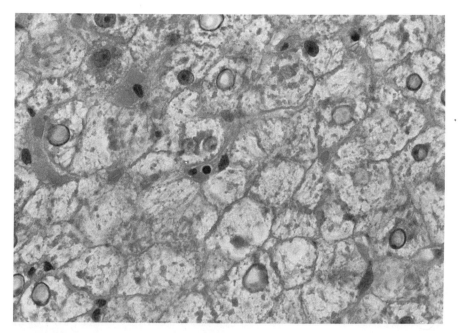

Figure 12.4A
Glycogen storage. Liver in glycogen storage disease, type III, is shown. Note glycogen-induced hepatocytomegaly with characteristic vacuolation of nuclei (nuclear glycogenosis).

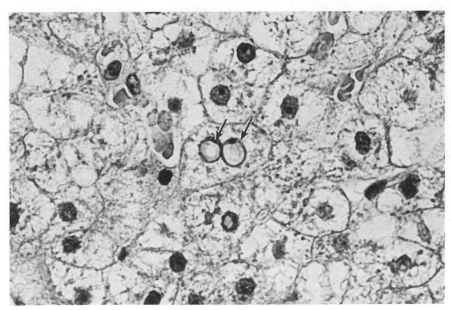

Figure 12.4B
Glycogen storage. Liver in severe juvenile-onset diabetes mellitus (Mauriac's syndrome) is shown. Hepatocytes are distended by glycogen, and glycogenated nuclei (arrows) are present also. Note the resemblance of the acquired glycogen deposition with genetic glycogen storage disease, as shown in Figure 12.4A.

characterized by a congenital deficiency of a related enzyme. More than 10 subtypes of this disease exist, all characterized by deficiencies of different enzymes.[35]

Morphologic features: Hepatocellular intracytoplasmic storage of glycogen or related substances (Figures 12.4A and 12.4B) is found in type I (glucose-6-phosphatase deficiency), III (amylo-1,6-glucosidase deficiency), IV (alpha-1,4-glucan-6-glycosyl transferase deficiency), and VI (glycogen phosphorylase deficiency). In glycogen storage disease, type IV (see also below under "Progressive Familial Myoclonic Epilepsy"), amylopectin is stored in the cytoplasm of the hepatocytes.[36] This substance imparts the features of groundglass hepatocytes and has the same staining characteristics as the Lafora bodies in progressive familial myoclonal epilepsy (see below). Periportal fibrosis may be observed in glycogen storage disease, type VI. For cirrhosis in glycogen storage disease, see Chapter 11. Intranuclear glycogen inclusions are found in glycogen storage disease, types I and III (Figure 12.4A). In type I, fatty changes and fibrosis may be present; in type III, fibrous septa may be found but little fat and no cirrhosis. In type VI, fibrous septa also may be present.[35] Finally, Mallory bodies have been found in glycogen storage disease, type Ia[37] (type Ib has normal in vitro activity of glucose-6-phosphatase); in this type, liver cell adenomas and hepatocellular carcinomas also have been observed.

Hepatic Allografts

Comments: The changes described below most commonly occur in association with rejection, but in some instances no unequivocal correlations can be found.

Morphologic features: Multinucleated giant cells occur primarily at the edges of centrilobular necroses, which are a rather common finding in allografts. The pathogenesis of these lesions is not clear.[38] Many allografts also contain megakaryocytes or foci of all erythropoietic elements (donor-derived?). Spotty hepatocellular calcifications of unknown cause also occur in allografts (unpublished observations).

Hepatocellular Carcinoma

Comments: The neoplasm may occur in otherwise normal livers but more often it is found in association with chronic viral hepatitis (see below) and posthepatitic cirrhosis. Indeed, cirrhosis of almost any etiology must be considered a preneoplastic condition. Findings in the tumor such as Mallory bodies have no relation to the underlying cirrhosis (except for the accumulation of hepatitis B antigen).

Morphologic features: Tumor cells may show groundglass features because of hepatitis B surface antigen in the cytoplasm. However, similar changes may be the result of oncocytic transformation (see above under "Alcoholic Liver Disease") or of fibrinogen storage (see "Hepatocellular Storage Cells" under "Morphologic Definitions"). Hyaline globules and "pale bodies" in malignant hepatocytes may represent alpha-1-antitrypsin, C-reactive protein, and other cell products, including fibrinogen as mentioned above.[34-39] Such inclusions are particularly common in a variant of hepatocellular carcinoma, namely fibrolamellar carcinoma of the liver.[40] Mallory bodies also are a common finding in hepatocellular carcinoma. Finally, multinucleated giant cells (Figure 12.5A) of hepatocellular type can be found in some tumors (giant cell hepatocellular carcinoma).

Herpes Simplex Hepatitis

For the intranuclear inclusions in herpes simplex hepatitis and for other clinical and morphologic features of this condition, see Chapter 9. For an illustration, see Figure 12.3B.

Hyperparathyroidism

Comments: Most patients with the hepatic changes described below had secondary hyperparathyroidism caused by chronic renal failure.

Morphologic features: Hepatic calcification has been observed; the changes occur primarily in or near centrilobular necroses and therefore are considered both metastatic and dystrophic.[41]

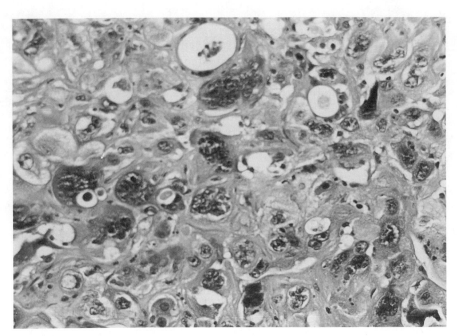

Figure 12.5A
Malignant giant cells in a hepatocellular carcinoma (giant cell hepatocellular carcinoma).

Hypoxia

Acidophilic globular intracytoplasmic inclusions occur in some hypoxic hepatocytes, but little further information is available.

I-Cell Disease (Mucolipidosis Type II)

Comments: A hereditary disorder of lipid, mucopolysaccharide, and glycoprotein metabolism characterized by a congenital deficiency of N-acetyl-glucosamine-1-phosphotransferase.

Morphologic features: The cytoplasm of hepatocytes, Kupffer cells, and macrophages is vacuolated due to deposition of sphingolipid and mucopolysaccharide.

Indian Childhood Cirrhosis

Mallory bodies and other morphologic features of this condition are described in Chapter 11.

Lead Poisoning

Comments: Children are particularly susceptible to lead poisoning, but it also occurs in adults, particularly after industrial exposure. Elevated lead levels in blood and urine confirm the diagnosis.

Morphologic features: Liver biopsy specimens may show eosinophilic, acid-fast inclusion bodies in the nuclei of hepatocytes; they appear to be composed of a lead-protein complex.[42] The inclusions are not membrane-bound. Intra-cytoplasmic inclusions also occur in lead poisoning, probably as a result of abnormal cell divisions.[43]

Mannosidosis

Comments: This is a hereditary disorder of glycoprotein metabolism, characterized by a congenital deficiency of alpha-mannosidase. This is a childhood disease with many systemic manifestations.

Morphologic features: Hepatocytes are vacuolated and contain PAS-negative membrane-bound amorphous and other material with alpha-D-mannose residues.

Mauriac's Syndrome

Comments: Patients with this syndrome have juvenile-onset diabetes mellitus with retarded growth, obesity, hypercholesterolemia, hepatomegaly, and other features. The hepatic changes in this condition also may occur in juvenile-onset diabetes without the syndrome.

Morphologic features: Hepatocytes show excessive intracytoplasmic glycogen deposition, and thus biopsy specimens closely resemble glycogen storage disease (Figure 12.4B). Fatty changes are mild. For other changes in diabetes mellitus, see below under "Nonalcoholic Fatty Changes or Nonalcoholic Steatohepatitis."

Mucolipidosis

Comments: This is a hereditary disorder of lipid, mucopolysaccharide, and glycoprotein metabolism characterized by a congenital deficiency of acid neuraminidase (type I) or N-acetylglucosamine-1-phosphotransferase (types II and III). Mucolipidosis type IV does not affect the liver.

Morphologic features: See above under "I-Cell Disease."

Mucopolysaccharidosis

See Chapter 11.

Neonatal Liver Disease

Comments: The main feature of neonatal hepatitis, namely, hepatocellular giant cell transformation, may be found in many cholestatic neonatal liver diseases, and therefore an extensive diagnostic workup is required in each case. If possible causes such as extrahepatic biliary atresia, paucity of intrahepatic bile ducts, and storage disease can be ruled out, "idiopathic neonatal hepatitis" can be diagnosed. For the relation between neonatal hepatitis and infantile obstructive cholangiopathy, see Chapter 15.

Morphologic features: The parenchyma is replaced by many multinucleated hepatocellular giant cells (Figure 12.5B). Causes other than neonatal hepatitis should be suspected if ductopenia (see Chapter 15), hemosiderosis (see Chapter 13), or features of storage disease are found (see above and below). Immunostains for alpha-1-antitrypsin should be prepared in all instances. Cytomegalovirus infection or herpes simplex infection also may present as neonatal hepatitis, but they have characteristic histologic features (see Chapter 9).

Niemann-Pick Disease

Comments: This is a hereditary disorder of lipid metabolism, characterized by diminished activity of sphingomyelinase. Five subtypes of this disease have been described; the condition may occur in infants, juveniles, and adults.

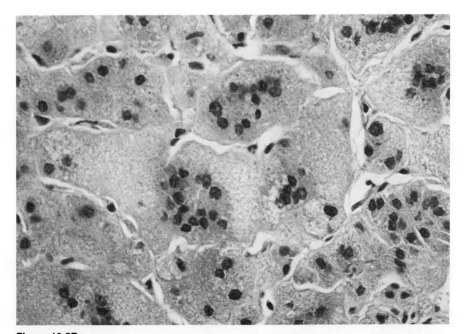

Figure 12.5B
Multinucleated hepatocellular giant cells in infant with biliary atresia. As shown in this example, such giant cells must not be interpreted as evidence of neonatal hepatitis.

Morphologic features: Hepatocytes and Kupffer cells show cytomegaly from intracytoplasmic accumulation of sphingomyelin. In infants, cholestasis may be present also. Cirrhosis is a rare complication of the disease.

Nonalcoholic Fatty Changes or Nonalcoholic Steatohepatitis

Comments: For clinical information and possible underlying or associated diseases, see Chapters 6 and 7.

Morphologic features: Specimens from patients with adult-onset diabetes mellitus often show lipid inclusions in the nuclei of hepatocytes. These inclusions are not membrane-bound; they can be demonstrated in frozen sections stained for fat. Pseudoinclusions may show similar features but are negative for fat. Lipid inclusions may be found in many conditions and also in normal specimens, particularly from young persons. For other morphologic changes, including Mallory bodies, see Figure 12.1B and Chapters 6 and 7.

Primary Sclerosing Cholangitis

This condition is a cause of prolonged cholestasis, leading to the formation of Mallory bodies. See also above under "Biliary Obstruction and Other Causes of Cholestasis." For further clinical and morphologic information on primary sclerosing cholangitis, see Chapters 2, 11, and 15.

Progressive Familial Myoclonic Epilepsy

Comments: This is a hereditary epilepsy characterized by the presence of Lafora bodies in the central nervous system and in the liver, among other organs. The condition probably is related to glycogen storage disease. The defective enzyme is unknown. Inclusions with features of Lafora bodies also have been observed in patients with presenile dementia but without epilepsy or myoclonus, and also in a patient without any neurologic symptoms.[44] The relation of these findings to progressive familial myoclonic epilepsy is not clear.

Morphologic features: Lafora bodies are stored in hepatocytes, primarily in the periportal regions. The intracytoplasmic inclusions characterizing this condition contain mucopolysaccharide (an unusual branched polyglucosan), which is the substrate of the groundglass features of the affected cells.[45] Lafora bodies can be stained with Hale's colloidal ferric oxide stain for acid mucopolysaccharides; they are weakly positive with PAS-D but the positivity can be abolished by pectinase digestion. Electron microscopically, the material appears fibrillar; it is not bound by a membrane.

Syncytial Giant Cell Hepatitis

Comments: Patients had been diagnosed as having active hepatitis non-A, non-B but biopsy features differed.

Morphologic features: Liver cords are replaced by syncytial giant cells with up to 30 nuclei. The condition probably is caused by a paramyxovirus.[46]

Thermal Injury

Comments: Patients in this group died from extensive third-degree burns involving between 35% and 78% of total body surface; death occurred between 5 and 31 days after the injury.[47]

Morphologic features: Large eosinophilic bodies may be found in the cytoplasm of hepatocytes but also in Kupffer cells and, most commonly, in sinusoids and spaces of Disse.[47] No specific stain for this material has been found. Electron microscopically, single membrane-bound structures with amorphous, moderately electron-dense material are seen. It appears likely that this material is a proteinaceous secretion product of hepatocytes.

Toxic Hepatitis

Comments: Exposure to vinyl chloride in the plastic industry has caused severe liver diseases, as described below.

Morphologic features: Multinucleated giant hepatocytes have been observed in this condition, but sinusoidal dilatation and transformation to angiosarcoma is the most important complication of vinyl chloride exposure.[33] Hepatocellular carcinoma also has been observed in these cases.[48]

Viral Hepatitis B and Non-A, Non-B (C, D)

Comments: For the clinical features and definitions of acute, unresolved, and chronic viral hepatitis, see Chapters 2 and 3.

Morphologic features: Degenerative changes of hepatocytes, as described above under "Morphologic Definitions," occur primarily in acute or unresolved viral hepatitis, the prototypes of lobular hepatitis (Chapter 3). Groundglass hepatocytes associated with hepatitis B (Figures 12.6A and 12.6B) occur primarily in unresolved or chronic viral hepatitis B (chronic persistent or chronic active) or in the carrier state for hepatitis B with near-normal histology. The affected hepatocytes are swollen and have an opaque, finely granular cytoplasm, which often is separated from the cell membrane by a space or halo (Figures 12.6A and 12.6B). Groundglass hepatocytes in hepatitis B are distributed at random, sometimes with clusters of positive cells in some areas and few such cells in other parts of the specimen. The groundglass changes are caused by the accumulation of filamentous hepatitis B surface antigen (HB_sAg) in proliferated smooth endoplasmic reticulum. Presence of HB_sAg can be confirmed in paraffin sections with Shikata's orcein stain (groundglass cytoplasm appears dark brown in positive stains: note that the orcein also stains granules of copper-associated protein [see Chapter 14] and elastic fibers), aldehyde thionine, aldehyde fuchsine, or Victoria blue (groundglass cytoplasm appears blue in positive stains). Immunoperoxidase staining for HB_sAg

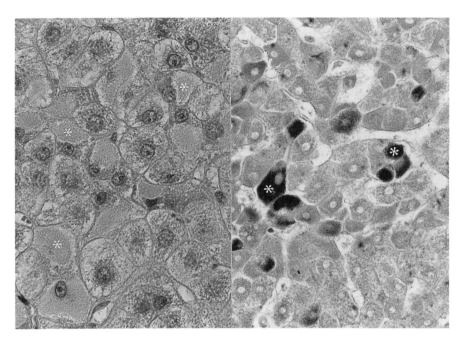

Figure 12.6A
Groundglass hepatocytes. Groundglass features associated with accumulation with hepatitis B surface antigen are shown. Note halo around the groundglass material (asterisks). This is a characteristic feature of this condition. The appearance in routine hematoxylin-eosin stains is shown in the left frame, and the features after staining with Shikata's orcein stain are shown in the right frame.

also can be done on paraffin sections and indeed may be more sensitive, yielding a better contrast between positive and negative cells.[49] However, it should be noted that not all commercial antisera are of equal specificity and sensitivity and that both false-positive and false-negative stains have been encountered.[50] Alternatively, electron microscopy and immunofluorescence can be used to identify hepatitis B antigen, but this is rarely done for routine purposes. Intranuclear inclusions also occur in hepatitis B infection. These inclusions have been described under "Sanded Nuclei" above; they consist of finely granular eosinophilic material that displaces the basophilic nuclear protein and the nucleoli. This material gives the nuclei an opaque or sanded appearance. The inclusions usually represent excess hepatitis B core antigen, but recently delta antigen has been found to cause similar nuclear changes.[51] Immunostaining with specific antisera is needed to distinguish the two antigens. On occasion, deposition of formalin pigment over hepatocellular nuclei (Figure 12.7) has been confused with immunostained core antigen. For light microscopic features of hepatitis non-A, non-B (hepatitis C), see Chapter 2. Presence of multinucleated giant hepatocytes is compatible with the diagnosis of viral hepatitis non-A, non-B.

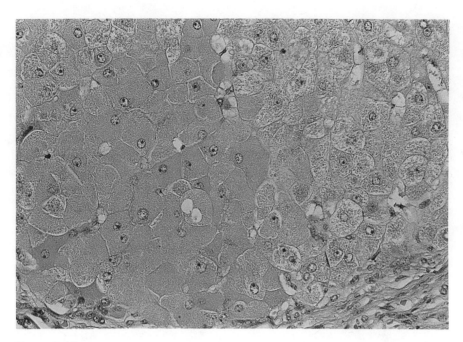

Figure 12.6B
Groundglass-like hepatocytes. Typical hepatocellular oncocytes are shown (mostly in the left half of the illustration) in a case of primary biliary cirrhosis. These cells resemble groundglass hepatocytes in hepatitis B infection but they lack the characteristic halo shown in Figure 12.6A. Oncocytes are more common in other types of cirrhosis, such as alcoholic cirrhosis.

However, some of these cases may represent syncytial giant cell hepatitis (see above). Giant cells of this type may also occur in autoimmune chronic active hepatitis or massive or submassive hepatic necrosis of any cause (see Chapter 9).

Wilson's Disease

Comments: For important clinical findings, see Chapters 2 and 14.

Morphologic features: Specimens from patients with precirrhotic Wilson's disease may show glycogenated nuclei (nuclear glycogen inclusions), primarily in periportal hepatocytes, together with fatty changes and Mallory bodies. In fulminant Wilson's disease, hepatocellular giant cells may be found. For additional histologic findings, see Chapter 2.

Wolman's Disease

Comments: This is a hereditary disorder of lipid metabolism characterized by a congenital deficiency of lysosomal acid lipase. The condition is more severe than

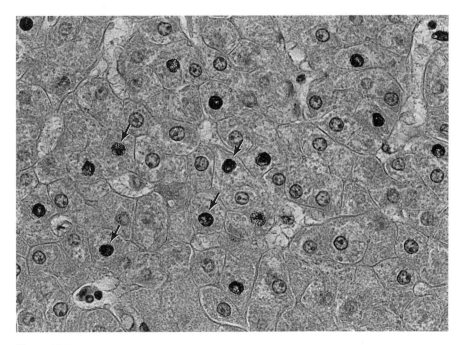

Figure 12.7
Fixation artifact. Formalin pigment over some hepatocellular nuclei (arrows) resembles positive immunostains for hepatitis B core antigen.

cholesteryl ester storage disease (see above) with which it is related. Wolman's disease always becomes symptomatic in childhood.

Morphologic features: Hepatocytes, Kupffer cells, and macrophages are stuffed with cholesteryl esters and triglycerides so that these two cell types become difficult to distinguish. Fibrosis and cirrhosis may develop.

References

1. Vieira WT, Gayotto LC, De Lima CP, et al: Histopathology of the human liver in yellow fever with special emphasis on the diagnostic role of the Councilman body. *Histopathology* 7:195-208, 1983.

2. Qizilbash A, Young-Pong O: Alpha₁-antitrypsin liver disease differential diagnosis of PAS-positive, diastase-resistant globules in liver cells. *Am J Clin Pathol* 79:697-702, 1983.

3. Ray MB: Distribution patterns of cytokeratin antigen determinants in alcoholic and nonalcoholic liver diseases. *Hum Pathol* 18:61-66, 1987.

4. Yoshioka K, Kakuma S, Tahara H, et al: Occurrence of immunohistochemically detected small Mallory bodies in liver disease. *Am J Gastroenterology* 84:535-539, 1989.

5. Koneru B, Jaffe R, Esquivel CO, et al: Adenoviral infections in pediatric liver transplant recipients. JAMA 258:489-492, 1987.

6. Uchida T, Kronborg I, Peters RL: Giant mitochondria in the alcoholic liver diseases— their identification, frequency and pathologic significance. Liver 4:29-38, 1984.

7. Junge J, Horn T, Christoffersen P: Megamitochondria as a diagnostic marker for alcohol induced centrilobular and periportal fibrosis in the liver. Virchows Arch [A] 410:553-558, 1987.

8. Gerber MA, Thung SN: Hepatic oncocytes: Incidence, staining characteristics, and ultrastructural features. Am J Clin Pathol 75:498-503, 1981.

9. Lindmark B, Millward-Sadler H, Callea F, et al: Hepatic inclusions of α_1-antichymotrypsin in a patient with partial deficiency of α_1-antichymotrypsin and chronic liver disease. Histopathology 16:221-225, 1990.

10. Carlson J: Endoplasmic reticulum storage disease. Histopathology 16:309-312, 1990.

11. Rakela J, Goldschmiedt M, Ludwig J: Late manifestations of chronic liver disease in adults with alpha-1-antitrypsin deficiency. Dig Dis Sci 32:1358-1362, 1987.

12. Pariente E-A, Degott C, Martin J-P, et al: Hepatocytic PAS-positive diastase-resistant inclusions in the absence of alpha-1-antitrypsin deficiency—high prevalence in alcoholic cirrhosis. Am J Clin Pathol 76:299-302, 1981.

13. Clausen PP, Linskov J, Gad I, et al: The diagnostic value of α_1-antitrypsin globules in liver cells as a morphologic marker of α_1-antitrypsin deficiency. Liver 4:353-359, 1984.

14. Callea F, Fevery J, Massi G, et al: Storage of alpha-1-antitrypsin in intrahepatic bile duct cells in alpha-1-antitrypsin deficiency (PiZ phenotype). Histopathology 9:99-108, 1985.

15. Thijs JC, Bosma A, Henzen-Logmans SC, et al: Postinfantile giant cell hepatitis in a patient with multiple autoimmune features. Am J Gastroenterol 80:294-297, 1985.

16. Zubair I, Herrera GA, Pretlow TG II, et al: Cytoplasmic inclusions in hepatocytes of bone marrow transplant patients: Light and electron microscopic characterization. Am J Clin Pathol 83:65-68, 1985.

17. Elleder M, Ledinová J, Cieslar P, et al: Subclinical course of cholesterol ester storage disease (CESD) diagnosed in adulthood: Report of two cases with remarks on the nature of the liver storage process. Virchows Arch [A] 416:357-365, 1990.

18. Klatt EC, Koss MN, Young TS, et al: Hepatic hyaline globules associated with passive congestion. Arch Pathol Lab Med 112:510-513, 1988.

19. Sacks SL, Freeman HJ: Cytomegalovirus hepatitis: Evidence for direct hepatic viral infection using monoclonal antibodies. Gastroenterology 86:346-350, 1984.

20. Naoumov NV, Alexander GJM, O'Grady JG, et al: Rapid diagnosis of cytomegalovirus infection by in-situ hybridization in liver grafts. Lancet 1:1361-1363, 1988.

21. Chehab FF, Xiao X, Kan YW, et al: Detection of cytomegalovirus infection in paraffin-embedded tissue specimens with the polymerase chain reaction. Mod Pathol 2:75-78, 1989.

22. Lewis JH, Mullick F, Ishak KG, et al: Histopathologic analysis of suspected amiodarone hepatotoxicity. Hum Pathol 21:59-67, 1990.

23. Pessayre D, Bichara M, Feldmann C, et al: Perhexiline maleate-induced cirrhosis. Gastroenterology 76:170-177, 1979.

24. Dienes HP, Gerharz C-D, Wagner R, et al: Accumulation of hydroxyethyl starch (HES) in the liver of patients with renal failure and portal hypertension. *J Hepatol* 3:223-227, 1986.

25. Jezequel AM, Libari ML, Mosca P, et al: Changes induced in human liver by long-term anticonvulsant therapy: Functional and ultrastructural data. *Liver* 4:307-330, 1984.

26. Pamperl H, Gradner W, Fridrich H, et al: Influence of long-term anticonvulsant treatment on liver ultrastructure in man. *Liver* 4:294-330, 1984.

27. Vazquez JJ, Pardo-Mindan J: Liver cell injury (bodies similar to Lafora's) in alcoholics treated with disulfiram (Antabuse). *Histopathology* 3:377-384, 1979.

28. Vazquez JJ, Guillen FJ, Zozaya J, et al: Cyanamide-induced liver injury: A predictable lesion. *Liver* 3:225-230, 1983.

29. Dubin HV, Harrell ER: Liver disease associated with methotrexate treatment of psoriatic patients. *Arch Dermatol* 102:498-503, 1970.

30. Simpson DG, Walker JH: Hypersensitivity to para-aminosalicylic acid. *Am J Med* 29:297-306, 1960.

31. Mellvanie SK, MacCarthy JD: Hepatitis in association with prolonged 6-mercaptopurine therapy. *Blood* 14:80-90, 1959.

32. Pessayre D, Degos F, Feldmann G, et al: Chronic active hepatitis and giant multinucleated hepatocytes in adults treated with clometacin. *Digestion* 22:66-72, 1981.

33. Berk PD, Martin JF, Young RS, et al: Vinyl chloride–associated liver disease. *Ann Intern Med* 84:717-731, 1976.

34. Ng IOL, Ng M, Lai ECS, et al: Endoplasmic storage disease of liver: Characterization of intracytoplasmic hyaline inclusions. *Histopathology* 15:473-481, 1989.

35. McAdams AJ, Hug G, Bove KE: Glycogen storage disease, types I to X. *Hum Pathol* 5:463-487, 1974.

36. Schochet SS Jr, McCormick WF, Zellweger H: Type IV glycogenosis (amylopectinosis): Light and electron microscopic observations. *Arch Pathol* 90:354-363, 1960.

37. Itoh S, Ishida Y, Matsuo S: Mallory bodies in a patient with type Ia glycogen storage disease. *Gastroenterology* 92:520-523, 1987.

38. Ludwig J, Gross JB, Perkins JD, et al: Persistent centrilobular necroses in hepatic allografts. *Hum Pathol* 21:656-661, 1990.

39. Stromeyer FW, Ishak KG, Gerber MA, et al: Ground-glass cells in hepatocellular carcinoma. *Am J Clin Pathol* 74:254-258, 1980.

40. Berman MA, Burnham JA, Sheahan DG: Fibrolamellar carcinoma of the liver: An immunohistochemical study of nineteen cases and a review of the literature. *Hum Pathol* 19:784-794, 1988.

41. Ladefoged C, Frifeldt JJ: Hepatocellular calcification. *Virchows Arch [A]* 410:461-463, 1987.

42. Goyer RA, Wilson MH: Lead-induced inclusion bodies. Results of ethylenediaminetetraacetic acid treatment. *Lab Invest* 32:149-156, 1975.

43. Klinge O: Hepatozelluläre Veränderungen im Leberpunktat bei der chronischen Bleivergiftung des Menschen. *Acta Hepato-Splenologica* 17:151-159, 1970.

44. Ng IOL, Sturgess RP, Williams R, et al: Ground-glass hepatocytes with Lafora body-like inclusions—histochemical, immunohistochemical and electronmicroscopic characterization. *Histopathology* 17:109-115, 1990.

45. Harriman DGF, Millar JHD, Stevenson AC: Progressive familial myoclonic epilepsy in three families: Its clinical features and pathologic basis. *Brain* 78:325-349, 1955.

46. Phillips MJ, Blendis LM, Poucell S, et al: Syncytial giant cell hepatitis: Sporadic hepatitis with distinctive pathological features, a severe clinical course, and paramyxoviral features. *N Engl J Med* 324:455-460, 1991.

47. Langlinais PC, Panke TW: Intrasinusoidal bodies in the livers of thermally injured patients. *Arch Pathol Lab Med* 103:499-504, 1979.

48. Evans DM, Williams WJ, Kung IT: Angiosarcoma and hepatocellular carcinoma in vinyl chloride workers. *Histopathology* 7:377-388, 1983.

49. Clausen PP, Thomsen P: Demonstration of hepatitis B-surface antigen in liver biopsies: A comparative investigation of immunoperoxidase and orcein staining on identical sections in formalin fixed, paraffin embedded tissue. *Acta Pathol Microbiol Scand* 86:383-388, 1978.

50. Goodman ZD, Langloss JM, Bratthauser GL, et al: Immunohistochemical localization of hepatitis B surface antigen and hepatitis B core antigen staining in tissue sections: A source of false positive staining. *Am J Clin Pathol* 89:533-537, 1988.

51. Moreno A, Ramón Y Cajal S, Marazuela M, et al: Sanded nuclei in delta patients. *Liver* 9:367-371, 1989.

Chapter 13

Iron-Positive Pigments

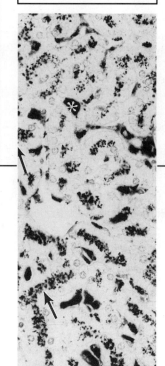

Morphologic and Chemical Definitions

Two types of stainable iron-containing pigments may be encountered, namely, ferritin and hemosiderin. Heme-iron also occurs[1] but appears to have no special staining characteristics.

Ferritin

Ferritin consists of protein subunits with central mycelia of ferric hydroxyphosphate. Crystalline ferritin is found free in the cytosol and thus imparts a diffuse blue discoloration ("diffuse iron") after the use of Perls' or Gomori's Prussian blue staining.

Hemosiderin

The other pigment, hemosiderin, consists of iron molecules from ferritin mycelia or other sources, bound to mucopolysaccharides. Hemosiderin is amorphous and is usually found in secondary lysosomes, where the noncrystalline material forms granules that are readily identifiable in iron stains. The presence of stainable hemosiderin in the liver is called hemosiderosis; the etiology of the hemosiderin deposition or its intensity is not considered in this context (see also below under "Genetic Hemochromatosis"). By convention, the name "hemosiderosis" is also used for specimens that contain only stainable ferritin. Any hepatic pigment that is stainable for iron is abnormal.

Table 13.1   Clinical Conditions Associated With Iron Pigmentation*

Alcoholic liver disease (hepatocytes and Kupffer cells)
Genetic (HLA-linked, primary) hemochromatosis (hepatocytes; later also Kupffer cells and
    other mesenchymal cells; biliary epithelium)
Transfusions (Kupffer cells; later also hepatocytes)
Transient hemolytic episodes (predominantly hepatocytes)
Viral hepatitis (ferritin in macrophages)
Uncommon causes:
    Cimetidine hemochromatosis (hepatocytes)
    Congenital atransferrinemia (hepatocytes)
    Dietary or medicinal iron ingestion (hepatocytes and Kupffer cells)
    Hemochromatosis after portacaval shunting (hepatocytes and Kupffer cells)
    Idiopathic perinatal hemochromatosis (hepatocytes and Kupffer cells)
    Parenteral iron administration (Kupffer cells; later also hepatocytes)
    Porphyria cutanea tarda (hepatocytes; later also Kupffer cells)
    Sideroblastic anemias (hepatocytes; later also Kupffer cells)
    Thalassemia major (hepatocytes; later also Kupffer cells)

*The main sites of iron deposition are shown in parentheses; unless otherwise stated, the pigment is hemosiderin.

Clinical Conditions

Alcoholic Liver Disease

Comments: In a small proportion of patients with alcoholic cirrhosis (see Chapter 11), hemosiderin accumulates in the liver. In instances with severe iron overload, clinical and biochemical findings as well as the frequency of HLA-A3 and HLA-B7 are essentially the same as in genetic (HLA-linked) hemo-chromatosis (see below). Only the mean hepatic iron concentration tends to be lower in alcoholic patients as compared to nonalcoholic patients with genetic hemochromatosis.[2] Nevertheless, hepatic iron stores in alcoholic cirrhosis may exceed the expected value by 15-fold (for normal values, see the Appendix), and in these cases findings most likely represent coexistent genetic hemochromatosis.[2] Alcohol appears to be a contributing factor in the homozygote.[3] In alcoholic cirrhosis with mild iron deposition, causes such as hemolysis must be considered.

Morphologic features: The liver shows the usual features of alcoholic cirrhosis (see Chapter 11); in addition, it also shows hemosiderin deposition in hepatocytes and often also in Kupffer cells, mesenchymal cells of portal tracts and fibrous septa, and bile duct epithelial cells. Fatty changes and inflammatory activity are important clues for the distinction between hemochromatosis of the alcoholic, and genetic hemochromatosis uncomplicated by alcoholism. After an alcoholic patient with hemochromatosis has stopped drinking for some time (usually several months), the two conditions become morphologically indistinguishable.

Cimetidine Hemochromatosis

Comments: One patient has been described who developed "hemo-chromatosis" after long-term cimetidine treatment.[4] An unexpected rise in serum iron levels and transferrin saturation prompted liver biopsy. The authors speculated that cimetidine interferes with the reduction of organic iron and its chelation.

Morphologic features: The liver biopsy specimens showed much hepa-tocellular hemosiderosis as well as portal and septal fibrosis. Cirrhosis was not described.

Congenital Atransferrinemia

Comments: This very rare congenital, autosomal-recessive disorder is characterized by the absence or quantitative deficiency of transferrin in the serum, leading to severe hypochromic anemia. Only six cases have been described. The long-term prognosis is uncertain.[5]

Morphologic features: Morphologic studies of the hepatic changes are not available. According to a recent general review, hemosiderin is found predominantly in hepatocytes.[1]

Dietary or Medicinal Iron Ingestion

Comments: Dietary iron overload is best known from the study of South African blacks (Bantu hemochromatosis).[6] In Europe and North America, consumption of oral iron medications or iron supplementation in the diet has led to hemosiderin deposition.[7]

Morphologic features: Hemosiderin deposition in hepatocytes and Kupffer cells, with or without fibrosis, are the only abnormalities. Cirrhosis would be a most unusual finding in a white patient with a history of excessive iron ingestion.

Genetic (HLA-Linked, Primary) Hemochromatosis

Comments: This hereditary disorder of iron metabolism is the prototype of iron storage diseases. Hepatomegaly, skin pigmentation, testicular atrophy, and arthropathy are prominent physical signs. Many patients develop diabetes mellitus. Biochemical abnormalities include increased serum transferrin-iron saturation and increased serum ferritin levels. HLA-typing is useful if first-degree relatives are available. The hepatic iron concentration is uniformly increased and increases with age. The hepatic iron index (hepatic iron [μmol/g dry weight]/age) allows a clear distinction between homozygotes, heterozygotes, and controls.[8] The tissue iron levels can be determined by flameless atomic absorption spectrophotometry, using fixed, paraffin-embedded liver biopsy tissue. Formalin fixation and paraffin embedding have no effect on the results.[2] In advanced genetic hemochromatosis, the hepatic iron content often is between 20,000 and 30,000 μg/g dry weight (normal, 200-2,000; for possible sex differences, see the Appendix).

Morphologic features: In precirrhotic stages of the disease, the liver may show only periportal hepatocellular hemosiderosis, without any other abnormalities (Figure 13.1). Unless iron stains are prepared routinely, the pigmentation may be

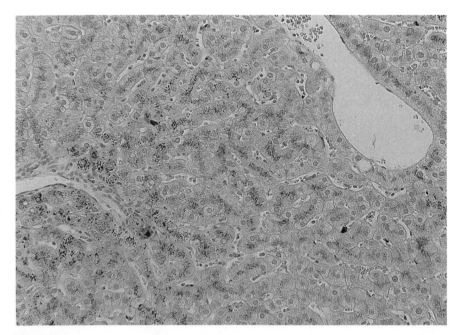

Figure 13.1
Hepatocellular hemosiderosis in precirrhotic genetic hemochromatosis. As always, the iron deposition is most pronounced in the periportal areas (left third of frame). Perls' stain for iron.

missed entirely. As the disease progresses, hemosiderin appears also in Kupffer cells, other mesenchymal cells, and bile duct epithelial cells. Some ferritin also may be seen. This accumulation of iron is accompanied by fibrosis and, eventually, by the development of pigment cirrhosis (Chapter 11). This type of cirrhosis characteristically lacks inflammatory activity or other complicating features such as cholestasis. It should be noted that the cirrhosis in genetic hemochromatosis appears to be reversible in some instances.[9] Whether such cases indeed represented cirrhosis or only fibrosis simulating cirrhosis is a matter of semantics. Of greater importance for clinical purposes is the observation that hepatocellular carcinoma develops in about 30% of patients with genetic hemochromatosis and pigment cirrhosis.[10] This type of malignancy may occur even after reversal of the cirrhosis[11] or prior to the development of cirrhosis.[12] During phlebotomy therapy, hemosiderin deposits gradually disappear. Prior to complete mobilization of the stainable iron, hemosiderin often is found in bile duct epithelium only. This feature appears to be diagnostic for incomplete iatrogenic removal of hepatic iron.

Hemochromatosis After Portacaval Shunting

Comments: After surgical portacaval shunting for cirrhosis, iron deposition may occur in the liver. Thus, by definition, the liver prior to shunt surgery should have been free of stainable iron. However, unexplained hemosiderosis in cirrhotic livers might be the result of spontaneous shunting. Increased iron absorption from the bowel and oral iron administration are other possible causes of this condition, and some patients also may have a predisposition to store excessive iron.[13]

Morphologic features: The cirrhotic livers contain large amounts of hemosiderin in hepatocytes and Kupffer cells. Depending on the features of the preexisting cirrhosis, the histologic changes may be indistinguishable from those of pigment cirrhosis in genetic hemochromatosis.

Idiopathic Perinatal Hemochromatosis

Comments: This is a rare neonatal iron storage disorder of unknown cause. Most affected infants die in the first months of life.

Morphologic features: Typically, the liver shows severe hepatocellular and Kupffer cell hemosiderosis and diffuse fibrosis with much ductular proliferation. Cholestasis also has been observed. The changes may resemble massive or submassive hepatic necrosis but true cirrhosis also may be present.[14] In rare instances, this type of iron deposition may be found in neonatal liver diseases of known cause—for instance, tyrosinemia.[15] In the idiopathic cases, other organs such as pancreas, kidneys, and thyroid are involved also.[14]

Parenteral Iron Administration

See below under "Transfusions."

Porphyria Cutanea Tarda

Comments: This disorder of porphyrin metabolism is encountered more commonly than others; it is characterized by a reduced hepatic activity of uroporphyrinogen decarboxylase, leading to accumulation of uroporphyrin I and other porphyrins. In some instances, the condition is familial but more often it appears to be acquired. Alcohol and drugs, among other factors, can trigger the expression of the disease. The relation between porphyria cutanea tarda and genetic hemochromatosis is controversial.[16,17]

Morphologic features: Moderate hemosiderin deposition is found in periportal hepatocytes and later also in Kupffer cells. Fatty changes provide an important etiologic clue. Nuclei of hepatocytes may be vacuolated and ceroid pigment may be found in mononuclear cells in the lobules. Portal tracts typically are inflamed. A specific histologic feature of porphyria cutanea tarda appears to be the presence of needle-shaped intracytoplasmic inclusions, which can be seen in hepatocytes after use of the ferric ferricyanide reduction test.[18] These acicular inclusions are best seen in rapidly stained or unstained sections, using polarizing microscopy.[19]

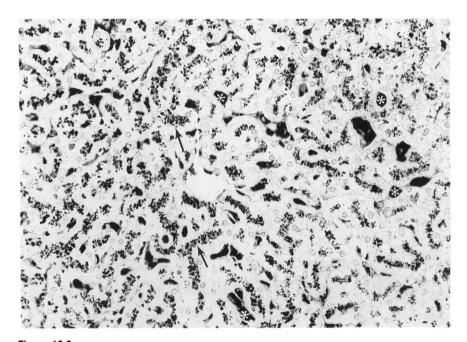

Figure 13.2
Combined hepatocellular (arrows) and Kupffer cell hemosiderosis in thalassemia major. Patchy iron deposits (asterisks) are created by the admixture of ferritin. Perls' stain for iron.

Sideroblastic Anemias and Thalassemia Major

Comments: Primary sideroblastic anemias may be acquired or hereditary; secondary sideroblastic anemias often are associated with other hematologic disorders but also with conditions such as alcoholism, carcinoma, malabsorption syndromes, and polyarthritis. Such secondary sideroblastic anemias also may be caused by drugs or lead poisoning. Pyridoxine-responsive sideroblastic anemia usually is considered separately. Thalassemia major (homozygous beta-thalassemia) is a severe hemolytic anemia of early infancy with jaundice and severe hepatosplenomegaly. A genetic association between HLA-linked hemochromatosis and idiopathic refractory sideroblastic anemia has been suggested.[20]

Morphologic features: Hemosiderin usually is found in both Kupffer cells and hepatocytes (Figure 13.2). Fibrosis or cirrhosis may be present also, making the specimens indistinguishable from those in genetic hemochromatosis. Interpretation often is difficult because most patients have received many transfusions, and thus the anemia-associated hemosiderosis may be complicated by transfusion

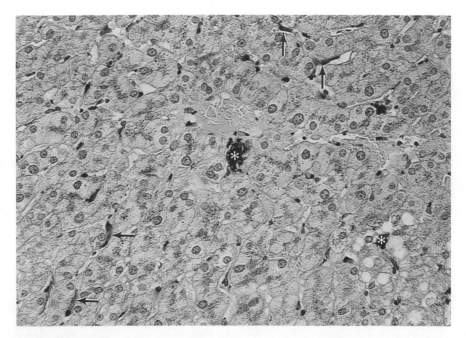

Figure 13.3
Kupffer cell hemosiderosis after blood transfusions. In contradistinction to hepatocellular hemosiderosis (see Figure 13.1), the iron-positive Kupffer cells do not have a zonal distribution. The Kupffer cells appear as elongated, slightly curved structures (arrows). If they also contain ferritin, the iron staining becomes patchy (asterisks). Perls' stain for iron.

hemosiderosis and by complications of acute or chronic non-A, non-B viral infections of the liver (hepatitis C infection).

Thalassemia Major

See above under "Sideroblastic Anemias and Thalassemia Major."

Transfusions

Comments: Repeated blood transfusions or one-time transfusion of large volumes of blood may lead to appreciable hemosiderosis in less than 1 week.

Morphologic features: Typically, after sudden influx of iron, hemosiderin is found only in Kupffer cells (Figure 13.3). However, with increasing iron deposition, hepatocytes become involved also. Unless complicated by hepatitis C infection (see above under "Sideroblastic Anemias and Thalassemia Major"), transfusions cause no other abnormalities.

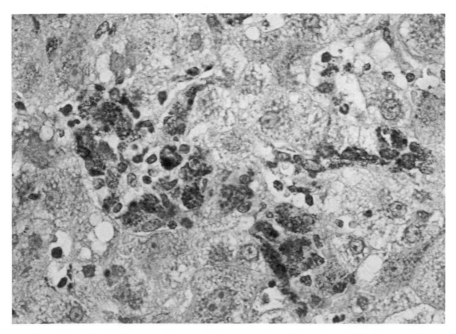

Figure 13.4
Viral hepatitis (chronic lobular hepatitis) with spotty necrosis in a lobule. The necrosis contains ferritin-laden macrophages. Perls' stain for iron.

Transient Hemolytic Episodes

Acquired hemolytic anemia and transient hemolytic episodes too mild to cause anemia may lead to hepatic hemosiderosis, indistinguishable from transfusion hemosiderosis (see above under "Transfusions").

Viral Hepatitis

Comments: For definitions of acute and unresolved viral hepatitis, see Chapter 3. Generally, hepatitis A, B, or non-A, non-B (C, D) are involved.

Morphologic features: Specimens show lobular hepatitis and spotty necroses with ferritin-laden macrophages ("diffuse iron"; Figure 13.4). The changes in these conditions have been described in Chapter 3. In rare instances, other types of hepatitis show similar features.

References

1. Tavill AS, Sharma BK, Bacon BR: Iron and the liver: Genetic hemochromatosis and other hepatic iron overload disorders. *Prog Liver Dis* 9:281-305, 1990.

2. LeSage GD, Baldus WP, Fairbanks VF, et al: Hemochromatosis: Genetic or alcohol-induced? *Gastroenterology* 84:1471-1477, 1983.

3. Milder MS, Cook JD, Stray S, et al: Idiopathic hemochromatosis, an interim report. *Medicine* 59:34-49, 1980.

4. Bodenheimer HC, Thayer WR: Hemochromatosis associated with cimetidine therapy? *J Clin Gastroenterol* 3:83-85, 1981.

5. Fairbanks VF, Beutler E: Congenital atransferrinemia and idiopathic pulmonary hemosiderosis. In Williams JW, Beutler E, Erslev AJ (eds): *Hematology*. 4th ed. New York, McGraw-Hill Inc, 1990, pp 506-510.

6. Bothwell TH, Abrahams C, Bradlow BA, et al: Idiopathic and Bantu hemochromatosis: Comparative histological study. *Arch Pathol* 79:163-168, 1965.

7. Olsson KS, Ritter B, Rosen U, et al: Prevalence of iron overload in central Sweden. *Acta Med Scand* 213:145-150, 1983.

8. Summers KM, Halliday JW, Powell LW: Identification of homozygous hemochromatosis subjects by measurement of hepatic iron index. *Hepatology* 12:20-25, 1990.

9. Perez-Tamayo R: Cirrhosis of the liver: A reversible disease? *Pathol Annu* 14:183-213, 1979.

10. Bassett ML, Halliday JW, Powell LW: Hemochromatosis and other iron storage disorders. *Surv Dig Dis* 2:73-84, 1984.

11. Blumberg RS, Chopra S, Ibrahim R, et al: Primary hepatocellular carcinoma in idiopathic hemochromatosis after reversal of cirrhosis. *Gastroenterology* 95:1399-1402, 1988.

12. Fellows IW, Stewart M, Jeffcoate WJ, et al: Hepatocellular carcinoma in primary hemochromatosis in the absence of cirrhosis. *Gut* 29:1603-1606, 1988.

13. Lombard CM, Strauchen JA: Postshunt hemochromatosis with cardiomyopathy. *Hum Pathol* 12:1149-1151, 1981.

14. Moerman P, Pauwels P, Vandenberghe K, et al: Neonatal hemochromatosis. *Histopathology* 17:345-351, 1990.

15. Witzleben CL, Uri A: Perinatal hemochromatosis: Entity or end result? *Hum Pathol* 20:335-340, 1989.

16. Kushner JP, Edwards CQ, Dadone MM, et al: Heterozygosity for HLA-linked hemochromatosis as a likely cause of the siderosis associated with sporadic porphyria cutanea tarda. *Gastroenterology* 88:1232-1238, 1985.

17. Beaumont C, Fauchet R, Phung LN, et al: Porphyria cutanea tarda and HLA-linked hemochromatosis: Evidence against a systematic association. *Gastroenterology* 92:1833-1838, 1987.

18. Fakan F, Chlumská A: Demonstration of needle-shaped hepatic inclusions in porphyria cutanea tarda using the ferric ferricyanide reduction test. *Virchows Arch [A]* 411:365-368, 1987.

19. Campo E, Bruguera M, Rodes J: Are there diagnostic histologic features of porphyria cutanea tarda in liver biopsy specimens? *Liver* 10:185-190, 1990.

20. Barron R, Grade ND, Sherwood G, et al: Iron overload complicating sideroblastic anemia: Is the gene for hemochromatosis responsible? *Gastroenterology* 96:1204-1206, 1989.

Chapter 14

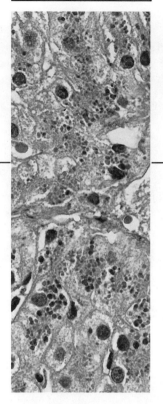

Iron-Negative Pigments and Abnormal Nonpigmented Substances

Morphologic and Chemical Definitions

A multitude of pigmented and nonpigmented iron-negative substances may appear in the liver; most can also be encountered in extrahepatic tissues.

Amyloid

This is a pathologic fibrillar proteinaceous substance, classified as AL (amyloid light chain) or AA (amyloid-associated).

Anthracotic Pigment

Anthracotic pigment is a black granular pigment consisting mainly of carbon; it is not birefringent. The pigment often is associated with silica (see below).

Barium Sulfate

Barium sulfate ($BaSO_4$) is a white powder that is insoluble in water and is used as a contrast medium in radiographic studies of the gastrointestinal tract. In tissues, the material is granular, light gray, and refractile. It has a characteristic appearance in scanning electron micrographs, and the barium can be unequivocally identified by energy-dispersive x-ray microanalysis.[1]

Bile

Bile is secreted by hepatocytes and contains bilirubin and other pigments that impart the typical greenish or golden-brown color; Fouchet's stain turns bile green (see Chapters 4 and 5).

Calcium

Calcium occurs in damaged tissue (dystrophic calcification) or in association with hypercalcemia in tissue with zones of high acidity (metastatic calcification). In von Kossa's stain, calcium is black.

Cellulose

Cellulose is a carbohydrate that forms a main structural component of plants and plant cells. Cellulose is used in the manufacture of tablets. This substance appears in multiple forms such as cotton, linen, and starch (see below).

Ceroid

Ceroid is an abnormal PAS-positive, diastase-resistant, acid-fast pigment, rich in oxidized lipids. In hematoxylin-eosin preparations, ceroid is brown and resembles lipofuscin (see below). In frozen sections, ceroid is sudanophilic. Acid-fastness is the main feature that distinguishes ceroid from lipofuscin.

Copper

Copper occurs in the liver primarily as a copper-protein complex. In this chemical form, the metal can be demonstrated with the rhodanine stain as a red granular pigment. The copper-associated protein forms dark brown granules in orcein-stained specimens. Stainable copper-protein complexes are always abnormal findings. It should be noted that copper cannot be stained after fixation in unbuffered or acid formalin, Zenker's fixative, or Lillie's B5 fixative. After prolonged fixation and storage in formalin, copper may leak from any specimen. Also, copper stains may be negative in some cases of Wilson's disease, despite high chemical copper contents (see Chapter 2).

Cystine

Cystine is a naturally occurring nonessential amino acid that can be found in most proteins; it can be formed by the oxidation of two molecules of cysteine. In cystinosis, colorless rectangular or hexagonal cystine crystals are found in tissues; they are birefringent in polarized light.[2]

Dubin-Johnson Pigment

Dubin-Johnson pigment shares features with both lipofuscin and melanin, but the granules in Dubin-Johnson syndrome are darker and more pleomorphic than lipofuscin, and they differ in some physiochemical properties from melanin.[3,4] The pigment is black in the Fontana-Masson silver stain; it sometimes can be stained with PAS-D. In frozen sections, the pigment can be shown to contain lipid, and ultraviolet microscopy reveals autofluorescence.[5] Electron microscopic studies may be helpful for the diagnosis.[6]

Formalin Pigment

Formalin pigment appears as dark brown, birefringent, granular material in hematoxylin-eosin sections. The pigment is acid formaldehyde hematin; it is formed when the fixative reacts with hemoglobin at a pH below 5.6. Formalin pigment can be removed from histologic sections—for instance, with a mixture of ammonia water, acetone, and hydrogen peroxide. (See also Figure 12.7.)

Hematoidin

Hematoidin is the name for bilirubin and other bile pigments when they are found as yellow or brown material at the site of old hemorrhages or infarcts. Fouchet's stain for bile is positive.

Hemozoin

Hemozoin is the malaria pigment. For further details, see below.

Lipochrome

Lipochrome is the collective name for a group of fat-soluble pigments such as carotenes that impart a yellow, yellow-orange, or orange-red color to lipid-containing tissues. In the liver, the name often is used as a collective term for ceroid, the Dubin-Johnson pigment (see above), and lipofuscin (see below).

Lipofuscin

Lipofuscin is a granular, PAS-negative pigment produced by lysosomal oxidation of lipids. Lipofuscin is brown in routine sections; it is a normal component of hepatocytes, particularly in elderly people.

Malaria Pigment

Malaria pigment in tissues consists of acid-fast, granular, insoluble ferriprotoporphyrin polymers (hemozoin) from trophozoites, which have broken-down hemoglobin from the host cell. In routine sections, the pigment is dark brown and not stainable for iron. However, the iron content of the pigment can be demonstrated after incineration. Hemozoin resembles formalin pigment (see above), and therefore formalin should not be used in suspected cases of malaria. The pigments of malaria and of schistosomiasis (see below) cannot be distinguished by light microscopy but differ ultrastructurally.[7]

Melanin

Melanin is a yellow, brown, or black pigment formed by the polymerization of tyrosine. Melanin does not occur in normal livers or non-neoplastic liver diseases; it differs from the Dubin-Johnson pigment (see above).

Povidone

Povidone is a polymer of 1-ethenyl-2-pyrrolidone, which forms a colloidal solution in water; it has been used as a dispersing and suspending agent and as a plasma volume expander. The material is not birefringent; it is stainable with Congo red.[2]

Protoporphyrin

Protoporphyrin accumulates in erythropoietic protoporphyria. In routine sections, dark brown deposits are found that show red fluorescence in frozen sections. Under polarized light, frozen sections reveal bright red and granular pigment, with a centrally located black Maltese cross.

Schistosomal Pigment

Schistosomal pigment is found in the vicinity of dead ova. The pigment has the same light microscopic features as malaria pigment (see above).

Silica

Silica is silicon dioxide (SiO_2), a crystalline (quartz and cristobalite) colorless substance. In tissues, needle-shaped birefringent crystals can be identified. Scanning electron microscopy reveals characteristic features.[1] Silica and anthracotic pigment (see above) usually occur together.

Silicone

Silicone is a collective name for any member of a large group of polymers, all of which contain silicon. Phase-contrast microscopy is needed to identify this colorless substance.

Silver

Silver compounds have been used in the past—for instance, in enemas for the treatment of chronic ulcerative colitis. In rare instances, the metal was demonstrated in the liver.[8]

Starch

Starch is the most common plant carbohydrate; it consists of amylose and amylopectine, two glucan chains. In tissues, starch is PAS-positive and birefringent, with a Maltese cross configuration.

Talc

Talc is hydrous magnesium silicate; it is used as a dusting powder. The crystals are colorless but are easily visible by their birefringence in polarized light. Talc has a characteristic "flake pastry" appearance in scanning electron micrographs.[1]

Thorotrast

Thorotrast was used as a radiological contrast medium; the name reveals its main component, radioactive thorium dioxide. In tissues, thorotrast can be identified as a brown, coarse, granular pigment. Autoradiographs show the characteristic tracks of the alpha particles. Positive identification of thorium requires energy-dispersive x-ray microanalysis in unstained thin sections.

Uroporphyrin

Uroporphyrin is an oxidation product of uroporphyrinogen; it accumulates in tissues in the form of needle-shaped crystals, which are difficult to see in routine sections but can be demonstrated well in polarized light, using unstained sections. In ultraviolet light, uroporphyrin has a red autofluorescence.[2]

Table 14.1   Clinical Conditions Associated With Iron-Negative Pigments and Abnormal Nonpigmented Substances*

Amyloid
   Amyloidosis
Anthracotic Pigment
   Anthracosis and anthracosilicosis
Barium Sulfate
   Previous radiographic studies
Bile
   Conditions listed in Chapters 4 and 5
Calcium
   Hepatocellular necrosis, all types
   Hypercalcemia
   Tumors and pseudotumors
Cellulose
   Intravenous substance abuse
Ceroid Pigment
   Hepatocellular necrosis, all types
   Total parenteral nutrition
   Unresolved viral hepatitis and other types of lobular hepatitis
Copper
   Alpha-1-antitrypsin deficiency
   Chronic cholestasis, any type
   Chronic nonsuppurative destructive cholangitis (syndrome of primary biliary cirrhosis)
   Copper storage disease
   Idiopathic adulthood ductopenia
   Idiopathic copper toxicosis
   Indian childhood cirrhosis
   Paucity of intrahepatic bile ducts and other types of infantile obstructive cholangiopathy
   Primary sclerosing cholangitis
   Total parenteral nutrition
   Tumors and pseudotumors
   Wilson's disease
Cystine
   Cystinosis
Dubin-Johnson Pigment
   Dubin-Johnson syndrome
Formalin Pigment
   Artifact of fixation, not directly related to any specific clinical condition but most
      common in tissues with high blood content. See also above under "Morphologic and
      Chemical Definitions."
Hematoidin
   Old hemorrhages and infarcts

continued on page 189

continued from page188
Hemozoin
    Malaria
Lipochrome
    See conditions listed under "Ceroid Pigment" and "Lipofuscin"
Lipofuscin
    Chronic granulomatous disease of childhood
    Drug idiosyncrasy and toxicity (Note: Pigments may only resemble lipofuscin)
    Dubin-Johnson syndrome (Note: Pigment only resembles lipofuscin)
    Gilbert's syndrome
    Hepatic atrophy
    Total parenteral nutrition
Malaria Pigment
    Malaria
Melanin
    Dubin-Johnson syndrome (Note: Pigment only resembles melanin)
    Malignant melanoma
Povidone (Polyvinylpyrrolidone)
    See below under "Povidone Administration." This substance is a pharmaceutical adjuvant
        and thus is not related to any specific clinical condition.
Protoporphyrin
    Erythropoietic protoporphyria
Schistosomal Pigment
    Schistosomiasis
Silica
    Silicosis and anthracosilicosis
Silicone
    See below under "Embolization of Silicone." The material may originate from damaged
        heart valve prostheses, antifoam agents, plastic tubing, or from silicone injections. Thus,
        silicone embolization is not related to any specific clinical condition.
Silver
    Argyria
Starch
    Intravenous substance abuse
    Previous surgery
Talc
    Intravenous substance abuse
    Previous surgery
Thorotrast
    Previous radiographic studies
Uroporphyrin
    Porphyria cutanea tarda

*Also see above under "Morphologic and Chemical Definitions."

Clinical Conditions

Alpha-1-Antitrypsin Deficiency

Comments: This hereditary disorder affects secretion of alpha-1-antitrypsin (alpha-1-proteinase inhibitor) from the liver and may lead to cirrhosis, hepatocellular carcinoma,[9] and other hepatic diseases.

Morphologic features: Presence of copper and copper-associated protein is a common finding in this condition. The typical rhodanine-positive and orcein-positive granules are found in periportal hepatocytes, together with the PAS-D–positive globules of alpha-1-antitrypsin. It has been suggested that copper metabolism also is disturbed in this condition.[10] There is also an association between alpha-1-antitrypsin deficiency and neonatal cholestatic jaundice,[11] including nonsyndromatic paucity of intrahepatic bile ducts. For additional descriptions, see the Index.

Amyloidosis

Comments: Hepatomegaly without major hepatic dysfunction is the main finding. Jaundice develops only rarely.

Morphologic features: Amyloid deposition is found most commonly in periportal and perisinusoidal areas; the amount varies from lobule to lobule. For vascular involvement by amyloid, see Chapter 16. In rare instances, globular amyloid has been observed.[12] In some cases of primary (AL or amyloid light [chain]) amyloidosis, cholestasis may be a prominent finding (see Chapter 5). Positive Congo red staining with green birefringence is the most important routine diagnostic criterion for amyloid. Diagnostic procedures do not differ from those used in amyloidosis of other organs.

Anthracosis and Anthracosilicosis

Comments: Most patients were coal workers, with a history of black lung disease.[13]

Morphologic features: Anthracotic pigment and silica are found in Kupffer cells and other macrophages, but fibrosilicotic nodules are a very rare finding in the liver.[14] For diagnostic features of the pigments, see above under "Morphologic and Chemical Definitions."

Argyria

Discoloration of skin and viscera occurs after parenteral administration of silver salts. For changes in the liver, see reference 8.

Chronic Cholestasis, Any Type

For clinical conditions and morphologic findings, see Chapters 4 and 5. The cholestatic conditions that are regularly associated with copper accumulation are listed below. In most other conditions listed in Chapters 4 and 5, copper is absent or inconspicuous.

Chronic Granulomatous Disease of Childhood

Comments: This congenital familial dysphagocytosis is characterized by recurrent infections related to severely decreased bactericidal and fungicidal capacity of neutrophils.

Morphologic features: The liver also may be affected in this disease; granulomas and microabscesses may be prominent findings. A characteristic finding in this condition is the accumulation of lipofuscin in Kupffer cells and other macrophages.[2]

Chronic Nonsuppurative Destructive Cholangitis (Syndrome of Primary Biliary Cirrhosis)

Comments: Clinical and laboratory findings usually reveal chronic cholestatic liver disease. High titers of antimitochondrial antibodies are characteristic.

Morphologic features: Special stains for copper (Figure 14.1) and copper-associated protein become positive as the disease progresses. In disease stages 3 and 4, some copper pigment can be identified in most instances; copper stains are always positive if periportal bile and Mallory bodies are present.[15] If primary sclerosing cholangitis (see below) can be ruled out, a strongly positive copper stain in a specimen from an adult patient with cholestatic liver disease supports the diagnosis of chronic nonsuppurative destructive cholangitis (syndrome of primary biliary cirrhosis). See also Chapter 11.

Copper Storage Disease (Exogenous Copper Toxicosis)

Comments: In the past, exogenous copper toxicosis was observed in vineyard sprayers.[16] In recent years, copper contamination of drinking water apparently has caused severe liver disease in at least three German infants, two of whom died.[17,18]

Morphologic features: The specimens showed lobular hepatitis or cirrhosis with ballooned hepatocytes, Mallory bodies, and strongly positive rhodanine stains for copper. Hepatocanalicular cholestasis, spotty necrosis, and ductular proliferation were associated findings in most specimens. The copper was found primarily in Kupffer cells and even in fibroblasts and sometimes in extrahepatic tissues such as hepatoduodenal lymph nodes[17] and spleen.[18] Thus, the copper distribution should allow a clear distinction between exogenous copper toxicoses and cholestasis-related copper accumulation. In copper storage disease, results of quantitative copper studies varied between approximately 200 and 2000 µg/g dry weight (controls, 60 µg/g dry weight).

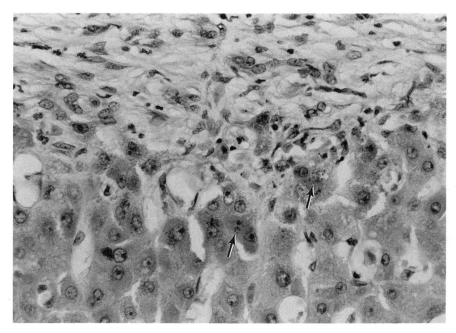

Figure 14.1
Copper granules in periportal hepatocytes in chronic nonsuppurative destructive cholangitis (syndrome of primary biliary cirrhosis). In the actual rhodanine-stained specimen, the granules (arrows) are bright red. If Shikata's orcein is used, similar granules can be stained in the same cells; they are dark brown and represent copper-associated protein.

Cystinosis

Comments: In this hereditary disorder of amino acid metabolism, L-cystine crystals accumulate in many organs and tissues, sometimes leading to renal failure in infancy. The specific enzyme deficiency or biochemical defect is unknown.

Morphologic features: Cystine crystals can be identified in Kupffer cells and portal macrophages. They are colorless, hexagonal, or rectangular as well as birefringent in polarized light.[2] Ultrastructural features of the L-cystine crystals in the liver also have been described.[19]

Drug Idiosyncrasy and Toxicity

Comments: The drug-induced hepatocellular pigment resembles lipofuscin and the Dubin-Johnson pigment (see below).[2] Therefore, the term lipochrome will be used in this instance. Accumulation of these pigments has been reported after use of acetaminophen and chlorpromazine. In other countries, lipochrome accumulation has been noted after use of aminopyrine and, in particular, after abuse of phenacetin. Phenacetin preparations are not dispensed in the United States, but reports in recent years from Italy[20] and Japan[21] have described the hepatic manifestations of the abuse of this analgesic. The drug was most popular several decades ago. Aminopyrine is hardly in use in the United States but still is administered in other countries.[22] (See also below under "Intravenous Substance Abuse.")

Morphologic features: In its mildest form, acetaminophen toxicity causes increased lipochrome deposition in centrilobular hepatocytes, inappropriate for the age of the patient.[23,24] Severe acetaminophen toxicity results in centrilobular necrosis; fulminant hepatic failure may ensue. Lipochrome accumulation also has been reported in chlorpromazine hepatitis.[2] After phenacetin abuse, the livers show prominent lipochrome deposition, which is most severe in zone 3 but may be found throughout the lobules. The pigmentation may be severe enough to render the liver slate gray or black.

Dubin-Johnson Syndrome

Comments: A hereditary chronic benign conjugated hyperbilirubinemia with characteristic histologic features is present. The pathogenesis of the hyperbilirubinemia is unknown.

Morphologic features: Typically, hepatocytes contain coarse, dark brown, iron-negative granules (Figure 14.2), primarily in zone 3 but often also involving hepatocytes in zones 2 and 1. For diagnostic features of the pigment, see above under "Morphologic and Chemical Definitions." Except for the pigmentation, liver biopsy samples in the Dubin-Johnson syndrome are normal. The intensity of the pigmentation in the Dubin-Johnson syndrome may vary considerably, both from patient to patient and over time in the same patient.[5]

Embolization of Silicone

Comments: The silicone may come from prosthetic heart valves that were implanted many years ago; current models do not contain silicone. During cardiopulmonary bypass surgery, silicone from antifoam agents may reach the liver, and patients undergoing hemodialysis may be exposed to such material from blood-pump tubing. Embolization during other surgical interventions also may be responsible.

Morphologic features: Silicone can be found in Kupffer cells and other macrophages as well as foreign body giant cells. The material is colorless and amorphous but easily identifiable by phase-contrast microscopy.[2]

Erythropoietic Protoporphyria

Comments: In this hereditary disorder of heme biosynthesis, the enzyme ferrochelatase is deficient. Cutaneous photosensitivity is the main clinical manifestation, but cirrhosis and liver failure may occur. In one such instance, liver

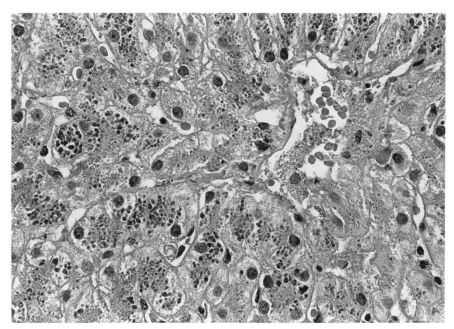

Figure 14.2
Dubin-Johnson pigment in a patient with the Dubin-Johnson syndrome. This dark coarse lipochrome-type hepatocellular pigment is most prominent in centrilobular (zone 3) hepatocytes but may involve the entire lobule.

transplantation has proved helpful.[25] To date, no clear indicators are known that would identify the patients who are at risk to develop liver disease.[26] Alcoholism appears to be one risk factor.[27]

Morphologic features: The main histologic feature is the presence of protoporphyrin, which accumulates as a reddish-brown pigment in hepatocytes, bile canaliculi, Kupffer cells, and cholangioles. Typically, the canaliculi contain brown concrements, with or without fracture lines. As stated, fibrosis and cirrhosis may be associated findings. See also Chapter 11.

Gilbert's Syndrome

Comments: A hereditary chronic benign unconjugated hyperbilirubinemia of unknown pathogenesis is present but with evidence of reduced uridine diphosphate glucuronyl transferase activity and reduced uptake of unconjugated bilirubin.

Morphologic features: Liver biopsy samples generally show normal histologic features, but increased lipofuscin deposition has been reported.[28]

Hepatic Atrophy

Comments: Loss of hepatic tissue in old age, starvation, wasting diseases, and related conditions usually has no appreciable hepatic manifestations.[29]

Morphologic features: The livers show increased lipofuscin granules in hepatocytes, primarily in zone 3 (Figure 14.3). Macroscopically, this change may render the parenchyma dark brown ("brown atrophy").

Hepatocellular Necrosis, All Types

Comments: For causes, types, and clinical manifestations, see Chapters 3 and 9.

Morphologic features: After hepatocellular necrosis, ceroid pigment can be identified in many macrophages. In specimens stained with hematoxylin-eosin, the pigment is pale brown and granular; the macrophages often are difficult to distinguish from hepatocytes. However, after staining with PAS-D, the bright-red pigment stands out clearly. This is an important finding, because it is characteristic for recent or partially resolved liver damage, usually in the context of lobular hepatitis. Normal livers do not contain stainable ceroid pigment. In rare instances, areas of hepatocellular necrosis may be the site of dystrophic or metastatic calcification.

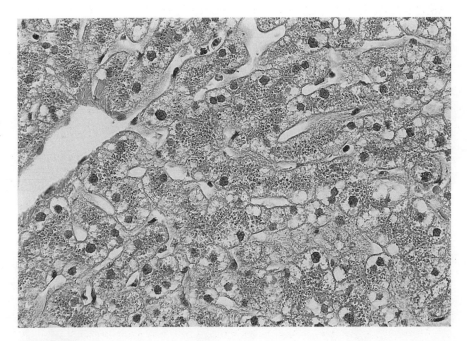

Figure 14.3
Age-related lipofuscin accumulation in zone 3 hepatocytes.

Hypercalcemia

See Chapter 16 under "Hyperparathyroidism." In rare instances, areas of hepatocellular necrosis may be the site of dystrophic or metastatic calcification.

Idiopathic Adulthood Ductopenia

See Chapter 15. As in other chronic cholestatic liver diseases, copper accumulation is a characteristic feature.

Idiopathic Copper Toxicosis

See above under "Copper Storage Disease" and below under "Indian Childhood Cirrhosis."

Indian Childhood Cirrhosis

Comments: This condition has been discussed in Chapter 11. The cause of Indian childhood cirrhosis still is obscure, but it might represent an exogenous copper toxicosis—for instance, after ingestion of copper-contaminated milk.[30] In early cases, penicillamine appears to be helpful.[31] Conditions with features of Indian childhood cirrhosis have been observed in Italy,[32] Germany (see above under "Copper Storage Disease"), and the United States.[33]

Morphologic features: Pericellular fibrosis, ballooning of hepatocytes with Mallory bodies, infiltrates of neutrophils, and spotty necroses are typical findings (see Chapter 11). Stains for copper and copper-associated protein are positive in all instances. Ductular proliferation and cholestasis are uncommon findings.

Intravenous Substance Abuse

Comments: An appropriate history may not have been volunteered, and therefore the histologic findings may provide an important clinical clue. A large array of more or less inert substances is used by dealers to dilute the active ingredients, and thus these fillers also enter the circulation. Many patients with the findings described here also have unresolved or chronic viral hepatitis.

Morphologic features: Cellulose crystals, starch granules, talc, and many other substances may be found in the liver, primarily in macrophages. Presence of foreign body giant cells or other unusual inflammatory changes in portal tracts may provide a clue. Study of specimens with polarized light is most helpful. See also under "Morphologic and Chemical Definitions."

Malaria

Comments: In malaria and the tropical splenomegaly syndrome, the liver is almost always involved but usually without appreciable clinical symptoms. In acute *Plasmodium falciparum* malaria, hepatomegaly is a common finding.

Morphologic features: In acute malaria, a characteristic finding is the sludging of erythrocytes in sinusoids.[34] Eventually, malaria pigment appears in all Kupffer cells. The pigment, hemozoin, has been described above under "Morphologic and Chemical Definitions." In the acute attack, Kupffer cells throughout the lobules contain pigment, but as the patients become increasingly immune, pigment is found primarily in periportal Kupffer cells and, eventually, in portal tracts only. In acute cases, some hemosiderin and centrilobular necrosis may be noted. Portal hepatitis and fibrosis also may be present.

Malignant Melanoma

Comments: Metastatic malignant melanoma in the liver can be found in any patient with widespread disease. However, a characteristic association exists between ocular melanoma and metastases from these tumors to the liver. The interval between enucleation of the eye and the development of hepatic metastases is approximately 4 to 5 years. Recent advances in hepatic arterial chemoembolization may have improved the prognosis somewhat.[35]

Morphologic features: Presence of metastatic melanotic malignant melanoma is the only situation in which melanin can be demonstrated in the liver. Histologic features and staining characteristics do not differ from malignant melanoma at other sites. The Fontana-Masson silver stain for argentaffin material can be used in the diagnosis of melanomas; the stain also is positive with carcinoid tumors and pheochromocytomas.

Old Hemorrhages and Infarcts

Comments: Intrahepatic hemorrhages associated with trauma, tumor, or other conditions are not always noted or evacuated while they are fresh. Biopsy material or surgical material from such lesions or from old infarcts sometimes is submitted to solve the diagnostic problem.

Morphologic features: Sections may show blood, granulation tissue, hemosiderin deposits (see Chapter 13), scar tissue, and iron-free pigment that is Fouchet-positive. This pigment is hematoidin (also see above under "Morphologic and Chemical Definitions").

Paucity of Intrahepatic Bile Ducts and Other Types of Infantile Obstructive Cholangiopathy

See Chapter 15. As in other chronic cholestatic liver diseases, copper accumulation is a characteristic feature.

Porphyria Cutanea Tarda

Comments: Photosensitivity is the main clinical feature of this disturbance of porphyrin metabolism. The condition is probably an acquired but genetically determined idiosyncrasy. Chronic liver disease with cirrhosis may develop. For further details, see Chapters 11 and 13.

Morphologic features: The characteristic needle-shaped inclusions in the hepatocytes consist of uroporphyrin[36] and appear to be specific for this condition. Staining of the inclusions is possible with the ferric ferricyanide reduction reaction.[37]

Povidone Administration

Comments: A history of parenteral drug administrations may bring this substance into diagnostic consideration. See also above under "Morphologic and Chemical Definitions."

Morphologic features: The material can be found in Kupffer cells. It is blue-gray, has a foamy appearance, and is stainable with Congo red.[2] It is not birefringent.

Previous Radiographic Studies

Comments: If barium sulfate is found in the liver, a history of gastrointestinal radiographic studies provides an explanation. If thorotrast is found in the liver, the contrast medium probably was administered between 1930 and 1953.

Morphologic features: Barium sulfate in the liver can be found in macrophages or granulomas. Barium sulfate embolization via the portal vein can lead to pylephlebitic abscesses and portal thrombosis.[2] For microscopic features of barium sulfate, see above under "Morphologic and Chemical Definitions." Thorotrast can be found in normal livers but more often it is seen in scar tissue, usually associated with cirrhosis, and in hepatocellular carcinoma,[38] cholangiocarcinoma,[39] and hemangiosarcoma.[40] Veno-occlusive disease and peliosis hepatis (see Chapter 16) also have been observed after thorotrast administration.[41] For the diagnostic features of thorotrast, see above under "Morphologic and Chemical Definitions."

Previous Surgery

Comments: During laparotomies, the liver surface may be exposed to talc and starch particles from surgical gloves.

Morphologic features: Biopsy specimens from the liver surface may show the particles in areas of inflammation and fibrosis. For further details, see above under "Morphologic and Chemical Definitions."

Primary Sclerosing Cholangitis

Comments: Clinical and laboratory findings usually reveal chronic cholestatic liver disease. Typical cholangiographic findings confirm the diagnosis. Most patients have chronic ulcerative colitis (see also Chapter 4).

Morphologic features: Special stains for copper and copper-associated protein become positive as the disease progresses. In disease stages 3 and 4, some copper pigment can be identified in most instances.[42] If chronic nonsuppurative destructive cholangitis can be ruled out, a strongly positive copper stain in a specimen from an adult patient with cholestatic liver disease supports the diagnosis of primary sclerosing cholangitis.

Schistosomiasis

Comments: The liver is the main target organ for *Schistosoma mansoni,* *Schistosoma mekongi,* and *Schistosoma japonicum.*

Morphologic features: Infected liver tissue shows portal granulomas with or without ova, portal phlebosclerosis, hepatic fibrosis, and deposition of a dark brown pigment in Kupffer cells and in portal and septal macrophages. With light microscopic methods, this pigment cannot be distinguished from malaria pigment (see also above under "Malaria").

Silicosis and Anthracosilicosis

Comments: A history of exposure to silica dusts can be obtained. Silicosis often is associated with anthracosis—for instance, in coal miners.

Morphologic features: See above under "Anthracosis and Anthracosilicosis."

Total Parenteral Nutrition

Comments: Patients often have been subjected to extensive intestinal resection and may be malnourished (see also above under "Hepatic Atrophy"). For chronic liver disease caused by total parenteral nutrition, see also Chapters 4 and 7.

Morphologic features: Steatohepatitis and cholestatic hepatitis with or without fibrosis may be present. In most cases, abnormal specimens contain much ceroid in macrophages, and in some instances, heavy periportal hepatocellular copper deposition may be encountered.[43] Hemosiderosis of Kupffer cells and hepatocytes also may be encountered. Finally, the lipofuscin content may be increased. After intravenous infusion of lipid emulsion in patients not receiving total parenteral nutrition, lipofuscin also has been found in Kupffer cells and macrophages.[44]

Unresolved Viral Hepatitis and Other Types of Lobular Hepatitis

Comments: For a definition of resolving or unresolved viral hepatitis and other types of lobular hepatitis, see Chapter 3.

Morphologic features: Specimens show lobular hepatitis as described for acute and unresolved viral hepatitis (Chapter 3). One important feature is the presence of ceroid-laden macrophages, which are strongly PAS-D positive. After resolution of the inflammatory process, this may be the only evidence of the previous disease.

Tumors and Pseudotumors

Copper can accumulate in hepatocellular carcinomas,[45] including fibrolamellar carcinomas,[46] as well as in focal nodular hyperplasia[47] and nodular transformation of the liver.[48] In rare instances, tumors may show dystrophic calcification.[49]

Wilson's Disease

The histologic changes of this hereditary disorder of copper metabolism have been described in Chapter 2. In the cirrhotic stage of this disease, presence of high copper levels may be the only feature with which Wilson's disease can be distinguished from posthepatitic cirrhosis. For methods of demonstrating copper, see above under "Morphologic and Chemical Definitions."

References

1. Ishak KG: Applications of scanning electron microscopy in the study of liver diseases. *Prog Liver Dis* 8:1-32, 1986.

2. Ishak KG: New developments in diagnostic liver pathology. In Farber E, Phillips MN, Kaufman N (eds): *Pathogenesis of Liver Diseases*. Baltimore, Williams & Wilkins, 1987, pp 223-273.

3. Varma RR, Sarna T: Hepatic pigments in Dubin-Johnson syndrome and mutant Corriedale sheep are not melanin. *Gastroenterology* 84:1401(A), 1983.

4. Wolkoff AW: Inheritable disorders manifested by conjugated hyperbilirubinemia. *Semin Liver Dis* 3:65-72, 1983.

5. Barone P, Inferrera C, Carrozza G: Pigments in the Dubin-Johnson syndrome. In Wolman M (ed): *Pigments in Pathology*. New York, Academy Press, 1969, pp 307-325.

6. Baba N, Ruppert RD: The Dubin-Johnson syndrome: Electron microscopic observation of hepatic pigment—a case study. *Am J Clin Pathol* 57:306-310, 1972.

7. Moore G, Homewood CA, Gilles HM: A comparison of pigment from *S. mansoni* and *P. berghei*. *Ann Trop Med Parasitol* 69:373-374, 1975.

8. Leodolter I, Stockinger L: Zur Lokalisation der Silbereinlagerungen bei Argyrose: Analyse von Leberpunktaten mit dem Electronenmikroskop. *Acta Hepato-Gastroenterol* 19:81-85, 1972.

9. Eriksson S, Carlson J, Valez R: Risk of cirrhosis and primary liver cancer in alpha$_1$-antitrypsin deficiency. *N Engl J Med* 314:736-739, 1986.

10. Callea F, Ray MB, Desmet VJ: Alpha-1-antitrypsin and copper in the liver. *Histopathology* 5:415-424, 1981.

11. Ghishan FZ, Greene HL: Liver disease in children with PiZZ α_1-antitrypsin deficiency. *Hepatology* 8:307-310, 1988.

12. Kanel GC, Uchida T, Peters RL: Globular hepatic amyloid—an unusual morphologic presentation. *Hepatology* 1:647-652, 1981.

13. Le Fevre MF, Green FHY, Joel DD, et al: Frequency of black pigment in livers and spleens of coal workers. *Hum Pathol* 13:1121-1126, 1982.

14. Slavin RE, Swedo JL, Brandes D, et al: Extrapulmonary silicosis: A clinical, morphologic, and ultrastructural study. *Hum Pathol* 16:393-412, 1985.

15. Ludwig J, McDonald GSA, Dickson ER, et al: Copper stains and the syndrome of primary biliary cirrhosis: Evaluation of staining methods and their usefulness for diagnosis and trials of penicillamine treatment. *Arch Pathol Lab Med* 103:467-470, 1979.

16. Pimentel JC, Menezes AP: Liver disease in vineyard sprayers. *Gastroenterology* 72:275-283, 1977.

17. Müller-Höcker J, Weiß M, Meyer U, et al: Fatal copper storage disease of the liver in a German infant resembling Indian childhood cirrhosis. *Virchows Arch [A]* 411:379-385, 1987.

18. Müller-Höcker J, Meyer U, Wiebecke B, et al: Copper storage disease of the liver and chronic dietary copper intoxication in two further German infants mimicking Indian childhood cirrhosis. *Pathol Res Pract* 183:39-45, 1988.

19. Scotto JM, Stralin HG: Ultrastructure of the liver in a case of childhood cystinosis. *Virchows Arch [A]* 377:43-48, 1977.

20. Faravelli A, Taccagni GL, Ferrari A: Lipofuscinosi epatocitaria da abuso di fenacetina. *Pathologica* 75:735-738, 1983.

21. Nagasaki Y, Kawasaki Y, Nishi S, et al: A case of black liver induced by phenacetin abuse [in Japanese]. *Nippon Shokakibyo Gakkai Zasshi* 78:932-936, 1981.

22. Gayotto LCC, Waitzberg VR, Almeida AV, et al: Long-term intake of aminopyrine leading to deposition of an orcein-positive lipofuscin in liver cells. *Hepatol Rapid Lit Rev* 14:9-10, 1984.

23. Portmann B, Talbot IC, Day DW, et al: Histopathological changes in the liver following a paracetamol overdose: Correlation with clinical and biochemical parameters. *J Pathol* 117:169-181, 1975.

24. James O, Lesna M, Roberts SH, et al: Liver damage after paracetamol overdose: Comparison of liver-function tests, fasting serum bile acids, and liver histology. *Lancet* 2:579-581, 1975.

25. Bloomer JR, Weimer MK, Bossenmaier IC, et al: Liver transplantation in a patient with protoporphyria. *Gastroenterology* 97:188-194, 1989.

26. Bloomer JR: The liver in protoporphyria. *Hepatology* 8:402-407, 1988.

27. Bonkovsky HL, Schned AR: Fatal liver failure in protoporphyria: Synergism between alcohol excess and the genetic defect. *Gastroenterology* 90:191-201, 1986.

28. Barth RF, Grimley PM, Berk PD, et al: Excess lipofuscin accumulation in constitutional hepatic dysfunction (Gilbert's syndrome). *Arch Pathol* 91:41-47, 1971.

29. Kintani K: Aging and the liver. *Prog Liver Dis* 9:603-623, 1990.

30. Tanner MS, Kantarjian AH, Bhave SA, et al: Early introduction of copper-contaminated animal milk feeds as a possible cause of Indian childhood cirrhosis. *Lancet* 2:992-995, 1983.

31. Tanner MS, Bhave SA, Pradhan AM, et al: Clinical trials of penicillamine in Indian childhood cirrhosis. *Arch Dis Child* 62:1118-1124, 1987.

32. Maggiore G, De Giacomo C, Sessa F, et al: Idiopathic hepatic copper toxicosis in a child. *J Pediatr Gastroenterol Nutr* 6:980-983, 1987.

33. Lefkowitch JH, Honig CL, King ME, et al: Hepatic copper overload and features of Indian childhood cirrhosis in an American sibship. *N Engl J Med* 307:271-277, 1982.

34. De Brito T, Barone AA, Faria RM: Human liver biopsy in *P. falciparum* and *P. vivax* malaria: A light and electron microscopic study. *Virchows Arch [A]* 348:220-229, 1969.

35. Mavligit GM, Charnsangavej C, Carrasco H, et al: Regression of ocular melanoma metastatic to the liver after hepatic arterial chemoembolization with cisplatin and polyvinyl sponge. *JAMA* 260:974-976, 1988.

36. Cortes JM, Oliva H, Paradinas FJ, et al: The pathology of the liver in porphyria cutanea tarda. *Histopathology* 4:471-485, 1980.

37. Fakan F, Chlumska A: Demonstration of needle-shaped hepatic inclusions in porphyria cutanea tarda using the ferric ferricyanide reduction test. *Virchows Arch [A]* 411:365-369, 1987.

38. Morgan AD, Jayne WHW, Marrack D: Primary liver cell carcinoma 24 years after intravenous injection of thorotrast. *J Clin Pathol* 11:7-18, 1958.

39. Rubel LR, Ishak KG: Thorotrast-associated cholangiocarcinoma: An epidemiologic and clinicopathologic study. *Cancer* 50:1408-1415, 1982.

40. Kojiro M, Nakashima T, Ito Y, et al: Thorium dioxide-related angiosarcoma of the liver: Pathomorphologic study of 29 autopsy cases. *Arch Pathol Lab Med* 109:853-857, 1985.

41. Dejgaard A, Krogsgaard K, Jabson N: Veno-occlusive disease and peliosis of the liver after thorotrast administration. *Virchows Arch [A]* 403:87-94, 1984.

42. Ludwig J, LaRusso NF, Wiesner RH: The syndrome of primary sclerosing cholangitis. *Prog Liver Dis* 9:555-566, 1990.

43. Bowyer BA, Fleming CR, Ludwig J, et al: Does long-term home parenteral nutrition in adult patients cause chronic liver disease? *JPEN* 9:11-17, 1985.

44. Passwell JH, David R, Katznelson R, et al: Pigment deposition in the reticuloendothelial system after fat emulsion. *Arch Dis Child* 51:366-368, 1976.

45. Haratake J, Horie A, Nakashima A, et al: Minute hepatoma with excessive copper accumulation: Report of two cases with resection. *Arch Pathol Lab Med* 110:192-194, 1986.

46. Teitelbaum DH, Tuttle S, Carey LC, et al: Fibrolamellar carcinoma of the liver: Review of three cases and presentation of a characteristic set of tumor markers defining this tumor. *Ann Surg* 202:36-41, 1985.

47. Vila MM, Haot J, Desmet VJ: Cholestatic features in focal nodular hyperplasia of the liver. *Liver* 4:387-395, 1984.

48. Stromeyer FW, Ishak KG: Nodular transformation (nodular "regenerative" hyperplasia) of the liver: A clinicopathologic study of 30 cases. *Hum Pathol* 12:60-71, 1981.

49. Meonandar IM: Extensive calcification in the stroma of a primary hepatic carcinoma. *J Pathol* 114:53-54, 1974.

Chapter 15

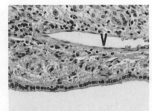

Abnormal Bile Ducts, Including Loss of Bile Ducts

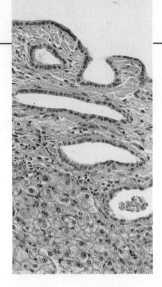

Morphologic Definition

Abnormalities of the biliary system at the biopsy level encompass (1) proliferation of ducts and ductules, including dilatation and formation of microcysts; (2) inflammation of ducts and ductules; and (3) postinflammatory states, degeneration, and loss of bile ducts. Proliferation and inflammation may affect both ducts and ductules (cholangioles). Whereas loss of bile ducts is an important feature, loss of ductules has not been documented; it probably occurs in inflammatory conditions but is hard to confirm and probably is of little consequence.

Proliferation of Bile Ducts (Ductal Proliferation)

This finding is characterized by the presence of an increased number of sections through bile ducts in portal tracts, mostly related to increased tortuosity of ducts. The proliferated ducts have the features of interlobular bile ducts or septal bile ducts, that is, they have the approximate size of the accompanying hepatic artery branches and they have a lumen and a basement membrane. Proliferated bile ducts usually are found near hepatic arteries and portal vein branches.

Proliferation of Bile Ductules (Ductular Proliferation, Cholangiolar Proliferation)

These structures arise from hepatic cell plates, ductules (cholangioles), or putative stem cells (ductular hepatocytes). The proliferated ductules are found most commonly in areas of periportal inflammation and necrosis; they often lack a clearly identifiable lumen and basement membrane.

Cholangiectases and Biliary Cysts

Cholangiectases usually are postinflammatory states (see below), and most cysts are hamartomatous lesions. Dilatation of bile ducts can be diagnosed if the diameters of the ducts appreciably exceed the diameters of the accompanying hepatic artery branches.

Inflammation of Ducts and Ductules (Cholangitis and Cholangiolitis)

If ducts or ductules are infiltrated by neutrophils, use of the terms *neutrophilic cholangitis* and *cholangiolitis* is appropriate; the terms *acute cholangitis* and *acute cholangiolitis* often are used for these conditions. However, lesions such as neutrophilic cholangiolitis also may be found in chronic diseases such as the syndrome of primary biliary cirrhosis. *Lymphoid cholangitis* (lymphocytic cholangitis) is characterized by lymphocytic aggregates or follicles, with or without germinal centers, in contact with the duct or surrounding the duct. Damage of the ductal epithelium may be present. If the inflammatory infiltrates consist of several types of inflammatory cells, such as lymphocytes, histiocytes, plasma cells, neutrophils, and eosinophils, the terms *mixed-cell* or *pleomorphic cholangitis* can be used. *Fibrous cholangitis* is characterized by the presence of a fibrous collar and interspersed inflammatory cells around the duct ("onion skin lesions"). If this condition is associated with degeneration and necrosis of the ductal epithelium or incomplete loss of the lumen, use of the term *fibrous-obliterative cholangitis* is recommended. Presence of a noncaseating epithelioid cell granuloma attached to a duct or replacing part of the duct represents *granulomatous cholangitis*. This type of cholangitis is best known under the name "florid duct lesion." *Nonsuppurative cholangitis* is the collective name for lymphoid, mixed-cell, fibrous, and granulomatous cholangitis. The name *chronic nonsuppurative destructive cholangitis* is currently used as a synonym for the syndrome of primary biliary cirrhosis.

Postinflammatory States, Degeneration, and Loss of Bile Ducts

These findings usually are features of advanced destructive cholangitis. Typical postinflammatory states without inflammation include some cases of cholangiectasis and periductal fibrosis. Degeneration of ducts involves primarily the epithelium; no specific names for such changes are available. Epithelial degenerative changes may accompany destructive suppurative or nonsuppurative cholangitis, but they also appear to occur in noncholangitic conditions such as ischemia, toxemia, or the vicinity of tumors. *Loss of bile ducts* is best described by the name *ductopenia*,[1] which is shorter than the older synonym, "paucity of intrahepatic bile ducts."[2] This condition can be diagnosed if the majority of portal tracts in a specimen appears to lack a bile duct. Ideally, 20 portal tracts should be reviewed and 10 of them should have no bile duct. However, ductopenia sometimes can be strongly suspected after study of only two or three portal tracts. Duct counts should be based on artery counts; 70% to 80% of all interlobular arteries should be accompanied by a bile duct.[3] It is important to note that ductules should not be counted because loss of bile ducts often is associated with proliferation of ductules. A helpful distinguishing feature is the location of the ducts. Interlobular and septal bile ducts tend to run with a hepatic artery branch, whereas ductules are found in the vicinity of the limiting plate.

Table 15.1   Clinical Conditions Associated With Abnormal Bile Ducts, Including Loss of Bile Ducts

---

Duct Proliferation and Cysts
Cholangiectases and Biliary Cysts or Microcysts
    Biliary cystadenoma, cystadenocarcinoma, and cholangiocarcinoma
    Biliary microhamartomas and other fibropolycystic liver diseases; bile duct adenomas
    Cystic fibrosis (mucoviscidosis of the liver)
    Obstruction of large (extrahepatic and perihilar intrahepatic) bile ducts
    Primary sclerosing cholangitis
    Solitary hepatic cysts
Proliferation of Bile Ducts (Ductal Proliferation)
    Chronic active hepatitis and other types of periportal hepatitis (see also Chapter 2)
    Drug-induced hepatitis (see below under "Drug-Induced and Toxic Hepatitis")
    Obstruction of large (extrahepatic and perihilar intrahepatic) bile ducts
    Primary sclerosing cholangitis
Proliferation of Bile Ductules (Ductular Proliferation)
    This is a nonspecific finding in both obstructive biliary diseases and inflammatory liver diseases, particularly in conditions associated with periportal hepatitis. Note: Ductal proliferation (see above) is an important diagnostic finding, whereas ductular (cholangiolar) proliferation only indicates damage to the limiting plate or to other parts of the hepatic parenchyma.

continued on page 206

continued from page 205
Cholangitis
Fibrous Cholangitis
  Chronic or healing stage of nonsuppurative cholangitis
  Graft-versus-host disease
  Obstruction of large (extrahepatic or perihilar intrahepatic) bile ducts
  Primary sclerosing cholangitis
  Schistosomiasis
Granulomatous Cholangitis (Florid Duct Lesions)
  Chronic intrahepatic cholestasis of sarcoidosis
  Hepatolithiasis (?) (see below under "Biliary Cystadenoma, Cystadenocarcinoma, and
    Cholangiocarcinoma")
  Syndrome of primary biliary cirrhosis
  Toxic oil syndrome (?)
Lymphoid and Mixed-Cell Cholangitis
  Drug-induced hepatitis (see below under "Drug-Induced and Toxic Hepatitis")
  Graft-versus-host disease
  Hepatic allograft rejection
  Primary sclerosing cholangitis
  Syndrome of primary biliary cirrhosis
  Systemic bacterial and viral infections (see below under "Systemic Bacterial Infections,
    Including the Toxic Shock Syndrome, and Systemic Viral Diseases")
  Toxic oil syndrome
  Viral hepatitis and idiopathic (autoimmune) chronic active hepatitis
Neutrophilic Cholangitis (Acute Cholangitis)
  Alcoholic hepatitis
  Drug-induced (sulindac) and toxic (paraquat) hepatitis (see below under "Drug-Induced and
    Toxic Hepatitis")
  Heat stroke
  Hepatic allograft rejection (?)
  Infective intra-abdominal conditions
  Mucocutaneous lymph node syndrome
  Obstruction of large (extrahepatic and perihilar intrahepatic) bile ducts
  Primary sclerosing cholangitis
  Recurrent pyogenic cholangitis
  Toxic shock syndrome and sepsis (see below under "Systemic Bacterial Infections,
    Including the Toxic Shock Syndrome, and Systemic Viral Diseases")
  Tumor-associated change
Neutrophilic Cholangiolitis (Acute Cholangiolitis)
  This is a nonspecific finding related to ductular proliferation (see above under "Proliferation
    of Bile Ductules"). Despite the abundance of neutrophils, this type of cholangiolitis often is
    not associated with an infectious process; ductular proliferation per se may be a
    leukotactic process.

continued on page 207

continued from page 206
Degeneration and Loss of Ducts
Degenerative Changes and Atypia of Ductal and Ductular Epithelium
    Hepatic allograft rejection
    Systemic bacterial infections (see below under "Systemic Bacterial Infections, Including the
      Toxic Shock Syndrome, and Systemic Viral Diseases")
    Tumor-associated changes
Loss of Bile Ducts (Ductopenia)
    Chronic active hepatitis (see below under "Viral Hepatitis and Idiopathic [Autoimmune]
      Chronic Active Hepatitis")
    Chronic intrahepatic cholestasis of sarcoidosis
    Drug-induced hepatitis (see below under "Drug-Induced and Toxic Hepatitis")
    Graft-versus-host disease
    Hepatic allograft rejection
    Idiopathic adulthood ductopenia
    Lymphoproliferative disorders
    Paucity of intrahepatic bile ducts (infantile obstructive cholangiopathy)
    Primary sclerosing cholangitis
    Syndrome of primary biliary cirrhosis
    Systemic viral infections (see below under "Systemic Bacterial Infections, Including the
      Toxic Shock Syndrome, and Systemic Viral Diseases")

Clinical Conditions

Alcoholic Hepatitis

Neutrophilic cholangitis occurred in a few patients with severe cholestasis associated with alcoholic hepatitis.[4]

Biliary Cystadenoma, Cystadenocarcinoma, and Cholangiocarcinoma

Comments: Biliary cystadenomas (hepatobiliary cystadenoma; intrahepatic bile duct cystadenoma) is a benign tumor of women; it has a high incidence of recurrence and malignant transformation.[5] The tumor also can arise from extrahepatic bile ducts, its official name—intrahepatic bile duct cystadenoma—notwithstanding.[6] Therefore, the term hepatobiliary cystadenoma also is in use. Biliary cystadenocarcinoma (bile duct cystadenocarcinoma) is a malignant cystic intrahepatic tumor of bile duct epithelium. The tumor may arise from biliary cystadenomas[5] but also from other lesions such as congenital cysts.[7] Cholangiocarcinoma (adenocarcinoma; cholangiocellular carcinoma; intrahepatic bile duct carcinoma) is the most common tumor of bile duct epithelium. It may occur combined with hepatocellular carcinomas, possibly from a common stem cell,[8] arise de novo, or develop in preexisting lesions such as primary sclerosing cholangitis and fibropolycystic liver disease.[9]

Morphologic features: Cystadenomas may resemble cystically dilated and proliferated bile ducts, but they usually form large, multiloculated cysts and mucinous tumors. The cysts are lined by columnar epithelia, which may be papillary, and they are surrounded by a mesenchymal cell layer, sometimes with features of ovarian stroma. The outer layer consists of connective tissue. Malignant transformation of the epithelial layer leads to cystadenocarcinoma. Malignant transformation of the mesenchymal layer also has been reported.[5] The neoplastic nature of fully developed cystadenocarcinomas is readily apparent, but for the recognition of early changes extensive sampling may be necessary. Cholangiocarcinomas may be confused with ductular proliferation (see also above under "Morphologic Definitions"); they also may cause diagnostic problems if they occur in preexisting lesions such as primary sclerosing cholangitis[10] and hepatolithiasis. The latter condition reportedly has been associated with both a granulomatous cholangitis and cholangiocarcinoma.[11]

Biliary Microhamartomas and Other Fibropolycystic Liver Diseases; Bile Duct Adenomas

Comments: Biliary microhamartomas (biliary hamartoma, cholangioma, von Meyenburg complex) usually are multiple; they are minute nodular hepatic lesions that are of no clinical significance unless they are confused with adenocarcinoma. These lesions belong to a group of hamartomatous liver diseases, collectively named fibropolycystic liver disease(s). In addition to the microhamartomas, the group comprises congenital hepatic fibrosis, cystic disease of the liver (two types; see below), and focal dilatation of intrahepatic bile ducts (Caroli's disease). Because fibropolycystic liver disease may be associated with extrahepatic biliary lesions such as choledochal cysts or multiple diverticula of the common bile duct, the term "fibropolycystic disease of the liver and biliary tract" has been coined.[12] The extrahepatobiliary lesions—in particular, polycystic renal disease—shall not be reviewed here. Most fibropolycystic diseases of the liver may be complicated by the development of cholangiocarcinoma (see previous entry). Bile duct adenomas are distinct from biliary microhamartomas,[13] but they also are asymptomatic nodules, albeit larger and single, which usually are discovered accidentally during abdominal surgery and which can be confused with adenocarcinoma.[14]

Morphologic features: Biliary microhamartomas rarely exceed 3 mm in diameter. They consist of small ducts or biliary microcysts, lined by cuboidal cells and set in a fibrous stroma (Figures 15.1A and 15.1B). Typically, these lesions are nodular and situated close to portal tracts. However, microhamartomas are not always distinct lesions but may consist merely of a group of microcystic ducts at the edge of a portal tract (forme fruste lesions). The presence of multiple biliary microhamartomas cannot be clearly distinguished from congenital hepatic fibrosis

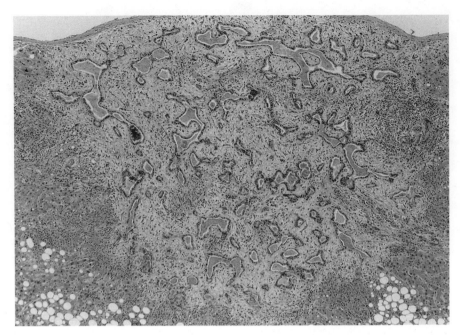

Figure 15.1A
Biliary microhamartomas. Note serpiginous microcystic ducts with secretions, embedded in abundant fibrous stroma. The subcapsular position of this lesion would be typical for a bile duct adenoma, but the appearance of the serpiginous microcystic glands is typical for a microhamartoma.

(see Figure 10.2). In this condition, fibrous septa with biliary ducts and microcysts may be so prominent that the liver appears cirrhotic. This impression may be reinforced clinically because some patients suffer from portal hypertension. However, the liver in congenital hepatic fibrosis is not cirrhotic because it lacks nodular regeneration; the portal hypertension probably is related to compression and possibly hypoplasia of portal veins, a common finding in congenital hepatic fibrosis. The dilated ducts in this condition may contain inspissated bile. Congenital hepatic fibrosis also may present as a localized lesion,[15] or it may occur together with idiopathic dilatation of intrahepatic bile ducts (see next paragraph). Histologically, congenital hepatic fibrosis cannot be clearly distinguished from autosomal-recessive cystic disease of the liver (infantile polycystic liver disease). If the microcystic ductal proliferations are widespread and permeate the lobules and if the fibrous component is rather inconspicuous, infantile polycystic liver disease probably is present.

In addition to the overlap with infantile polycystic liver disease, the features of congenital hepatic fibrosis also may merge with those of idiopathic dilatation of intrahepatic bile ducts (Caroli's disease).[16] Evidence of ascending infection with neutrophilic cholangitis is the main indicator of such an association (Figure 15.2).

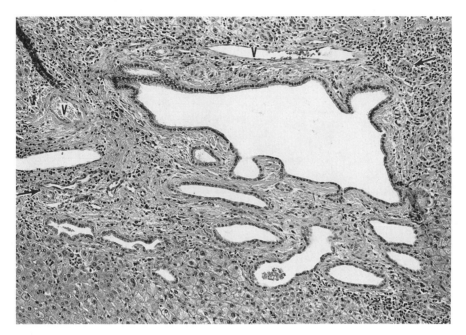

Figure 15.1B
Biliary microhamartoma adjacent to a portal tract (on left side of frame and top right) with portal vein (V), bile ducts, and arteries (arrows).

A patient can have congenital hepatic fibrosis in one lobe and Caroli's disease in another. The extent of the bile duct dilatations in Caroli's disease cannot be appreciated in biopsy specimens, but the disease should be considered if neutrophilic cholangitis, cholangitic abscesses, and related complications are found. Hepatolithiasis may occur in Caroli's disease. Adenocarcinoma may arise from any of the aforementioned conditions.[9,17] Single hepatic cysts or cysts in autosomal-dominant cystic disease of the liver (adult polycystic liver disease) do not differ appreciably from cysts in other organs. Biliary microhamartomas may coexist with autosomal-dominant polycystic liver disease.

Cholangiocarcinoma

See above under "Biliary Cystadenoma, Cystadenocarcinoma, and Cholangio-carcinoma."

Chronic Active Hepatitis and Other Types of Periportal Hepatitis

See below under "Viral Hepatitis and Idiopathic (Autoimmune) Chronic Active Hepatitis."

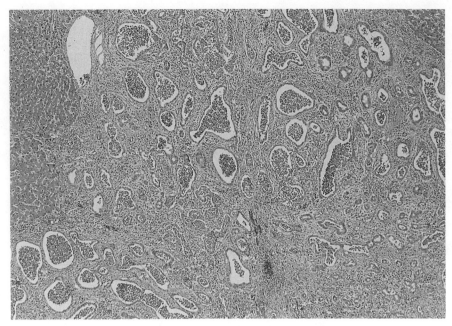

Figure 15.2
Caroli's disease (idiopathic dilatation of intrahepatic bile ducts). In this low-power illustration, multiple cystically dilated bile ducts are stuffed with neutrophils. Abscesses cannot be appreciated in this specimen.

Chronic Intrahepatic Cholestasis of Sarcoidosis

Comments: This is a rare chronic liver disease associated with sarcoidosis that resembles the syndrome of primary biliary cirrhosis.[18] Typically, patients show biochemical evidence of cholestasis, together with clinical and laboratory features of sarcoidosis such as a positive Kveim-Siltzbach test, elevated levels of serum angiotensin-converting enzyme, and increased lysozyme activities. Tests for antimitochondrial antibodies are negative. However, sarcoidosis and the syndrome of primary biliary cirrhosis may coexist, and in these instances antimitochondrial antibodies will be present.

Morphologic features: Specimens show typical noncaseating sarcoid-type epithelioid cell granulomas, but in contradistinction to the "usual" cases of hepatic sarcoidosis, granulomas are attached to or surround interlobular and septal bile ducts, which they destroy (see Figures 8.3A and 8.3B). This type of granulomatous cholangitis is indistinguishable from some florid duct lesions seen in the syndrome of primary biliary cirrhosis. Biliary fibrosis and cirrhosis may be found, usually together with prominent ductopenia.[19] Cholestasis rarely is a prominent morphologic feature. Thus, a clear distinction between chronic intrahepatic cholestasis of sarcoidosis and the syndrome of primary biliary cirrhosis cannot always be made.

Chronic or Healing Stage of Nonsuppurative Cholangitis

In the syndrome of primary biliary cirrhosis but also in most other types of nonsuppurative cholangitis described in this chapter, fibrous cholangitis or periductal fibrosis may be found, representing chronic or healing stages—for instance, of lymphocytic cholangitis in chronic active hepatitis or the syndrome of primary biliary cirrhosis.[20]

Cystic Fibrosis (Mucoviscidosis) of the Liver

Comments: Cystic fibrosis (mucoviscidosis) is a hereditary, autosomal-recessive disorder that affects multiple organs and tissues, including the liver and the extrahepatic bile ducts. Clinical symptoms may be related to cholangiographically demonstrable biliary strictures,[21] or to intrahepatic small-duct disease. Systemic amyloidosis has been another complication of the disease.[22]

Morphologic features: Small bile ducts may contain inspissated eosinophilic material or eosinophilic concretions, associated with proliferation of ducts and ductules as well as biliary fibrosis. The fibrotic changes may vary considerably from one site to the next, and therefore the terms *focal biliary fibrosis* and *multilobular biliary fibrosis* have been coined. Beyond the neonatal period, bile stasis is quite uncommon.[23] The liver also may show just nonspecific changes, evidence of large-duct obstruction (usually in the presence of extrahepatic strictures[21]), or severe fatty changes. In the absence of inspissated material in bile ducts, cystic fibrosis usually cannot be diagnosed from liver specimens alone.

Drug-Induced and Toxic Hepatitis

Comments: The diagnosis can be suggested if an appropriate history has been provided. For drugs that can cause nonsuppurative cholangitis, see below and Table 15.2.

Morphologic features: Ductal proliferation is a common feature of drug-induced periportal hepatitis (see Chapter 2) or multilobular (submassive or massive) necrosis (see Chapter 9). Lymphoid or mixed-cell cholangitis and related features of nonsuppurative cholangitis, including ductopenia, have been reported after ingestion of the drugs listed in Table 15.2. Neutrophilic cholangitis ("acute cholangitis") has been observed after the use of sulindac.[24] Also, neutrophilic cholangitis or degenerative changes or necrosis of bile duct epithelial cells can result from paraquat (a herbicide) poisoning[25] and methylenediamine poisoning[26] (an epoxy resin hardener; first reported in this context as the cause of "Epping jaundice," named after the town where it first appeared); similar changes were observed in the Spanish toxic oil syndrome[27] (see below).

Graft-Versus-Host Disease

Comments: Most patients with hepatic graft-versus-host disease (GVHD) have undergone bone marrow transplantation for hematologic malignancies or aplastic anemia. Customarily, the term acute GVHD is used if the condition develops during the first 100 days after bone marrow transplantation. Subsequently, the name chronic GVHD is applied. This appears justified because two different pathogenetic mechanisms may be involved.[28]

Morphologic features: Nondestructive or destructive lymphocytic or mixed-cell cholangitis with degeneration and necrosis of bile duct epithelium is the hallmark of acute GVHD. These findings are encountered most commonly between days 35 and 90.[29] Lobular changes with many acidophilic bodies also may be found but they appear to be most prominent prior to day 35.[29] Acute GVHD often is followed by chronic GVHD, and in that condition, ductopenia, biliary fibrosis, and cholestasis usually prevail. Biliary cirrhosis has developed in a few instances.[30] Recently, fibrous-obliterative cholangitis and other features resembling primary sclerosing cholangitis have been described after bone marrow transplantation.[31]

Heatstroke

Neutrophilic cholangitis has been found in fatal exertional heatstroke; the affected patients survived more than 12 hours (for references and additional information, see Chapter 6).

Hepatic Allograft Rejection

Comments: In contradistinction to graft-versus-host disease (see that entry above), hepatic allograft rejection is the result of an immune response of the host against the graft. Customarily, three types of rejection are recognized— hyperacute,[32] acute, and chronic.[33-36] In the context of bile duct changes, only acute and chronic rejection need consideration. Controversy exists about definitions, but the following statements would probably be accepted by most experts.

Acute rejection is defined by the presence of the histologic features of cellular rejection, as described below, unrelated to duration and clinical findings. Chronic rejection also is defined by the presence of certain histologic features, primarily ductopenia with or without rejection arteriopathy. In contradistinction to acute rejection, chronic rejection has the added connotation of irreversibility. Again, onset and duration of the condition are no longer considered. Thus, it appears reasonable to use only a morphologic term (see below). In any event, the features of these two types of rejection overlap considerably, and therefore biopsy findings in rejection are more important than these terminologic distinctions.

Morphologic features: If the rejection is clinically acute, biopsy specimens typically show portal or periportal hepatitis with lymphoid or mixed-cell cholangitis (Figure 15.3). Immunocytes often are found inside the basement membrane of the bile ducts, together with pyknoses, vacuolation, and other degenerative changes of bile duct epithelial cells. In some instances, features of neutrophilic cholangitis and cholangiolitis are seen. However, in such cases, associated bile flow impairment (including bile leak) should be strongly considered. Ischemic necrosis of major bile ducts, strictures, and bile leaks often

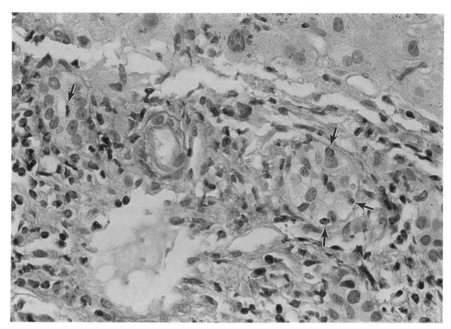

Figure 15.3
Hepatic allograft rejection with mixed-cell cholangitis, 3 weeks after orthotopic liver transplantation. Note immunocytes (arrows) in wall of bile ducts.

appear to trigger rejection episodes. Portal or periportal hepatitis with rejection cholangitis and endotheliitis of portal and hepatic vein branches (see Chapter 16) are the hallmark of *cellular rejection*, the morphologic counterpart to acute rejection. However, cellular rejection is not always acute; it may be persistent, recurrent, or asymptomatic. Thus, cellular rejection and acute rejection in a clinical sense do not correspond completely.

Persistent, treatment-unresponsive rejection cholangitis, with or without rejection arteriopathy (see Chapter 16), and other factors may lead to extensive duct destruction, ductopenia, and cholestatic graft failure (vanishing bile duct syndrome). Centrilobular necrosis (see Chapter 9) and cholestatic lobular hepatitis often accompany these changes. These findings are the hallmark of *ductopenic rejection*, the morphologic counterpart of chronic rejection. Again, ductopenic rejection is not always chronic; it may have a rather acute course.[36] Thus, ductopenic rejection and chronic rejection in a clinical sense do not correspond completely.

Idiopathic Adulthood Ductopenia

Comments: Adult patients with unexplained chronic nongranulomatous cholestatic liver disease and with histologic evidence of ductopenia may qualify for this diagnosis.[37] Cholangiograms should be normal, antimitochondrial antibodies should be absent, and colonoscopic findings should be negative for inflammatory bowel disease. Exposure to drugs and chemicals that might cause ductopenia (see "Postinflammatory States, Degeneration, and Loss of Bile Ducts" under "Morphologic Definitions" above) should be ruled out. A history of (early-onset) infantile obstructive cholangiopathy (see below under "Paucity of Intrahepatic Bile Ducts [Infantile Obstructive Cholangiopathy]") is another exclusion criterion. Possible causes include isolated small-duct primary sclerosing cholangitis, chronic active hepatitis C, and late-onset infantile obstructive cholangiopathy.[38] Of course, antimitochondrial antibody–negative primary biliary cirrhosis without histologic evidence of granulomas (see next paragraph) would also fall into this category.

Morphologic features: The liver shows periportal hepatitis, septal fibrosis, or biliary cirrhosis, with ductopenia (Figure 15.4) and cholestatic features, including copper deposition. Histologic exclusion criteria include granulomatous cholangitis (florid duct lesions), histiocytosis X, lymphoma, or other neoplastic diseases, as well as neutrophilic suppurative or nonsuppurative cholangitis.[37]

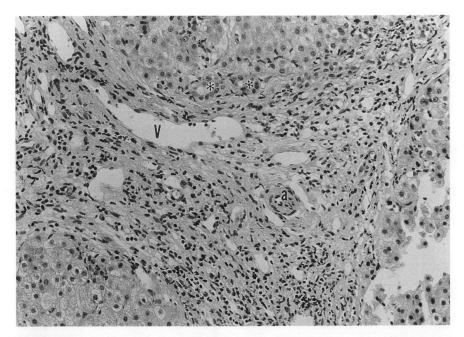

Figure 15.4
Idiopathic adulthood ductopenia. Branches of the portal vein (V) and of the hepatic artery (a) can be clearly identified, but an interlobular bile duct cannot be found. The duct-like structures in the adjacent parenchyma (asterisks) represent ductules (cholangioles), not ducts. Ductopenia as shown here has many possible causes. The diagnostic criteria for idiopathic adulthood ductopenia are listed in the text.

Infective Intra-abdominal Conditions

Comments: Peritonitis, infective intestinal disorders, and pancreatitis appear to cause nonspecific-reactive hepatitis and, sometimes, ascending cholangitis. This association has not been documented properly in the literature, possibly because pathogenetic mechanisms are difficult to elucidate; they may be linked to bacterial toxemia and related mechanisms that are presented below. (See below under "Systemic Bacterial Infections, Including the Toxic Shock Syndrome, and Systemic Viral Diseases.") In pancreatitis, bile duct lesions may develop by direct extension,[19] leading to cholangitis.

Morphologic features: Neutrophilic cholangitis, sometimes associated with other changes suggesting obstruction of large bile ducts (see below), are present. If these features are accompanied by normal cholangiographic findings, intra-abdominal or systemic infections should be considered.

Lymphoproliferative Disorders

Neoplastic infiltrates of this type sometimes can obscure or destroy small bile ducts,[40,41] leading to ductopenia. Jaundice associated with lymphoproliferative

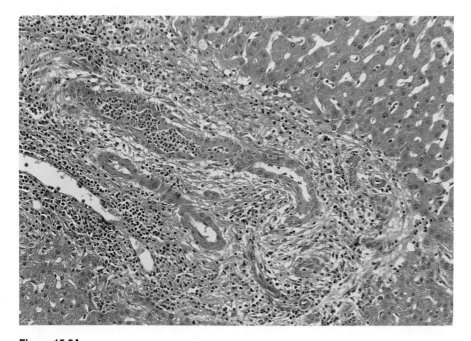

Figure 15.5A
Obstruction of extrahepatic bile ducts. Portal edema with long, slightly tortuous intralobular bile duct is shown. Tortuosity may lead to the appearance of multiple cross-sections through bile ducts in one portal tract (see also Figure 15.6). Note neutrophils in lumen of duct (see also Figure 15.5B).

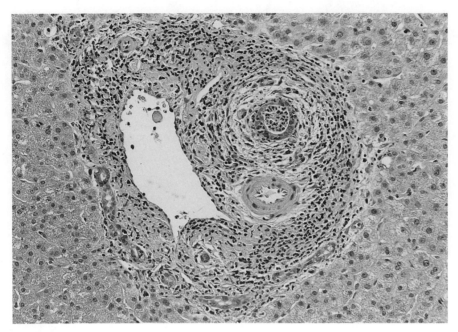

Figure 15.5B
Obstruction of extrahepatic bile ducts. Interlobular bile duct with neutrophils in wall and lumen (neutrophilic cholangitis) is shown. This is an unusual finding in biliary obstruction and generally indicates ascending infection.

hepatic infiltrates and duct destruction must be distinguished from jaundice associated with paraneoplastic cholestasis (see Chapter 5).

Mucocutaneous Lymph Node Syndrome

In this rare pediatric condition, which is also known under the name "Kawasaki disease," hydrops of the gallbladder is a common finding. A possible liver biopsy finding is neutrophilic and eosinophilic cholangitis.[42]

Obstruction of Large (Extrahepatic and Perihilar Intrahepatic) Bile Ducts

Comments: Biopsy is often done because of negative cholangiographic or ultrasound studies. In many instances, parenchymal liver disease is suspected.

Morphologic features: If the obstruction is acute or associated with infection, neutrophilic cholangitis may be a prominent finding (Figures 15.5A, 15.5B, and 15.5C). Experience with allografts suggests that bile leaks or drains in the bile duct may cause neutrophilic cholangitis, ductal proliferation, and other features that

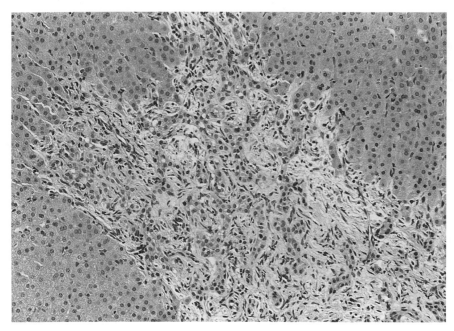

Figure 15.5C
Obstruction of extrahepatic bile ducts. Prominent ductular proliferation is apparent. This feature occurs not only in large-duct biliary obstruction but also in the syndrome of primary biliary cirrhosis and many other chronic liver diseases. See also Figures 4.7A and 4.7B.

usually are associated with actual obstruction. Thus, any type of bile flow impairment may be sufficient to cause these duct changes. Periductal fibrosis and fibrous cholangitis develop in prolonged obstruction (Figure 15.6). Cholangiectases also may be the result of biliary obstruction, but this feature usually is associated with primary sclerosing cholangitis only. Periductal fibrosis or inflammation also may occur in the vicinity of hepatic tumors, probably because of stretching and stricturing of intrahepatic bile ducts. The process may simulate sclerosing cholangitis.[43]

Paucity of Intrahepatic Bile Ducts (Infantile Obstructive Cholangiopathy)

Comments: In the past, this condition was named "intrahepatic biliary atresia"; it is now recognized as part of a large disease family with the collective designation "infantile obstructive cholangiopathy."[44] Paucity of intrahepatic bile ducts may occur in the absence of other abnormalities or in nonobligatory association with conditions such as alpha-1-antitrypsin deficiency or Down's syndrome (nonsyndromatic paucity of intrahepatic bile ducts).[45] The liver condition also may occur in obligatory linkage with cardiovascular and other extrahepatic malformations (Alagille's syndrome, arteriohepatic dysplasia, syndromatic paucity of intrahepatic bile ducts).[46] The conditions—particularly the nonsyndromatic disease—may lead to fatal biliary cirrhosis.

Morphologic features: The hallmark of the condition is severe ductopenia, often associated with ductular proliferation, biliary fibrosis, and cholestasis. The last feature is found primarily in early infancy, sometimes together with giant cell transformation. The presence of hepatocellular giant cells in this setting should not be misinterpreted as self-limited neonatal hepatitis. As in other chronic cholestatic conditions, rhodanine stains for copper may become positive.

Primary Sclerosing Cholangitis

Comments: Clinical and laboratory findings usually reveal chronic cholestatic liver disease. Typical cholangiographic findings confirm the diagnosis. Most patients also have chronic ulcerative colitis. See also Chapter 4, under "Chronic Hepatitis Associated With Primary Sclerosing Cholangitis."

Morphologic features: The main morphologic findings have been described in Chapter 4. Lymphocytic or mixed-cell cholangitis also may be found in this

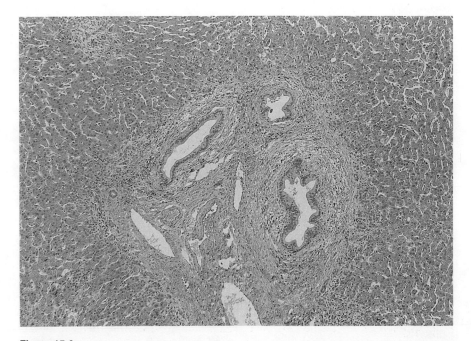

Figure 15.6
Chronic obstruction of extrahepatic bile ducts (choledocholithiasis). Ductal proliferation and periductal fibrosis are conspicuous findings.

condition. Fibrous cholangitis (Figure 15.7) is the most common finding, but cholangiectases and ductal obliteration also are rather constant features of primary sclerosing cholangitis (PSC). However, these lesions (Figures 15.8A and 15.8B) usually are not found in liver biopsy samples. The biopsy features in PSC reflect small-duct PSC, and the pathologist cannot predict from them whether the patient also has classic or large-duct PSC with cholangiographically demonstrable lesions. Small-duct PSC may occur in patients with chronic ulcerative colitis, cholestatic liver disease, and normal cholangiograms.[47] In the past, this lesion was named "pericholangitis." If neutrophilic cholangitis is found, large-duct involvement with ascending infection is the most likely cause.

Recurrent Pyogenic Cholangitis

Comments: This disease is common in East Asia. Intrahepatic calcium bilirubinate stones and biliary strictures lead to recurrent biliary infections. This condition is also known under the name "Oriental cholangiohepatitis"; it is seen in an increasing number of patients who have immigrated from endemic areas. A history of infestations with *Ascaris lumbricoides* or *Clonorchis sinensis* often is obtained.[48]

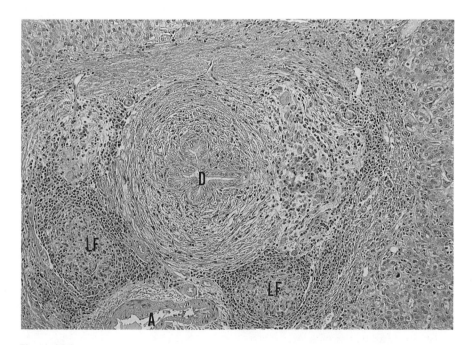

Figure 15.7
Fibrous cholangitis in primary sclerosing cholangitis. Note resemblance with duct changes in cholelithiasis (see Figure 15.6). D, septal bile duct surrounded by collar of connective tissue and chronic inflammatory cells; A, hepatic artery; LF, lymphoid follicles.

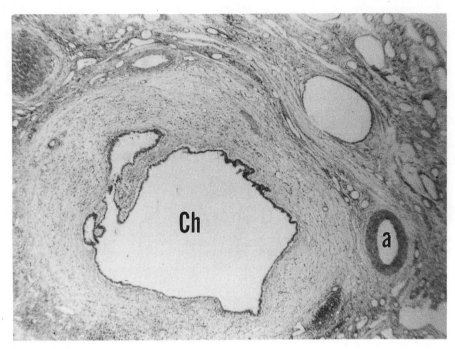

Figure 15.8A
Cholangiectasis and duct obliteration in primary sclerosing cholangitis. Cholangiectasis with prominent fibrous cholangitis of wall is shown. Compare the diameter of the cholangiectasis (Ch) with that of the artery (a). Normally, bile duct and artery have the same size. (Reprinted, with permission, from Ludwig J, MacCarty RL, LaRusso NF, et al: Intrahepatic cholangiectases and large-duct obliteration in primary sclerosing cholangitis. *Hepatology* 6:560-568, 1986.)

Morphologic features: Biopsy changes do not differ from those seen in other types of large-duct obstruction (see Chapter 4). During episodes of biliary infection, neutrophilic cholangitis is the main finding.

Schistosomiasis

For bile duct changes in this condition, see Chapter 10.

Solitary Hepatic Cyst

This is an incidental finding, usually without clinical consequence. Cysts of this type are lined by cuboidal, biliary-type epithelium; they are unilocular in most instances but may be multilocular. Solitary hepatic cysts are not typically associated with cysts in other organs.

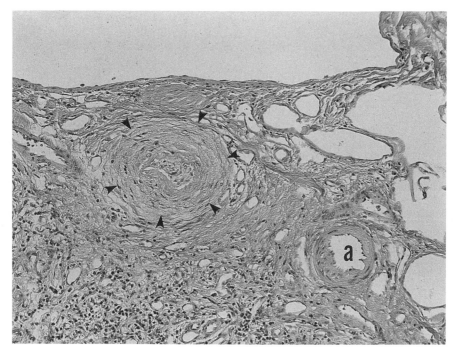

Figure 15.8B
Cholangiectasis and duct obliteration in primary sclerosing cholangitis. An obliterated bile duct is shown (arrowheads). The duct is represented by a round scar, approximately twice as large as the hepatic artery (a), suggesting that periductal fibrosis had been present also.

Syndrome of Primary Biliary Cirrhosis (Chronic Nonsuppurative Destructive Cholangitis)

Comments: Clinical and laboratory findings usually reveal chronic cholestatic liver disease. High titers of antimitochondrial antibodies are characteristic.

Morphologic features: In the early stages of the disease, lymphocytic, mixed-cell, and granulomatous cholangitis are the most important manifestations (Figures 15.9A, 15.9B, and 15.9C). The nonsuppurative lymphocytic and mixed-cell cholangitis may be destructive or nondestructive; the granulomatous cholangitis (florid duct lesion) probably is destructive in most instances. Fibrous cholangitis also may be found in this condition, probably representing a healing stage of any of the other types of cholangitis.[20] In later stages of the disease, ductopenia prevails. A distinction between the nonsuppurative cholangitis of the syndrome of primary biliary cirrhosis and small-duct primary sclerosing cholangitis (chronic hepatitis associated with primary sclerosing cholangitis; see Chapter 4) may be impossible. For cholestasis, Mallory bodies, and copper in the syndrome of primary biliary cirrhosis, see Chapters 4, 12, and 14, respectively.

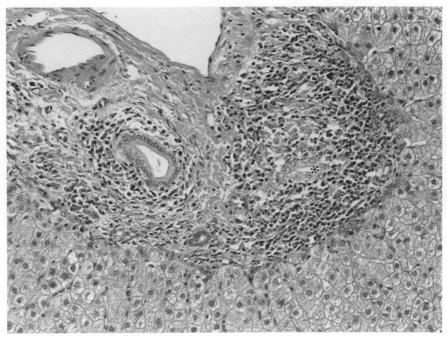

Figure 15.9A
Cholangitis in the syndrome of primary biliary cirrhosis. Lymphocytic cholangitis in early chronic nonsuppurative destructive cholangitis is shown. Duct destruction is not yet apparent. Note very early granuloma formation at interlobular bile duct on the right (asterisk).

Systemic Bacterial Infections, Including the Toxic Shock Syndrome, and Systemic Viral Diseases

Comments: The association between cholangitis with or without cholestasis (see Chapter 4) and bacteremia or septicemia, not originating from infections in the hepatobiliary system, still is controversial.[49,50] Published documentations include *Escherichia coli* septicemia.[49] In that instance, endotoxemia was thought to have caused the biliary damage. In acute cholangitis associated with toxic shock syndrome, the toxin of *Staphylococcus aureus* or other bacteria appears to be the responsible agent.[50] The toxic shock syndrome may develop if highly absorbent tampons, suture material, and other special conditions provide a suitable culture medium. The patients have fever, multiorgan dysfunction, and shock. The clinical features of systemic viral diseases are determined by the type of virus.

Morphologic features: In bacterial infections, interlobular bile ducts show degenerative changes with pyknotic nuclei, epithelial vacuolation, and other changes, which may lead to segmental duct necrosis.[49] The inflammatory changes are mild but some lesions could be described as necrotizing mixed-cell cholangitis.

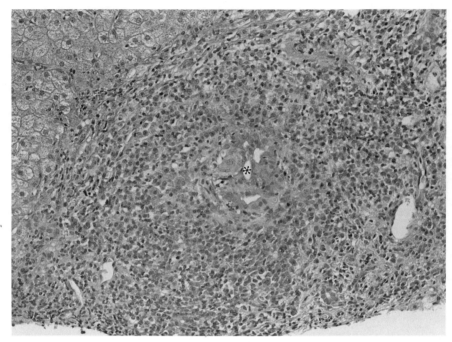

Figure 15.9B
Cholangitis in the syndrome of primary biliary cirrhosis. Mixed-cell cholangitis in chronic nonsuppurative destructive cholangitis is shown. Inflammatory destruction of the duct is in progress. Note that the outlines of the interlobular bile duct (asterisk) cannot be discerned clearly.

Portal edema, ductular proliferation, and neutrophilic cholangiolitis are accompanying features (Figure 15.10). In the toxic shock syndrome, neutrophilic cholangitis has been described,[50] with or without thrombosis of some portal vein branches. Most specimens also showed microvesicular fatty changes; they indeed appear to be a more constant finding than the neutrophilic cholangitis.

Among the systemic viral infections, cholangitis most commonly is caused by cytomegalovirus (CMV) infection. In infancy, it may cause obliterative cholangitis and thus might be a precursor of paucity of intrahepatic bile ducts[51] (see above). CMV cholangitis also occurs in many hepatic allografts, after bone marrow transplantation, and in some patients with the acquired immune deficiency syndrome (AIDS).[52,53] In the last group, the characteristic CMV inclusions also were found at the ampulla of Vater[52]; the portal tracts showed fibrosis, lymphocytic and fibrous cholangitis with degenerative epithelial changes, and focal ductopenia. In patients with AIDS, cholangiographic features of sclerosing cholangitis also may be found,[52,53] probably related to large-duct infection with CMV, *Cryptosporidium*, or bacteria such as *Salmonella*.[53]

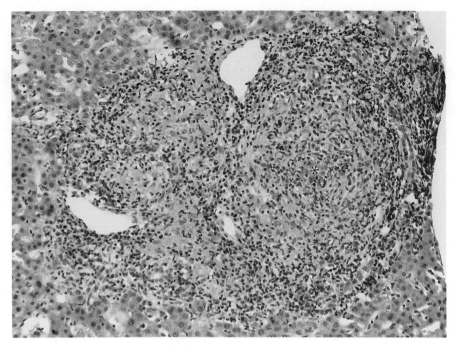

Figure 15.9C
Cholangitis in the syndrome of primary biliary cirrhosis. Destructive granulomatous cholangitis is shown. Three poorly defined clusters of epithelioid cells can be seen. An interlobular bile duct (asterisk) is in the center of the granuloma on the right. This is near-diagnostic for the syndrome of primary biliary cirrhosis. See also Figures 2.3A, 2.3B, 8.1A, and 8.1B.

Toxic Oil Syndrome

Comments: This multisystem disorder appeared in Spain in 1981; it was caused by adulterated rapeseed oil. A considerable number of patients with this condition developed liver diseases.[54] The observations from that episode are important because other hitherto unknown substances might cause similar lesions in the future.

Morphologic features: Mixed-cell cholangitis was found, sometimes with epithelioid cells, imparting features of granulomatous cholangitis (the illustrations of the latter lesions are not very convincing). The most common early-phase liver disease was cholestatic hepatitis. Later complications included nonalcoholic steatohepatitis, periportal (chronic active) hepatitis, nodular regenerative hyperplasia, liver cell adenoma, and biliary cirrhosis.[54] Some of the complications may have been coincidental, but in other instances the etiologic association with the toxic oil syndrome appeared convincing.

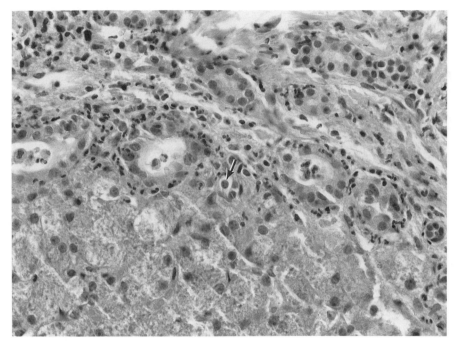

Figure 15.10
Neutrophilic cholangiolitis in a case of *Pseudomonas* septicemia. Bile (arrow) is inconspicuous here but may be another prominent finding.

Tumor-Associated Changes

Portal edema, neutrophilic cholangitis, and ductular proliferation with degeneration and reactive changes of the ductular epithelium are characteristic of the changes in the vicinity of metastatic intrahepatic lymphomas or carcinomas.[55] In the ductules, large hyperchromatic nuclei are found, together with eosinophilic cytoplasm and irregular arrangement and multilayering of the epithelial cells. Congestive changes with distortion of liver cell plates may be found in zone 1. Necrosis of single hepatocytes surrounded by mononuclear cells is another common finding in this condition. In contradistinction to large-duct biliary obstruction, cholestasis is usually absent in these cases. In patients with extrahepatic tumors,[56] ductular epithelial cells and hepatocytes may show hyperchromatism of nuclei and dysplastic changes. Such malignancy-associated changes with nonspecific changes in the liver may lead to hepatic dysfunction, best documented under the name "Stauffer's syndrome" in patients with renal cell carcinoma.[57]

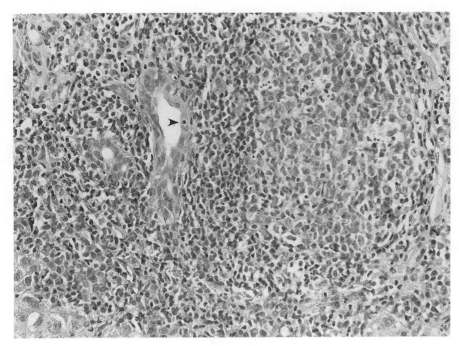

Figure 15.11A
Cholangitis in unresolved viral hepatitis (probably hepatitis C). Lymphoid cholangitis is shown, with lymphocytes surrounding interlobular bile duct and lymphoid follicle at right side of frame. Note lymphocyte (arrowhead) within bile duct epithelium.

Viral Hepatitis and Idiopathic (Autoimmune) Chronic Active Hepatitis

Comments: For the clinical features of acute, unresolved, and chronic viral hepatitis, as well as idiopathic (autoimmune) chronic active hepatitis, see Chapters 2 and 3, respectively.

Morphologic features: Lymphoid, mixed-cell (Figures 15.11A and 15.11B), and fibrous cholangitis[20] may be found in acute, unresolved, and chronic viral hepatitis,[58,59] particularly in non-A, non-B (hepatitis C) infection[60] but also in other types—for instance, acute cholestatic viral hepatitis A (see Chapter 4). These types of cholangitis—in particular, lymphoid cholangitis—also may be found in idiopathic (autoimmune) chronic active hepatitis. In rare cases, chronic active viral hepatitis appears to be associated with destructive nonsuppurative cholangitis, leading to ductopenia. This may be the etiology of some cases of idiopathic adulthood ductopenia (see above). Presence of nonsuppurative cholangitis may indicate progressive disease in both acute and chronic active hepatitis.[59] Most of these cases appear to represent hepatitis C. However, in most cases of unresolved and chronic active viral hepatitis or idiopathic (autoimmune) chronic active hepatitis, ducts and ductules are proliferated and not inflamed.

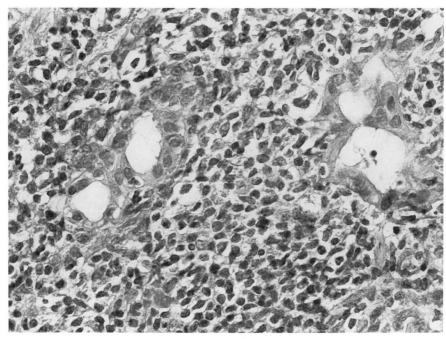

Figure 15.11B
Cholangitis in unresolved viral hepatitis (probably hepatitis C). Mixed-cell cholangitis is shown, with lymphocytes, plasma cells, and other mononuclear inflammatory cells surrounding the bile ducts.

Table 15.2   Drugs That May Cause Nonsuppurative Cholangitis and Ductopenia*

Generic or Chemical Name	Product Classification
Acetaminophen	Analgesic and antipyretic
Ampicillin[61]	Antibiotic
Chlorpromazine	Tranquilizer: phenothiazine
Cromolyn sodium	Antasthmatic
Diazepam	Sedative and hypnotic: benzodiazepine
Haloperidol	Antipsychotic
Imipramine	Antidepressant
Methyltestosterone	Androgen
Phenylbutazone	Anti-inflammatory
Prochlorperazine[62]	Tranquilizer: phenothiazine
Thiabendazole[63]	Anthelmintic
Tolbutamide	Oral hypoglycemic
Trifluoperazine hydrochloride	Tranquilizer: phenothiazine

*This list does not include drugs that are unavailable in the United States. For further information, see
  reference 64.

References

1. Pérez-Soler A: The inflammatory and atresia-inducing disease of the liver and bile ducts. *Monogr Pediatr* 8:1-245, 1976.

2. Sharp HL, Carey JB Jr, White JG, et al: Cholestyramine therapy in patients with a paucity of intrahepatic bile ducts. *J Pediatr* 71:723-736, 1967.

3. Nakanuma Y, Ohta G: Histometric and serial section observations of the intrahepatic bile ducts in primary biliary cirrhosis. *Gastroenterology* 76:1326-1332, 1979.

4. Afshani P, Littenberg GD, Wollman J, et al: Significance of microscopic cholangitis in alcoholic liver diseases. *Gastroenterology* 75:1045-1050, 1978.

5. Akwari OE, Tucker A, Seigler HF, et al: Hepatobiliary cystadenoma with mesenchymal stroma. *Ann Surg* 211:18-27, 1990.

6. Marcial MA, Hauser SC, Cibas ES, et al: Intrahepatic biliary cystadenoma: Clinical, radiological, and pathological findings. *Dig Dis Sci* 31:884-888, 1986.

7. Devine P, Ucci AA: Biliary cystadenocarcinoma arising in a congenital cyst. *Hum Pathol* 16:92-94, 1985.

8. Sell S, Dunsford HA: Evidence for the stem cell origin of hepatocellular carcinoma and cholangiocarcinoma. *Am J Pathol* 134:1347-1363, 1989.

9. Ludwig J, Wiesner RH, LaRusso NF: Focal dilatation of intrahepatic bile ducts (Caroli's disease), cholangiocarcinoma, and sclerosis of extrahepatic bile ducts: A case report. *J Clin Gastroenterol* 4:53-57, 1982.

10. Wee A, Ludwig J, Coffey RC Jr, et al: Hepatobiliary carcinoma associated with primary sclerosing cholangitis and chronic ulcerative colitis. *Hum Pathol* 16:719-726, 1985.

11. Ohta G, Nakanuma Y, Terada T: Pathology of hepatolithiasis: Cholangitis and cholangiocarcinoma. In Okuda K, Nakayama F, Wong J (eds): *Intrahepatic Calculi*. New York, Alan R. Liss Inc, 1984, pp 91-113.

12. Sherlock S: Fibro-polycystic disease of the liver and biliary tract. In Sherlock S (ed): *Diseases of the Liver and Biliary System*. 8th edition. Cambridge, Mass, Blackwell Scientific Publications Inc, 1989.

13. Govindarajan S, Peters RL: The bile duct adenoma: A lesion distinct from Meyenburg complex. *Arch Pathol Lab Med* 108:922-924, 1984.

14. Allaire GS, Rabin L, Ishak KG, et al: Bile duct adenoma: A study of 152 cases. *Am J Surg Pathol* 12:708-715, 1988.

15. Hausner RJ, Alexander RW: Localized congenital hepatic fibrosis presenting as an abdominal mass. *Hum Pathol* 9:473-476, 1978.

16. Nakanuma Y, Terada T, Ohta G, et al: Caroli's disease in congenital hepatic fibrosis and infantile polycystic disease. *Liver* 2:346-354, 1982.

17. Chen KTK: Adenocarcinoma of the liver: Association with congenital hepatic fibrosis and Caroli's disease. *Arch Pathol Lab Med* 105:294-295, 1981.

18. Pereira-Lima J, Schaffner F: Chronic cholestasis in hepatic sarcoidosis with clinical features resembling primary biliary cirrhosis. *Am J Med* 83:144-148, 1987.

19. Murphy JA, Sjogren MH, Kikendall JW, et al: Small bile duct abnormalities in sarcoidosis. *J Clin Gastroenterol* 12:555-561, 1990.

20. Ludwig J, Czaja A, Dickson ER, et al: Manifestations of nonsuppurative cholangitis in chronic hepatobiliary diseases: Morphologic spectrum, clinical correlations and terminology. *Liver* 4:105-116, 1984.

21. Gaskin KJ, Waters DLM, Howman-Giles R, et al: Liver disease and common-bile-duct stenosis in cystic fibrosis. *N Engl J Med* 318:340-346, 1988.

22. McGlennen RC, Burke BA, Dehner LP: Systemic amyloidosis complicating cystic fibrosis: A retrospective pathology study. *Arch Pathol Lab Med* 110:879-884, 1986.

23. Park RW, Grand RJ: Gastrointestinal manifestations of cystic fibrosis: A review. *Gastroenterology* 81:1143-1161, 1981.

24. Lerche A, Vyberg M, Kirkegaard E: Acute cholangitis and pancreatitis associated with sulindac (Clinoril). *Histopathology* 11:647-653, 1987.

25. Mullick FG, Ishak KG, Mahabir R, et al: Hepatic injury associated with paraquat toxicity in humans. *Lab Invest* 42:138-139, 1980.

26. McGill DB, Mott JD: An industrial outbreak of toxic hepatitis due to methylenediamine. *N Engl J Med* 291:278-282, 1974.

27. Solis-Herruzo JA, Castellano G, Colina F, et al: Hepatic injury in the toxic epidemic syndrome caused by ingestion of adulterated cooking oil (Spain 1981). *Hepatology* 4:131-139, 1984.

28. Snover DC: Acute and chronic graft versus host disease: Histopathological evidence for two distinct pathogenetic mechanisms. *Hum Pathol* 15:202-205, 1984.

29. Shulman HM, Sharma P, Amos D, et al: A coded histologic study of hepatic graft-versus-host disease after human bone marrow transplantation. *Hepatology* 8:463-470, 1988.

30. Stechschulte DJ Jr, Fishback JL, Emami A, et al: Secondary biliary cirrhosis as a consequence of graft-versus-host disease. *Gastroenterology* 98:223-225, 1989.

31. Geubel AP, Cnudde A, Ferrant A, et al: Diffuse biliary tract involvement mimicking primary sclerosing cholangitis after bone marrow transplantation. *J Hepatol* 10:23-28, 1990.

32 Bird G, Friend P, Donaldson P, et al: Hyperacute rejection in liver transplantation: A case report. *Transplant Proc* 21:3742-3744, 1989.

33. Klintmalm GBG, Nery JR, Husberg BS, et al: Rejection in liver transplantation. *Hepatology* 10:978-985, 1989.

34. Adams DH, Neuberger JM: Pattern of graft rejection following liver transplantation. *J Hepatol* 10:113-119, 1990.

35. Snover DC, Freese DK, Sharp HL, et al: Liver allograft rejection: An analysis of the use of biopsy in determining outcome of rejection. *Am J Surg Pathol* 11:1-10, 1987.

36. Wiesner RH, Ludwig J, Van Hoek B, et al: Current concepts in cell-mediated hepatic allograft rejection leading to ductopenia and liver failure. *Hepatology* 14:721-729, 1991.

37. Ludwig J, Wiesner RH, LaRusso NF: Idiopathic adulthood ductopenia: A cause of chronic cholestatic liver disease and biliary cirrhosis. *J Hepatol* 7:193-199, 1988.

38. Zafrani ES, Metreau J-M, Douvin C, et al: Idiopathic biliary ductopenia in adults: A report of five cases. *Gastroenterology* 99:1823-1828, 1990.

39. Di Bisceglia AM, Paterson AC, Segal I: The liver in biliary obstruction due to chronic pancreatitis. *Liver* 5:189-195, 1985.

40. Leblanc A, Hadchouel M, Jehan P, et al: Obstructive jaundice in children with histiocytosis X. *Gastroenterology* 80:134-139, 1981.

41. Lefkowitch JH, Falkow S, Whitlock RT: Hepatic Hodgkin's disease simulating cholestatic hepatitis with liver failure. *Arch Pathol Lab Med* 109:424-426, 1985.

42. Edwards KM, Glick AD, Greene HL: Intrahepatic cholangitis associated with mucocutaneous lymph node syndrome. *J Pediatr Gastroenterol Nutr* 4:140-142, 1985.

43. Vilgrain V, Erlinger S, Belghiti J, et al: Cholangiographic appearance simulating sclerosing cholangitis in metastatic adenocarcinoma of the liver. *Gastroenterology* 99:850-853, 1990.

44. Landing BH: Considerations of the pathogenesis of neonatal hepatitis, biliary atresia and choledochal cyst: The concept of infantile obstructive cholangiopathy. *Prog Pediatr Surg* 6:113-139, 1974.

45. Kahn E, Daum F, Markowitz J, et al: Nonsyndromatic paucity of interlobular bile ducts: Light and electron microscopic evaluation of sequential liver biopsies in early childhood. *Hepatology* 6:890-901, 1986.

46. Deprettere A, Portmann B, Mowat AP: Syndromic paucity of the intrahepatic bile ducts: Diagnostic difficulty; severe morbidity throughout early childhood. *J Pediatr Gastroenterol Nutr* 6:865-871, 1987.

47. Ludwig J: Small-duct primary sclerosing cholangitis. *Semin Liver Dis* 11:11-17, 1991.

48. Bonar S, Burrell M, West B, et al: Recurrent cholangitis secondary to Oriental cholangiohepatitis. *J Clin Gastroenterol* 11:464-468, 1989.

49. Vyberg M, Poulsen H: Abnormal bile duct epithelium accompanying septicemia. *Virchows Arch [Pathol Anat]* 402:451-458, 1984.

50. Ishak KG, Rogers WA: Cryptogenic acute cholangitis—association with toxic shock syndrome. *Am J Clin Pathol* 76:619-626, 1981.

51. Finegold MJ, Carpenter RJ: Obliterative cholangitis due to cytomegalovirus: A possible precursor of paucity of intrahepatic bile ducts. *Hum Pathol* 13:662-665, 1982.

52. Viteri A, Greene JF Jr: Bile duct abnormalities in the acquired immune deficiency syndrome. *Gastroenterology* 92:2014-2018, 1987.

53. Roulot D, Valla D, Brun-Vezinet F, et al: Cholangitis in the acquired immunodeficiency syndrome: Report of two cases and review of the literature. *Gut* 28:1653-1660, 1987.

54. Solis-Herruzo JA, Vidal JV, Colina F, et al: Clinico-biochemical evolution and late hepatic lesions in the toxic oil syndrome. *Gastroenterology* 93:558-568, 1987.

55. Gerber MA, Thung SN, Bodenheimer HC Jr, et al: Characteristic histologic triad in liver adjacent to metastatic neoplasm. *Liver* 6:85-88, 1986.

56. Nieburgs HE, Parets AD, Perez V, et al: Cellular changes in liver tissue adjacent and distant to malignant tumors. *Arch Pathol* 80:262-272, 1965.

57. Utz DC, Warren MM, Gregg JA, et al: Hepatic dysfunction with hypernephroma. *Mayo Clin Proc* 45:161-169, 1970.

58. Poulsen H, Christoffersen P: Abnormal bile duct epithelium in liver biopsies with histological signs of viral hepatitis. *Acta Pathol Microbiol Scand* 76:383-390, 1969.

59. Poulsen H, Christoffersen P: Abnormal bile duct epithelium in chronic aggressive hepatitis and cirrhosis: A review of morphology and clinical, biochemical, and immunologic features. *Hum Pathol* 3:217-225, 1972.

60. Schmid M, Pirovino M, Altorfer J, et al: Acute hepatitis non-A, non-B: Are there any specific light microscopic features? *Liver* 2:61-67, 1982.

61. Cavanzo FJ, Garcia CF, Botero RC: Chronic cholestasis, paucity of bile ducts, red cell aplasia, and the Stevens-Johnson syndrome. *Gastroenterology* 99:854-856, 1990.

62. Lok ASF, Ng JOL: Prochlorperazine-induced chronic cholestasis. *J Hepatol* 6:369-373, 1988.

63. Manivel JC, Bloomer JR, Snover DC: Progressive bile duct injury after thiabendazole administration. *Gastroenterology* 93:245-249, 1987.

64. Ludwig J, Axelson R: Drug effects on the liver: An updated tabular compilation of drugs and drug-related hepatic diseases. *Dig Dis Sci* 28:651-666, 1983.

Chapter 16

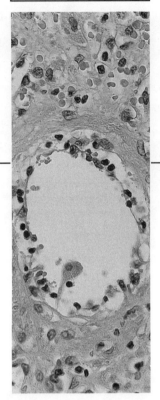

Abnormal Blood Vessels and Hemorrhages

Morphologic Definition

Hepatic artery branches are found in portal tracts, but their most distal segments also may be seen within the lobules where they eventually connect with sinusoids. In biopsy specimens, these vessels are named "arteries," although they often have the caliber of arterioles. Portal vein branches, by definition, run in portal tracts, together with hepatic arteries. For the tributaries of the hepatic veins, two terminologies are in use. The traditional names are "central veins" (the smallest tributaries that connect to the sinusoids), "sublobular veins," "collective veins," and "hepatic veins." Currently, the following terms are preferred: "terminal hepatic veins" (corresponding to "central veins"), "intercalated veins," "interlobular veins" (or "collecting veins"), and "hepatic veins." Definitions that would correlate a size range of intrahepatic arteries and veins with a specific name do not exist.

**Table 16.1   Clinical Conditions Associated With Abnormal Blood
Vessels and Hemorrhages***

Abnormal Hepatic Arteries (Including Loss of Arteries)
   Amyloidosis
   Arteriosclerosis
   Arteritis (focal or systemic)
   Drug effect (contraceptive-induced intimal hyperplasia)
   Hepatic allograft rejection (arteritis, arteriopathy, obliteration of arteries, loss of arteries)
   Hyperparathyroidism (calcification)
   Idiopathic arterial calcification of infancy
   Thrombi and emboli
   Toxic shock syndrome (arteritis)
Abnormal Portal Veins
   Congenital hepatic fibrosis (compression or hypoplasia of portal veins)
   Graft-versus-host disease (endotheliitis/phlebitis)
   Hepatic allograft rejection (endotheliitis/phlebitis)
   Idiopathic portal hypertension (phlebosclerosis, obliteration)
   Infectious intra-abdominal processes (pylephlebitis)
   Schistosomiasis (intimal proliferation, parasites, thrombi)
   Thrombi and emboli
   Toxic shock syndrome (pylephlebitis)
Abnormal Dilated Sinusoids
   Centrilobular or both centrilobular and midzonal:
      Budd-Chiari syndrome
      Congestive heart failure
      Granulomatous diseases
      Hepatic venous outflow obstruction of unknown cause
      Hypervitaminosis A
      Malignant lymphoma (extrahepatic Hodgkin's lymphoma)
      Normal specimens (biopsy artifact?)
      Rheumatoid arthritis
      Tumor-associated change (abdominal carcinomas)
      Veno-occlusive disease
   Midzonal:
      Tumor-associated change (renal cell carcinoma)
   Periportal:
      Disseminated intravascular coagulation (nongestational)
      Drug effect
      Hypervitaminosis A
      Preeclampsia or eclampsia
      Pregnancy
   Irregular or diffuse:
      Acquired immune deficiency syndrome
      Arsenic poisoning
      Disseminated intravascular coagulation (nongestational)

continued on page 235

continued from page 234
  Drug effect
  Granulomatous diseases
  Idiopathic portal hypertension
  Infarcts of Zahn
  Liver cell adenoma, hepatocellular carcinoma, and regenerative nodules
  Rheumatoid arthritis
  Thorotrast administration
  Tumor-associated change
  Vascular tumors or pseudotumors (angiosarcoma, epithelioid
    hemangioendothelioma, visceral bacillary epithelioid angiomatosis)
  Vinyl chloride poisoning
Abnormal Hepatic Veins (Central or Terminal Hepatic Veins, Intercalated Veins,
  and Interlobular Veins)
  Acute, unresolved or chronic active hepatitis, primary biliary cirrhosis, and primary
    sclerosing cholangitis (endotheliitis/phlebitis)
  Alcoholic liver disease (phlebosclerosis and fibrous obliteration, endotheliitis)
  Budd-Chiari syndrome (thrombosis or fibrous obliteration)
  Conditions associated with centrilobular necrosis (see Chapter 9)
  Drug effects (thrombosis)
  Graft-versus-host disease (endotheliitis/phlebitis)
  Hepatic allograft rejection (endotheliitis/phlebitis)
  Hepatotoxins (fibrous obliteration, thrombosis)
  Hypervitaminosis A (phlebosclerosis and fibrous obliteration)
  Idiopathic portal hypertension (phlebosclerosis)
  Malignant lymphoma (pseudoendotheliitis)
  Nonalcoholic steatohepatitis (endotheliitis)
  Sarcoidosis (endotheliitis)
  Syndromes of primary biliary cirrhosis and primary sclerosing cholangitis (see below
    under "Acute, Unresolved, or Chronic Active Hepatitis; Syndromes of Primary Biliary
    Cirrhosis and Primary Sclerosing Cholangitis")
  Thorotrast administration (fibrous obliteration)
  Thrombi (see below under "Thrombi and Emboli")
  Veno-occlusive disease (nonthrombotic fibrous obliteration)
Peliosis Hepatis
  Acquired immune deficiency syndrome
  Angioimmunoblastic lymphadenopathy with hypoxemia
  Arteritis (necrotizing vasculitis)
  Arsenic poisoning
  Bacterial endocarditis
  Diabetes mellitus
  Drug effects
  Hypervitaminosis A
  Liver cell adenoma
  Marasmus
  Multiple myeloma (see below under "Waldenström's
    Macroglobulinemia and Multiple Myeloma")

continued on page 236

continued from page 235
    Renal transplantation and chronic hemodialysis
    Sprue
    Thorotrast administration
    Vinyl chloride poisoning
    Waldenström's macroglobulinemia and multiple myeloma
Hemorrhages and Rupture
    Liver cell adenoma
    Preeclampsia and eclampsia
    Streptokinase administration
    Trauma
    Vascular tumors

*Morphologic findings and other explanatory remarks are in parentheses.

Clinical Conditions

Acquired Immune Deficiency Syndrome

Comments: Among the many manifestations of acquired immune deficiency syndrome (AIDS) in the liver,[1] non-neoplastic vascular lesions as described below are quite rare. The association between these lesions and Kaposi's sarcoma in the livers of patients with AIDS is not clear. For the association with cutaneous bacillary angiomatosis, see next paragraph and below under "Vascular Tumors and Pseudotumors."

Morphologic features: Although sinusoidal dilatation has been found in many autopsy cases[2] (the affected zones were not stated), it is not a regular biopsy finding. Peliosis hepatis also has been described in AIDS[3] but appears to be quite rare; the condition is said to have led to progressive hepatocellular dysfunction. The lesions also involved lymph nodes in the porta hepatis and the spleen. Bacillary peliosis hepatis has been observed in several patients with AIDS who also had cutaneous bacillary angiomatosis. This type of peliosis represents a treatable opportunistic infection.[4]

Acute, Unresolved, or Chronic Active Hepatitis; Syndromes of Primary Biliary Cirrhosis and Primary Sclerosing Cholangitis

Comments: The clinicopathologic features of acute and unresolved viral hepatitis have been described in Chapter 3 and of chronic active hepatitis in Chapter 2. For features of the syndromes of primary biliary cirrhosis and primary sclerosing cholangitis, see the Index.

Morphologic features: In addition to the morphologic features described in Chapters 2 and 3, endotheliitis or phlebitis of hepatic vein branches may be a prominent finding in acute, unresolved (Figure 16.1), and chronic active hepatitis, particularly in cases complicated by multilobular (submassive) necrosis (see also Chapter 9). We also have observed endotheliitis in patients with the syndromes of primary biliary cirrhosis and primary sclerosing cholangitis.

Alcoholic Liver Disease

As stated in Chapter 7, alcoholic hepatitis may be associated with lymphocytic phlebitis, phlebosclerosis (Figure 16.2), or fibrous obliteration of the central (terminal hepatic) veins. Such fibrous obliterative changes indicate chronicity. However, endotheliitis without phlebosclerosis may also occur in chronic alcoholic liver disease, including alcoholic cirrhosis.

Amyloidosis

Amyloid deposition in hepatic arteries and portal veins is found in both primary (AL, amyloid light [chain]) and secondary (AA, amyloid-associated)

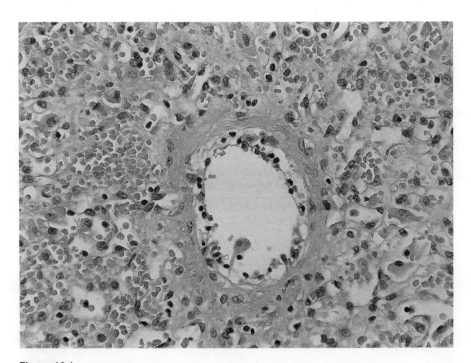

Figure 16.1
Endotheliitis and phlebitis of interlobular vein in patient with subfulminant viral hepatitis.

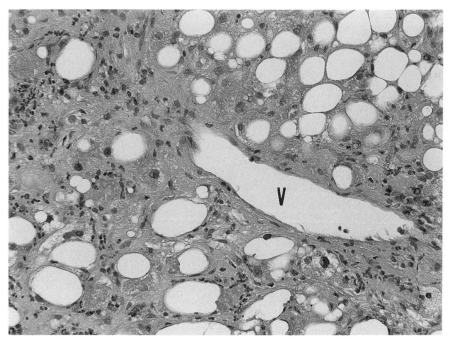

Figure 16.2
Phlebitis and phlebosclerosis in patient with acute and chronic alcoholic hepatitis. Because of the presence of acute alcoholic liver disease, some neutrophils can be found in the area of phlebosclerosis. V, central vein.

amyloidosis.[5] Exclusive vascular involvement is not proof of secondary amyloidosis, as suggested by some authors.

Angioimmunoblastic Lymphadenopathy

Peliosis hepatis and nodular regenerative hyperplasia have been observed in a case of angioimmunoblastic lymphadenopathy with severe hypoxemia.[6]

Arsenic Poisoning

See below under "Vinyl Chloride Poisoning."

Arteriosclerosis

Features of arteriosclerosis and arteriolosclerosis are common findings in biopsy specimens. Hyaline arteriosclerosis may be a cause of nodular regenerative hyperplasia, similar to obliteration of portal vein branches (see below under "Thrombi and Emboli").

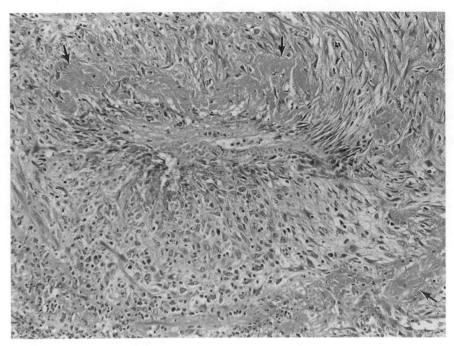

Figure 16.3
Polyarteritis nodosa affecting small branch of hepatic artery. Note mixed inflammatory infiltrates and fibrinoid necrosis (arrows) surrounding the artery.

Arteritis

Systemic arteritis rarely affects the liver appreciably, but in a few instances such lesions can be encountered, usually in patients with polyarteritis nodosa (Figure 16.3). Although arteritis can be found in needle biopsy specimens,[7] it is identified more often in wedge specimens. An important distinction must be made between reactive arteritis in the vicinity of abscesses or other inflammatory lesions, and manifestations of systemic arteritis. In the first instance the arteritis is merely an unimportant complication, whereas in the second instance it may be the cause of the liver disease. For peliosis hepatis in necrotizing arteritis, see below under "Marasmus."

Bacterial Endocarditis

Peliosis hepatis has been described in rare instances.

Budd-Chiari Syndrome

Comments: The following definition has been proposed[8]: "Budd-Chiari syndrome (BCS) consists of hepatic venous outflow obstruction and its manifestations, regardless of cause, the obstruction being either within the liver or in the inferior vena cava between the liver and the right atrium. Functional hepatic venous outflow obstruction caused by congestive heart failure is not part of BCS." A common clinical manifestation is the sudden onset of ascites, and the most common cause is thrombotic occlusion of the hepatic veins. Hematologic disorders and the use of oral contraceptives most often are the underlying conditions, but idiopathic thrombosis also is common.[8] For drugs that may cause hepatic venous outflow obstruction or BCS, see Table 16.2. Veno-occlusive disease (small-vein obstruction) can be considered a special type of BCS, caused by a rather well-defined group of chemicals such as pyrrolizidine. It recently has been encountered after use of comfrey herb tea[9] and intra-arterial hepatic infusions of 5-fluoro-2'-deoxyuridine.[10]

Morphologic features: Biopsy specimens show severe sinusoidal dilatation, primarily in zone 3. Early in the disease, the spaces of Disse usually are filled with erythrocytes, and the hepatic cell plates appear compressed. Later, major portions of the hepatic parenchyma may have dropped out and may have been replaced by blood lakes. In the most severe cases, rims of hepatocytes around the portal tracts are the only remnants of the parenchyma. If the disease has been survived long enough, centrilobular and midzonal fibrosis (congestive fibrosis) may become a prominent feature (Figure 16.4). Whether congestive cirrhosis can develop is controversial. The central (terminal hepatic), intercalated, and interlobular veins often are merely dilated, but fresh or organized thrombi sometimes can be identified, with or without centrilobular necrosis. In rare instances, features of a nonthrombotic, obliterative venopathy may be encountered, and then veno-occlusive disease in its traditional meaning can be diagnosed.[8,10]

Congenital Hepatic Fibrosis

As mentioned in Chapter 15, compression and possibly hypoplasia of portal vein branches may be prominent features of congenital hepatic fibrosis, and indeed may be the cause of portal hypertension. See also Chapter 10.

Congestive Heart Failure

Comments: Most patients have hepatomegaly, but severe liver dysfunction secondary to heart failure is rare although it has been documented[11,12]; most patients had biventricular failure with reduced systemic arterial pressure.

Morphologic features: Centrilobular sinusoidal dilatation, sometimes with compression of hepatic cell plates, small centrilobular necroses,[13] and fatty changes, is the main finding. Presence of centrilobular fibrosis indicates chronicity. Published cases or "cardiac cirrhosis" usually represent examples of potentially reversible congestive fibrosis.[14] (See also Chapter 11.)

Diabetes Mellitus

See below under "Marasmus."

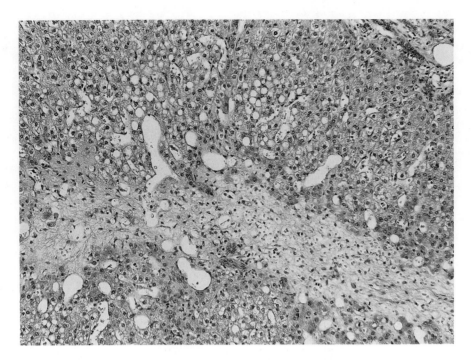

Figure 16.4
Obliteration of the central vein with centrilobular fibrosis in case of protracted hepatic venous outflow obstruction (Budd-Chiari syndrome). Note sinusoidal dilatation in the vicinity of the obliterated vein. A portion of an intact portal tract is visible in the right upper corner of the illustration.

Disseminated Intravascular Coagulation (Nongestational)

Most patients with this condition have advanced neoplastic or severe infectious diseases. Experiences are based largely on autopsy material.[15] Periportal or diffuse nonpatterned sinusoidal dilatation is a common histologic finding. The diagnosis of disseminated intravascular coagulation can be confirmed by the demonstration of intrasinusoidal microthrombi, with or without evidence of organization.[15] For related findings, see below under "Preeclampsia and Eclampsia (Toxemia of Pregnancy)."

Drug Effects

Comments: The diagnosis can be suggested if an appropriate history has been provided. Most drugs that cause vascular changes as described below belong to the steroids group (see also Table 16.3). Drug-induced vasculitis may also occur in the liver.[16]

Morphologic features: Periportal sinusoidal dilatation, with or without midzonal involvement, may be observed after long-term use of oral contraceptives.[17] The same drugs also may induce prominent arterial changes,[16] characterized primarily by intimal hyperplasia; medial hypertrophy also may occur. These arterial changes often are found in the vicinity of liver cell adenomas and thus may be the cause of infarctions with hemorrhages from these tumors.[16] Hepatic infarction not related to a tumor also has been observed after oral contraceptive use[18]; this probably is related to rupture of the liver in such patients. For hemorrhages and other complications associated with streptokinase administration, see below under that heading. For drugs that may cause hepatic vein thrombosis, see Table 16.2 and under "Budd-Chiari Syndrome" above.

Peliosis hepatis also can be caused by steroids, albeit only rarely by oral contraceptives.[19] Most of the drugs in this group are estrogens, androgens, or anabolic steroids; they are listed in Table 16.3. Arteriovenous shunting, characterized by irregular slit-like blood vessels around the central veins, and arteriographic evidence of hemangiomatosis have been observed after administration of metoclopramide.[20]

Eclampsia

See below under "Preeclampsia and Eclampsia (Toxemia of Pregnancy)."

Graft-Versus-Host Disease

Comments: For the clinical background of graft-versus-host disease (GVHD) and possible pathogenetic features, see Chapter 15.

Morphologic features: Attachment of lymphocytes and other immunocytes to the endothelium of portal and central (terminal hepatic) veins is a rather specific but not very sensitive feature of acute GVHD.[21] (See also below under "Hepatic Allograft Rejection.") For other conditions showing this type of endotheliitis or phlebitis, see above under "Acute, Unresolved, or Chronic Active Hepatitis; Syndromes of Primary Biliary Cirrhosis and Primary Sclerosing Cholangitis."

Granulomatous Diseases

Sinusoidal dilatation has been observed in patients with pulmonary tuberculosis, with or without hepatic involvement, but also in other granulomatous diseases (brucellosis, Crohn's disease).[22] The sinusoidal dilatation involved either zones 2 and 3 or the entire lobule. The pathogenesis of these lesions is not clear.

Hepatic Allograft Rejection

Comments: For the clinical background and classification of hepatic allograft rejection, see Chapter 15.

Morphologic features: Attachment of lymphocytes and other immunocytes to the endothelium of portal and central (terminal hepatic) veins is a common feature of cellular rejection. Typically, immunocytes also are found underneath the damaged endothelium (Figures 16.5A and 16.5B), sometimes together with a few neutrophils and eosinophils. The entire wall of the veins may be inflamed in this setting. Endothelial attachment and subendothelial infiltration represent endotheliitis[23]; involvement of all wall layers can be described as endotheliitis/phlebitis. The condition tends to disappear rather quickly, either spontaneously or after onset of antirejection treatment. The same process that leads to portal and central vein endotheliitis might lead to a comparable interaction between immunocytes and sinusoidal endothelial cells (sinusoidal endotheliitis).[23]

Medium-sized hepatic artery branches may be the site of a rejection-related arteritis, leading to intimal accumulation of cholesterol-laden macrophages (Figure 16.5C). At that stage, inflammatory cells may have completely disappeared, and then the condition is best named "rejection arteriopathy." These arterial changes have been used as a major diagnostic criterion for chronic rejection.[24] Cholesterol-laden macrophages also may appear in sinusoids of these patients.[25]

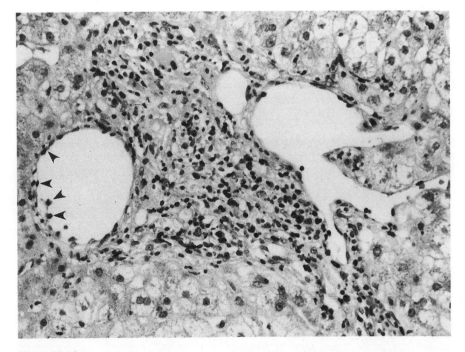

Figure 16.5A
Vascular changes in hepatic allograft rejection. Rejection endotheliitis in a case of ductopenic (chronic) rejection is shown. Note immunocytes underneath and attached to the luminal site of the portal vein endothelium (arrowheads). Portal hepatitis is present also; it is a feature of persistent cellular rejection. The bile duct has been destroyed.

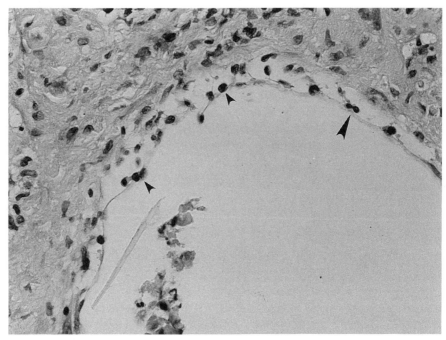

Figure 16.5B
Vascular changes in hepatic allograft rejection. Rejection endotheliitis in interlobular vein is shown. Note immunocytes (short arrowheads) and neutrophils (long arrowhead) underneath the endothelial cell layer, which has been lifted from the remaining intima.

An uncommon but also highly specific vascular feature of rejection is the loss of small artery branches that may occur in some cases of ductopenic rejection (usually in the clinical setting of chronic irreversible rejection). The loss of arteries (arterioles) appears to follow the loss of bile ducts (see Chapter 15), with only portal veins remaining.[26]

Hepatic Venous Outflow Obstruction of Unknown Cause

This diagnosis is recommended if histologic study shows features of severe sinusoidal congestion without any clues as to the cause of the condition. Congestive heart failure, obstruction of the hepatic and suprahepatic inferior vena cava, and obstruction of the small or large hepatic veins must be considered in this context. See also above under "Budd-Chiari Syndrome."

Hepatotoxins

See above under "Budd-Chiari Syndrome" and below under "Veno-occlusive Disease."

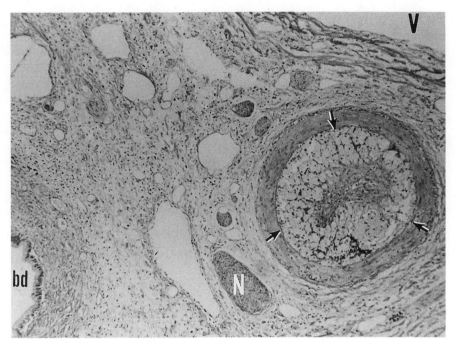

Figure 16.5C
Vascular changes in hepatic allograft rejection. Rejection arteriopathy with foam cells in the intima
(arrows) leads to almost complete occlusion of the lumen. The muscularis is intact. V, portal vein; bd, bile
duct; N, nerve.

Hodgkin's Disease

See below under "Malignant Lymphoma."

Hyperparathyroidism

Severe hypercalcemia in hyperparathyroidism may lead to hepatic artery
calcification[16] but also to hepatocellular calcification, particularly in areas of
hepatocellular necrosis.[27]

Hypervitaminosis A

Comments: Prolonged and excessive ingestion of vitamin A often is the
result of a food fadism but sometimes also occurs when the vitamin is taken
because of a skin condition, for cancer prevention, or for other perceived
benefits.[28] Typically, hypervitaminosis A causes skin and hair changes, among
other symptoms. Hepatomegaly and manifestations of portal hypertension may be
leading features of chronicity.[29]

Morphologic features: Vacuolated lipid-laden Ito cells (perisinusoidal lipocytes) are a sensitive feature of hypervitaminosis A. Patchy inflammatory infiltrates often are present also, imparting the changes of steatohepatitis. Presence of specific vitamin A fluorescence helps to confirm the diagnosis in doubtful cases.

Vascular changes involve the central (terminal hepatic) veins, which become fibrosed and sometimes obliterated (veno-occlusive disease), sometimes associated with centrilobular fibrosis. Hence, sinusoids in zones 2 and 3 usually are dilated also. Portal fibrosis and sinusoidal dilatation in zone 1 also have been observed.[30] Peliosis hepatis may be another manifestation. Perisinusoidal fibrosis develops around the vacuolated Ito cells. Cirrhosis is an uncommon feature but it has been documented.[31]

Idiopathic Arterial Calcification of Infancy

This unusual condition was described in newborn siblings[32]; a disturbed iron metabolism may be involved. Hepatic artery calcification may be part of this condition.[16]

Idiopathic Portal Hypertension

Comments: Idiopathic or primary portal hypertension is rare in Western countries[33] but common in India and Japan.[34] The diagnosis requires exclusion of diseases that can produce portal hypertension in the absence of cirrhosis—for instance, alcoholic liver disease, chronic active hepatitis, hypervitaminosis A, myeloproliferative disorders, and the early stages of the syndrome of primary biliary cirrhosis.[35] Some cases of hepatoportal sclerosis in childhood may be a complication of portal vein thrombosis.[36]

Morphologic features: Liver biopsy specimens may be normal, but frequently hepatoportal sclerosis is noted, characterized by portal tract fibrosis as well as portal phlebosclerosis with much intimal thickening (Figure 16.6). Elastic stains often are needed to appreciate these changes. The lesions are irregularly distributed, which may explain why some specimens appear to be normal. Periductal fibrosis or fibrosis of only parts of portal tracts can be observed. Thrombi or emboli also may be found in portal vein branches, with or without evidence of recanalization. Atrophy of hepatic lobules, perisinusoidal fibrosis, and nodular regenerative hyperplasia are commonly associated features. These secondary parenchymal changes lead to a markedly disturbed architecture of the affected livers. The apparent proximity of portal tracts to central veins (terminal hepatic veins, THV) or THV-like structures is a near diagnostic but unexplained feature of idiopathic portal hypertension. In Asian (Japanese) cases, additional changes can be observed, such as dilatation of portal veins, dilated sinusoids, formation of abnormal vascular channels between portal tracts and central veins, and hepatic phlebosclerosis.[37]

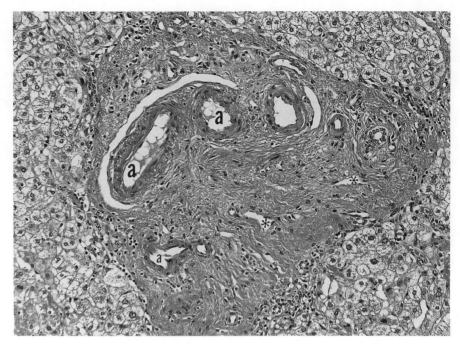

Figure 16.6
Hepatoportal sclerosis in case of Oriental idiopathic portal hypertension. The patient was a Japanese woman in her sixties. Note severe fibrosis of portal tract with extreme narrowing of the portal vein branches (asterisks). a, hepatic artery branches.

Infarcts of Zahn

Thrombosis of portal vein branches leads to atrophy of hepatic cell plates and secondary sinusoidal dilatation. There is no tissue necrosis. Changes of this type also may be found in the vicinity of tumors.

Infectious Intra-abdominal Processes

Suppurative pylephlebitis, with or without thrombi or emboli, is a rare but important complication of intra-abdominal bacterial infections—for instance, perforated diverticulitis.[38] Multiple pylephlebitic abscesses may develop. Acute omphalitis in infants has led to similar complications.[16]

Liver Cell Adenoma, Hepatocellular Carcinoma, and Regenerative Nodules

Irregular sinusoidal dilatation may be observed in liver cell adenomas, sometimes associated with peliosis of the tumor.[39] In addition, intimal proliferation of arteries, primarily in the vicinity of the adenomas, has been observed.[16] These changes may be responsible for infarctions, hemorrhages, and rupture of adenomas. With rare exceptions,[40] patients with these lesions are women who had been taking oral contraceptives. Irregular sinusoidal dilatation sometimes also may be found in hepatocellular carcinomas or regenerative nodules.

Malignant Lymphoma

In patients with intrahepatic or extrahepatic Hodgkin's lymphoma, sinusoidal dilatation has been found, primarily in zones 2 and 3. An alteration of the sinusoidal barrier has been implicated.[41] Peliosis hepatis also may occur in such patients (Figure 16.7).[42] Involvement of veins by neoplastic cells in any type of lymphoma may result in "pseudoendotheliitis" (Figure 16.8). In patients with treated lymphoma, endotheliitis has been observed, which probably was associated with drug-induced hepatitis.[23]

Marasmus

Peliosis hepatis has been reported in marasmus, uncomplicated by conditions that have been implicated in the past—primarily malignancies and tuberculosis.[43] It is possible that pathogenetic mechanisms related to rapid weight loss are the common denominator. This might also pertain to the cases of peliosis hepatis in

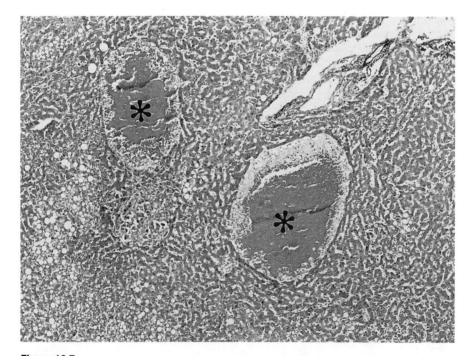

Figure 16.7
Peliosis hepatis (asterisks) in a patient with extrahepatic malignant lymphoma and septicemia.

the acquired immune deficiency syndrome (see above) and to the rare cases of peliosis in diabetes mellitus,[44] sprue,[45] necrotizing vasculitis,[46] and bacterial endocarditis.[47]

Nonalcoholic Steatohepatitis

Endotheliitis of central (terminal hepatic) or intercalated and interlobular veins can be found in rare instances. For other features of this condition, see Chapter 7.

Normal Specimens

Centrilobular sinusoidal dilatation sometimes is noted in otherwise normal specimens or in specimens from patients with liver disease but without any evidence of congestion. In these instances, the sinusoidal dilatation probably is an artifact (biopsy suction?). Compression of hepatic cell plates is not noted in this situation.

Preeclampsia and Eclampsia (Toxemia of Pregnancy)

Dilated periportal sinusoids, fibrin deposition, and periportal hemorrhagic

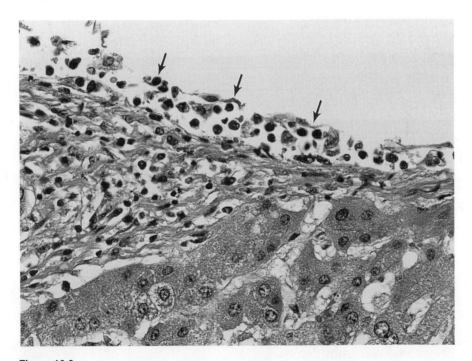

Figure 16.8
Pseudoendotheliitis in a patient with non-Hodgkin's lymphoma. Note accumulation of lymphoma cells underneath endothelial membrane (arrows).

necrosis in eclampsia have been described in Chapter 9. In both eclampsia and preeclampsia, hemorrhages from these lesions may lead to large subcapsular hematomas[48] or to rupture of the liver.[49] Hepatic infarction also may occur in such cases.[50] It should be noted that periportal sinusoidal dilatation also may occur in uncomplicated pregnancy.[51] The diagnosis of preeclampsia or eclampsia requires the presence of fibrin deposits and of other features as described above.

Pregnancy

See above under "Preeclampsia and Eclampsia (Toxemia of Pregnancy)."

Renal Cell Carcinoma

See below under "Tumor-Associated Change."

Renal Transplantation and Chronic Hemodialysis

Peliosis hepatis has been described in both conditions.[52]

Rheumatoid Arthritis

In a review of patients with adult-onset rheumatoid arthritis, patchy nonzonal, midzonal, or centrilobular sinusoidal dilatation was found, without other major morphologic abnormalities.[53] The patients had been taking many different drugs, but it is unclear whether the medications were responsible for the lesions.

Sarcoidosis

The features of this condition are described in Chapter 8. We have observed endotheliitis of hepatic vein branches in rare cases of sarcoidosis.

Schistosomiasis

Specimens may show intimal proliferation of portal veins, thrombi in portal vein branches, or parasites in the lumens of these vessels (see also Chapter 10).

Sprue

See above under "Marasmus."

Streptokinase Administration

Streptokinase can cause transient liver function abnormalities,[54] but the main complication is the development of hematomas,[55] which may lead to rupture of the liver.[56]

Thorotrast Administration

The identification of thorotrast and the main complications of past use have been described in Chapter 14. The main neoplastic complication, angiosarcoma, may be preceded by irregular sinusoidal dilatation[57] and peliosis hepatis.[58] Veno-occlusive disease also has been found in such cases.[58]

Thrombi and Emboli

Hepatic artery and portal vein branches may both be the sites of emboli or thrombi. For thrombi in hepatic vein branches, see above under "Budd-Chiari Syndrome." Portal vein thrombosis is sometimes found in cirrhosis and often in the vicinity of malignant hepatic tumors. In cases of hepatocellular carcinoma, the thrombi may consist partly or entirely of tumor. Conditions that may cause hepatic vein thrombosis, such as hematologic disorders or oral contraceptives, also may cause portal vein thrombosis. For portal vein thrombosis in disseminated intravascular coagulation, see Chapter 9. For portal vein thrombosis in trauma, see below under "Trauma." Portal vein thrombi and emboli may complicate infectious intra-abdominal processes (see above), and portal vein thrombosis also may be found in hepatoportal sclerosis (see above under "Idiopathic Portal Hypertension"). Arterial emboli in the liver do not differ from those in other organs. Arterial thrombosis may be a complication of arteritis (see above). Hepatic atrophy and nodular regenerative hyperplasia appear to be common complications of small-vessel disease, primarily postembolic or post-thrombotic portal vein obliteration.[59]

Toxic Shock Syndrome

Liver disease—in particular, acute cholangitis—in toxic shock syndrome has been described in Chapter 15. In some cases, pylephlebitis and portal arteritis were found also.[60]

Trauma

Biopsy specimens from the vicinity of post-traumatic lesions, usually intrahepatic arterial ruptures, show hemorrhage, necrosis, and vascular or extravascular thrombi. More commonly, pathologists receive lobectomy specimens or sublobular resection specimens containing the entire traumatic lesion.[61]

Tumor-Associated Change

Focal midzonal sinusoidal dilatation may be a paraneoplastic manifestation of renal cell carcinoma. Some but not all of the affected patients had Stauffer's syndrome (hepatic dysfunction associated with renal cell carcinoma).[62] Generalized sinusoidal dilatation or sinusoidal dilatation in zones 2 and 3 has been observed in association with other neoplasms—for instance, carcinomas of the colon or uterus.[22] These changes were found in the presence of hepatic metastases but also in the absence of hepatic tumor involvement. Characteristically, hepatic tissue obtained from liver adjacent to hepatic metastases shows focal sinusoidal dilatation and congestion with compression and distortion of hepatic cell plates. The portal tracts in these specimens are edematous and contain neutrophils around bile ducts and ductules.[63] The bile ductules are proliferated and show pleomorphism and hyperchromatism of epithelial cells. For sinusoidal dilatation associated with Hodgkin's lymphoma, see above under "Malignant Lymphoma."

Vascular Tumors and Pseudotumors

Benign vascular tumors include cavernous hemangiomas and infantile hemangioendothelioma, which has a guarded prognosis. The most important malignant vascular tumor, angiosarcoma, has been associated with exposure to thorotrast (see above under that heading), arsenic, and vinyl chloride (see below under that heading). However, in many cases no specific etiology is recognized. A malignant vascular tumor with a better prognosis is the epithelioid hemangioendothelioma. For an excellent recent synopsis, see reference 64. Hepatic hemorrhage and rupture may complicate angiosarcomas. A recently described condition in HIV-infected and other immunosuppressed patients is visceral bacillary epithelioid angiomatosis.[65] The hepatic lesions resemble epithelioid hemangioendothelioma except for the presence of neutrophils between the vascular spaces and pyknotic nuclear debris.

Veno-occlusive Disease

Historically, only cases with nonthrombotic obliterative endophlebitis of centrilobular (terminal hepatic) veins or intercalated and interlobular veins qualified for this diagnosis. The prototype was observed after pyrrolizidine alkaloid poisoning. Recently, many other conditions were considered in this context,[9,10] as described above under "Budd-Chiari Syndrome." Centrilobular sinusoids are dilated in all instances. Chemicals such as dimethylnitrosamine and aflatoxin cause veno-occlusive lesions together with centrilobular necrosis. Arsenic can cause veno-occlusive disease with perisinusoidal fibrosis.

Vinyl Chloride Poisoning

Similar to arsenic and thorotrast, vinyl chloride also can cause irregular sinusoidal dilatation and peliosis, prior to the development of angiosarcoma.[57]

Waldenström's Macroglobulinemia and Multiple Myeloma

Peliosis hepatis has been observed in both conditions.[66,67] In a patient with Waldenström's macroglobulinemia, nodular regenerative hyperplasia and light-chain deposits in sinusoidal walls also were found.[66]

Table 16.2   Drugs That May Cause Large-Vein Thrombotic Hepatic Outflow Obstruction (Budd-Chiari Syndrome) or Veno-occlusive Disease*

Generic or Chemical Name	Product Classification
Adriamycin	Antineoplastic
Azathioprine	Antineoplastic (antimetabolite) and immunosuppressant
Carmustine (BCNU)	Antineoplastic
Cysteamine[68]	(For the treatment of cystinosis)
Cytosine arabinoside	Antineoplastic (cytotoxic agent)
Dacarbazine	Antineoplastic
Daunorubicin hydrochloride	Antineoplastic
Ethinyl estradiol	Oral contraceptive
5-Fluoro-2'-deoxyuridine[†]	Antineoplastic (antimetabolite)
Mestranol	Oral contraceptive
Methyltestosterone	Anabolic steroid and androgen
Mitomycin	Antineoplastic
Norethindrone	Oral contraceptive
6-Thioguanine	Antineoplastic (antimetabolite)
Valproic acid	Anticonvulsant
Vinblastine sulfate	Antineoplastic

*This list does not include drugs that are unavailable in the United States. For further information, see reference 69. For additional substances, see above under "Alcoholic Liver Disease," "Hypervitaminosis A," "Thorotrast Administration," and "Veno-occlusive Disease."

†Veno-occlusive lesions in both central vein and portal vein branches have been observed after intra-arterial infusion in the treatment of hepatic metastases.[10]

Table 16.3   Drugs That May Cause Peliosis Hepatis*

Generic or Chemical Name	Product Classification
Azathioprine	Antineoplastic (antimetabolite and immunosuppressant)
Corticosteroids	Anti-inflammatory and hormone
Danazol[70]	Antiestrogen
Diethylstilbestrol diphosphate	Estrogen
Fluoxymesterone	Androgen
Methandrostenolone	Anabolic steroid
Methyltestosterone	Anabolic steroid and androgen
Oxymetholone	Androgen
Tamoxifen[71]	Antiestrogen
6-Thioguanine[72]	Antineoplastic (antimetabolite)

*This list does not include drugs that are unavailable in the United States. For further information, see reference 69. For peliosis hepatis after thorotrast administration or in hypervitaminosis A, see above under those headings. Chemicals that may cause peliosis hepatis include arsenic[57] and copper sulfate.[73]

References

1. Schaffner F: The liver in HIV infection. *Prog Liv Dis* 9:505-522, 1990.

2. Welch K, Finkbeiner W, Alpers CE, et al: Autopsy findings in the acquired immune deficiency syndrome. *JAMA* 252:1152-1159, 1984.

3. Czapar CA, Weldon-Linne CM, Moore DM, et al: Peliosis hepatis in the acquired immune deficiency syndrome. *Arch Pathol Lab Med* 110:611-613, 1986.

4. Perkocha LA, Geaghan SM, Yen TSB, et al: Clinical and pathological features of bacillary peliosis hepatis in association with human immunodeficiency virus infection. *N Engl J Med* 323:1581-1586, 1990.

5. Chopra S, Rubinow A, Koff RS, et al: Hepatic amyloidosis: A histopathologic analysis of primary (AL) and secondary (AA) forms. *Am J Pathol* 115:186-193, 1984.

6. Cadranel J-F, Cadranel J, Buffet C, et al: Nodular regenerative hyperplasia of the liver, peliosis hepatis, and perisinusoidal fibrosis: Association with angioimmunoblastic lymphadenopathy and severe hypoxemia. *Gastroenterology* 99:268-273, 1990.

7. Rousselet M-Ch, Kettani S, Rohmer V, et al: A case of temporal arteritis with intrahepatic arterial involvement. *Pathol Res Pract* 185:329-331, 1989.

8. Ludwig J, Hashimoto E, McGill DB, et al: Classification of hepatic venous outflow obstruction: Ambiguous terminology of the Budd-Chiari syndrome. *Mayo Clin Proc* 65:51-55, 1990.

9. Bach N, Thung SN, Schaffner F: Comfrey herb tea–induced hepatic veno-occlusive disease. *Am J Med* 87:97-99, 1989.

10. Nakhleh RE, Wesen C, Snover DC, et al: Venoocclusive lesions of the central veins and portal vein radicles secondary to intraarterial 5-fluoro-2'-deoxyuridine infusion. *Hum Pathol* 20:1218-1220, 1989.

11. Ross RM: Hepatic dysfunction secondary to heart failure. *Am J Gastroenterol* 76:511-518, 1981.

12. Hoffman BJ, Pate MB, Marsh WH, et al: Cardiomyopathy unrecognized as a cause of hepatic failure. *J Clin Gastroenterol* 12:306-309, 1990.

13. Kanel GC, Ucci AA, Kaplan MM, et al: A distinctive perivenular hepatic lesion associated with heart failure. *Am J Clin Pathol* 73:235-239, 1980.

14. Lemmer JH, Coran AG, Behrendt DM, et al: Liver fibrosis (cardiac cirrhosis) five years after modified Fontan operation for tricuspid atresia. *J Thorac Cardiovasc Surg* 86:757-760, 1983.

15. Shimamura K, Oka K, Nakazawa M, et al: Distribution patterns of microthrombi in disseminated intravascular coagulation. *Arch Pathol Lab Med* 107:543-547, 1983.

16. Ishak KG: New developments in diagnostic liver pathology. In Farber E, Phillips MJ, Kaufman N (eds): *Pathogenesis of Liver Diseases*. Baltimore, Williams & Wilkins, 1987, pp 223-373.

17. Balázs M: Sinusoidal dilatation of the liver in patients on oral contraceptives: Electron microscopical study of 14 cases. *Exp Pathol* 35:231-237, 1988.

18. Jacobs MB: Hepatic infarction related to oral contraceptive use. *Arch Intern Med* 144:642-643, 1984.

19. Van Erpecum KJ, Janssens AR, Kreuning J, et al: Generalized peliosis hepatis and cirrhosis after long-term use of oral contraceptives. *Am J Gastroenterol* 83:572-575, 1988.

20. Feurle GE: Arteriovenous shunting and cholestasis in hepatic hemangiomatosis associated with metoclopramide. *Gastroenterology* 99:258-262, 1990.

21. Snover DC: Acute and chronic graft versus host disease: Histopathological evidence of two distinct pathogenetic mechanisms. *Hum Pathol* 15:202-205, 1984.

22. Bruguera M, Aranguibel F, Ros E, et al: Incidence and clinical significance of sinusoidal dilatation in liver biopsies. *Gastroenterology* 75:474-478, 1978.

23. Ludwig J, Batts KB, Ploch M, et al: Endotheliitis in hepatic allografts. *Mayo Clin Proc* 64:545-554, 1989.

24. Adams DH, Neuberger JM: Patterns of graft rejection following liver transplantation. *J Hepatol* 10:113-119, 1990.

25. Grond J, Gouw ASH, Poppema S, et al: Chronic rejection in liver transplants: A histopathologic analysis of failed grafts and antecedent serial biopsies. *Transplant Proc* 18:128-135, 1986.

26. Ludwig J, Wiesner RH, Batts KP, et al: The acute vanishing bile duct syndrome (acute irreversible rejection) after orthotopic liver transplantation. *Hepatology* 7:476-483, 1987.

27. Ladefoged C, Frifelt JJ: Hepatocellular calcification. *Virchows Arch [A]* 410:461-463, 1987.

28. Minuk GY, Kelly JK, Hwang W-S: Vitamin A hepatotoxicity in multiple family members. *Hepatology* 8:272-275, 1988.

29. Russell RM, Boyer JL, Bagheri SA, et al: Hepatic injury from chronic hypervitaminosis A resulting in portal hypertension and ascites. *N Engl J Med* 291:435-440, 1974.

30. Bioulac-Sage P, Quinton A, Saric J, et al: Chance discovery of hepatic fibrosis in patient with asymptomatic hypervitaminosis A. *Arch Pathol Lab Med* 112:505-509, 1988.

31. Le Marchand P, Benatre A, Metman E-H, et al: Cirrhose induite par la vitamine A. *Gastroenterol Clin Biol* 8:116-120, 1984.

32. Anderson KA, Burbach JA, Fenton LA, et al: Idiopathic arterial calcification of infancy in newborn siblings with unusual light and electron microscopic manifestations. *Arch Pathol Lab Med* 109:838-842, 1985.

33. Scully RE, Mark EJ, McNeely WF, et al: Case records of the Massachusetts General Hospital (Case 30-1989). *N Engl J Med* 321:246-253, 1989.

34. Okuda K, Nakashima T, Okudeira M, et al: Liver pathology of idiopathic portal hypertension. Comparison with non-cirrhotic portal fibrosis of India. The Japan Idiopathic Portal Hypertension Study. *Liver* 2:176-192, 1982.

35. Lebrec D, Benhamou J-P: Noncirrhotic intrahepatic portal hypertension. *Semin Liver Dis* 6:332-340, 1986.

36. Maksoud JG, Mies S, da Costa Gayotto LC: Hepatoportal sclerosis in childhood. *Am J Surg* 151:484-488, 1986.

37. Hashimoto E, Ludwig J, Obata H, et al: Clinicopathologic conference on idiopathic portal hypertension. *Hepatology*. In press.

38. Navarro C, Clain DJ, Kondlapoodi P: Perforated diverticulum of the terminal ileum: A previously unreported cause of suppurative pylephlebitis and multiple hepatic abscesses. *Dig Dis Sci* 29:171-177, 1984.

39. Kerlin P, Davis GL, McGill DB, et al: Hepatic adenoma and focal nodular hyperplasia: Clinical, pathologic, and radiologic features. *Gastroenterology* 84:994-1002, 1983.

40. McInerney PD, Van Dessel MG, Berstock DA: Spontaneous haemoperitoneum from rupture of a primary hepatic adenoma in an adult man. *Gut* 28:1170-1172, 1987.

41. Bruguera M, Caballero T, Carreras E, et al: Hepatic sinusoidal dilatation in Hodgkin's disease. *Liver* 7:76-80, 1987.

42. Carulli N, Ponz de Leon M, Di Marco G, et al: Peliosis hepatis in a case of Hodgkin's disease: One year follow-up. *Ital J Gastroenterol* 10:112-115, 1978.

43. Simon DM, Krause R, Galambos JT: Peliosis hepatis in a patient with marasmus. *Gastroenterology* 95:805-809, 1988.

44. Hamilton FT, Lubitz JM: Peliosis hepatis: Report of three cases, with discussion of pathogenesis. *Arch Pathol* 54:546-572, 1952.

45. Zak FG: Peliosis hepatis. *Am J Pathol* 26:1-15, 1950.

46. Delas N, Faurel JP, Wechsler B, et al: Association d'une péliose à une vascularite nécrotisante. *Nouv Presse Med* 11:2787, 1982.

47. Molle D, Benoit P, Labrousse J, et al: Endocardite bactérienne compliquée de péliose hépatique. *Nouv Presse Med* 8:2481, 1979.

48. Manas KJ, Welsh JD, Rankin RA, et al: Hepatic hemorrhage without rupture in preeclampsia. *N Engl J Med* 312:424-426, 1985.

49. Bis KA, Waxman B: Rupture of the liver associated with pregnancy: A review of the literature and a report of two cases. *Obstet Gynecol Surg* 31:763-773, 1976.

50. Krueger KJ, Hoffman BJ, Lee WM: Hepatic infarction associated with eclampsia. *Am J Clin Gastroenterol* 85:588-592, 1990.

51. Fisher MR, Neiman HL: Periportal sinusoidal dilatation associated with pregnancy. *Cardiovasc Interventional Radiol* 7:299-302, 1984.

52. Hankey GJ, Saker BM: Peliosis hepatis in a renal transplant recipient and in a hemodialysis patient. *Med J Aust* 146:102-105, 1987.

53. Laffón A, Moreno A, Gutierrez-Bucero A, et al: Hepatic sinusoidal dilatation in rheumatoid arthritis. *J Clin Gastroenterol* 11:653-657, 1989.

54. Sallen MK, Efrusy ME, Kniaz JL, et al: Streptokinase-induced hepatic dysfunction. *Am J Gastroenterol* 78:523-524, 1983.

55. Willis SM, Bailey SR: Streptokinase-induced subcapsular hematoma of the liver. *Arch Intern Med* 144:2084-2085, 1984.

56. Eklöf BO, Gjöres JE, Lohi A, et al: Spontaneous rupture of liver and spleen during streptokinase treatment of deep venous thrombosis [in Swedish]. *Lakartidningen* 75:777-778, 1978.

57. Popper H, Thomas LB, Telles NC, et al: Development of hepatic angiosarcoma in man induced by vinyl chloride, thorotrast, and arsenic. *Am J Pathol* 92:349-376, 1978.

58. Dejgaard A, Krogsraard K, Jacobson M: Veno-occlusive disease and peliosis hepatis after thorotrast administration. *Virchows Arch [Pathol Anat]* 403:87-94, 1984.

59 Wanless IR: Micronodular transformation (nodular regenerative hyperplasia) of the liver: A report of 64 cases among 2,500 autopsies and a new classification of benign hepatocellular nodules. *Hepatology* 11:787-797, 1990.

60. Ishak KG, Rogers WA: Cryptogenic acute cholangitis—association with toxic shock syndrome. *Am J Clin Pathol* 76:619-626, 1981.

61. Mays ET: Hepatic trauma. *N Engl J Med* 288:402-405, 1973.

62. Aoyagi T, Mori I, Ueyama Y, et al: Sinusoidal dilatation of the liver as a paraneoplastic manifestation of renal cell carcinoma. *Hum Pathol* 20:1193-1197, 1989.

63. Gerber MA, Thung SN, Bodenheimer HC, et al: Characteristic histologic triad in liver adjacent to metastatic neoplasm. *Liver* 6:85-88, 1986.

64. Craig J, Peters RL, Edmondson HA: Tumors of the liver and intrahepatic bile ducts. *Atlas of Tumor Pathology*, 2nd series, Fascicle 26. Washington, DC, Armed Forces Institute of Pathology, 1989.

65. Kemper CA, Lombard CM, Deresinski SC, et al: Visceral bacillary epithelioid angiomatosis: Possible manifestations of disseminated cat scratch disease in the immunocompromised host: A report of two cases. *Am J Med* 89:216-220, 1990.

66. Voinchet O, Degott C, Scoazec J-Y, et al: Peliosis hepatis, nodular regenerative hyperplasia of the liver, and light chain deposition in a patient with Waldenström's macroglobulinemia. *Gastroenterology* 95:482-486, 1988.

67. Caroli J, Julien C, Albano O: Péliose hépatique et plasmosarcomatose splénique: Première observation reconnue in vivo. *Semin Hop Paris* 40:1709-1720, 1964.

68. Avner ED, Ellis D, Jaffe R: Veno-occlusive disease of the liver associated with cysteamine treatment of nephropathic cystinosis. *J Pediatr* 102:793-796, 1983.

69. Ludwig J, Axelson R: Drug effects on the liver: An updated tabular compilation of drugs and drug-related hepatic diseases. *Dig Dis Sci* 28:651-666, 1983.

70. Nesher G, Dollberg L, Zimran A, et al: Hepatosplenic peliosis after danazol and glucocorticoids for ITP. *N Engl J Med* 312:242-243, 1985.

71. Loomus GN, Aneja P, Bota RA: A case of peliosis hepatis in association with tamoxifen therapy. *Am J Clin Pathol* 80:881-883, 1983.

72. Larrey D, Fréneaux E, Berson A, et al: Peliosis hepatis induced by 6-thioguanine administration. *Gut* 29:1265-1269, 1988.

73. Pimentel JC, Menezes AP: Liver diseases in vineyard sprayers. *Gastroenterology* 72:275-283, 1977.

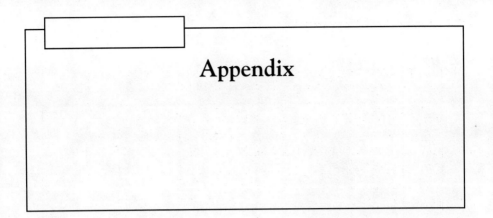

Appendix

Normal Test Values for the Evaluation of Liver Diseases*

Substance or Test	Normal Serum Values			Conventional Units (Conversion Factor)	Common Test Abnormalities
	Age	M	F		
Alanine aminotransferase (ALT)	6-14 y	14-27	12-25 U/L	U/L (1)	Increased levels in many liver diseases; 5-10x or more in chronic active hepatitis; 10-500x or more in fulminant hepatitis (massive or submassive hepatic necrosis).
	5-18 y	12-25	10-22 U/L	U/L (1)	
	>18 y	10-32	9-24 U/L	U/L (1)	
Albumin	>1 y	31-43	31-43 g/L	g/dL (0.1)	Decreased in chronic active hepatitis, fulminant hepatitis, and cirrhosis.
Alkaline phosphatase (AP)	>18 y	90-239 U/L	—	U/L (1)	Normal or slightly increased levels in chronic acive hepatitis; increased 2-10x or more in the syndrome of primary biliary cirrhosis, primary sclerosing cholangitis, and other cholestatic diseases. May be decreased in Wilson's disease.
	≤45 y	—	76-196 U/L	U/L (1)	
	>45 y	—	87-250 U/L	U/L (1)	
AP liver isoenzyme	Adults	20-130	20-130 U/L	U/L (1)	
Alpha-1-antitrypsin (A₁AT)	All ages	1.26-2.26	1.26-2.26 g/L	mg/dL (100)	Decreased levels suggest alpha-1-antitrypsin deficiency.
Alpha-fetoprotein (AFP)	>6 mo	15	15 µg/L	ng/mL (1)	Levels increased 5-10x or more in chronic active hepatitis and cirrhosis; rapid additional rise in hepatocellular carcinoma.

Normal Test Values for the Evaluation of Liver Diseases*

Substance or Test	Age	Normal Serum Values M	F	Conventional Units (Conversion Factor)	Common Test Abnormalities
Antihepatitis antigens and antibodies					See "Serologic Findings in Viral Hepatitis" table below.
Antimitochondrial antibodies (AMA)					Present in high titers in the syndrome of primary biliary cirrhosis; low titers may be present in viral or alcoholic hepatitis, autoimmune hepatitis and other liver diseases.
Aspartate aminotransferase (AST)	All ages	12-31	12-31 U/L	U/L (1)	Similar to alanine aminotransferase (ALT).
Bilirubin Total	All ages	18	18 µmol/L	mg/dL (0.05848)	Levels increased 5-50x or more in fulminant hepatitis and 2-20x or more in the syndrome of primary biliary cirrhosis, primary sclerosing cholangitis, and other cholestatic diseases. Slight increase in chronic active hepatitis.
Direct	All ages	0-6	0-6 µmol/L	mg/dL (0.05848)	
Ceruloplasmin	All ages	230-430	230-430 mg/L	mg/dL (0.1)	Decreased levels in Wilson's disease.
Cholesterol	See right column				Cholesterol and triglyceride values show age and sex dependence throughout life. Consult appropriate tables.[1] Abnormalities tend to be similar to those of albumin levels.

Normal Test Values for the Evaluation of Liver Diseases*

Substance or Test	Normal Serum Values Age	M	F	Conventional Units (Conversion Factor)	Common Test Abnormalities
Copper	Adults	11.8-22.8	11.8-22.8 μmol/L	μg/mL (0.0635)	Increased in Wilson's disease.
Ferritin	Adults	200-300	20-120 μg/L	ng/mL (1)	Levels increased 4-30x or more in genetic (primary) hemochromatosis. Increased levels also observed in autoimmune chronic active hepatitis and in alcoholic hepatitis.
Gamma globulin	All ages	7-16	7-16 g/L	g/dL (0.1)	Levels increased 2-4x in autoimmune chronic active hepatitis but sometimes also in viral or alcoholic hepatitis and chronic cholestatic liver diseases.
Gamma-glutamyl transferase (GGT)	≥1 y	—	6-29 U/L	U/L (1)	Levels increased in chronic cholestatic liver diseases and alcoholic hepatitis.
	≤45 y	7-37 U/L		U/L (1)	
	>45 y	10-48 U/L		U/L (1)	
Iron	All ages	13-31	12-30 μmol/L	μg/dL (5.58)	Levels increased in genetic (primary) hemochromatosis. Increased levels also observed in viral or alcoholic hepatitis and in autoimmune chronic active hepatitis. See also below under "Total iron-binding capacity."

Normal Test Values for the Evaluation of Liver Diseases*

Substance or Test	Normal Serum Values			Conventional Units (Conversion Factor)	Common Test Abnormalities
	Age	M	F		
Lactate dehydrogenase (LDH)	>18 y	48-115	48-115 U/L	U/L (1)	Increased levels in viral and chronic active hepatitis.
Mitochondrial antibodies					See "Antimitochondrial antibodies."
Prothrombin time (PT)	All ages	10.9-12.8	10.9-12.8 s	s (1)	Changes parallel to albumin: prolonged in chronic cholestatic liver diseases (primary biliary cirrhosis, primary sclerosing cholangitis) and in viral or alcoholic hepatitis.
Smooth muscle antibodies (SMA)					Present in autoimmune chronic active hepatitis; sometimes found in primary biliary cirrhosis, primary sclerosing cholangitis, and in viral or alcoholic hepatitis.
Total iron-binding capacity (TIBC)	All ages	43-81	43-81 µmol/L	µg/dL (5.58)	See "Iron."
Uric acid	All ages	0.26-0.48	0.14-0.36 mmol/L	mg/dL (16.8)	Decreased levels in Wilson's disease.
Vitamin A (retinol)	All ages	1.25-4.20	1.25-4.20 µmol/L	µg/dL (28.7)	See "25-Hydroxy-vitamin D."

Normal Test Values for the Evaluation of Liver Diseases*

Substance or Test	Normal Serum Values			Conventional Units (Conversion Factor)	Common Test Abnormalities
	Age	M	F		
25-Hydroxy-vitamin D					Levels decreased in chronic cholestatic liver diseases (primary biliary cirrhosis, primary sclerosing cholangitis) and in hemochromatosis.
Winter	All ages	0.46-1.39	0.46-1.39 μmol/L	ng/mL (30)	
Summer	All ages	0.50-2.64	0.50-2.64 μmol/L	ng/mL (30)	
Vitamin E (alpha-tocopherol)	Adults	0.13-0.39	0.13-0.39 mmol/L	mg/L (43.1)	As in 25-hydroxy-vitamin D.

Substance or Test	Normal Urine Values			Conventional Units (Conversion Factor)	Common Test Abnormalities
	Age	M	F		
Copper	All ages	0.2-1.2	0.2-1.2 μmol/d	μg/d (63.53)	1.6 μmol/d or more in Wilson's disease.

Substance or Test	Normal Tissue Values†			Conventional Units (Conversion Factor)	Common Test Abnormalities
	Age	M	F		
Copper	All ages	0.16-0.56	0.16-0.56 μmol/g	μg/g (63.53)	4 μmol/g dry weight or more in Wilson's disease: similar increase in chronic cholestatic liver diseases (primary biliary cirrhosis, primary sclerosing cholangitis)
Iron	All ages	3.58-39.38	3.58-28.64 μmol/g	μg/g (55.83)	180 μmol/g dry weight or more in genetic (primary) hemochromatosis, depending on stage of disease.

* Some normal test values differ slightly from laboratory to laboratory. For most test results in pediatric patients, additional tables must be consulted.
† All tissue values are expressed as gram dry weight.

Serologic Findings in Viral Hepatitis*

HBsAg	Anti-HBs	Anti-HBc	Anti-HBc (IgM)	HBeAg	Anti-HBe	HBV-DNA	Anti-HD	Anti-HAV	Anti-HAV (IgM)	Anti-HCV	Interpretation
−	−	−	−	−	−	−	−	+	+	−	Recent acute hepatitis A
−	−	−	−	−	−	−	−	+	−	−	Recovery from hepatitis A
+	−	−	−	+/−	−	+/−	−	−	−	−	Early (presymptomatic) acute type B hepatitis
+	+/−	+	+	+/−	+/−	+/−	−	−	−	−	Acute or unresolved type B hepatitis
−	−	+	+	−	−	+/−	−	−	−	−	Recent hepatitis B infection in "window" period
−	+	+	+/−	−	+/−	−	−	−	−	−	Recovery from type B hepatitis
−	+/−	+	−	−	−	−	−	−	−	−	Late-recovery hepatitis B
+	−	+	−	+/−	+/−	+/−	−	−	−	−	Chronic type B hepatitis
−	+	−	−	−	−	−	−	−	−	−	Hepatitis B vaccine recipient

Serologic Findings in Viral Hepatitis*

HBsAg	Anti-HBs	Anti-HBc	Anti-HBc (IgM)	HBeAg	Anti-HBe	HBV-DNA	Anti-HD	Anti-HAV	Anti-HAV (IgM)	Anti-HCV	Interpretation
+	−	+	−	+/−	+/−	+/−	+	−	−	−	Chronic type D hepatitis
−	−	−	−	−	−	−	−	−	−	−	Early acute type C hepatitis or non A, B, C, D hepatitis
−	−	−	−	−	−	−	−	−	−	+	Late acute, unresolved, or chronic hepatitis C

* HBsAg, hepatitis B surface antigen; Anti-HBs, hepatitis B surface antibody; Anti-HBc, hepatitis B core antibody; Anti-HBc (IgM), hepatitis B core antibody, immunoglobulin M; HBeAg, hepatitis B e antigen; Anti-HBe, hepatitis B e antibody; HBV-DNA, hepatitis B virus deoxyribonucleic acid; Anti-HD, hepatitis D antibody; Anti HAV, hepatitis A viral antibody; Anti-HAV (IgM), hepatitis A viral antibody, immunoglobulin M; Anti-HCV, hepatitis C viral antibody.

Reference

1. *Clinical Diagnosis & Management by Laboratory Methods.* 18th ed. Henry JB (ed). Philadelphia, WB Saunders, 1991.

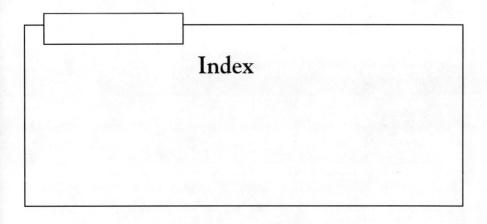

Index

Unless otherwise specified, all entries pertain to the liver. Thus, only a few entries begin with "Liver…" or "Hepatic…." Numbers in **boldface** refer to pages on which figures appear; numbers in *italics* refer to pages on which tables appear.

A

Abetalipoproteinemia, morphologic features, 63, 73, 75
Abnormal bile ducts
    as tumor-associated change, 7, 252
    associated clinical conditions, *205-207*
    definition, 203
Abnormal hepatocytes, definition, 143
Abnormal nonpigmented substances
    associated clinical conditions, *188-189*
    definition, 183
Abnormal vascular channels in idiopathic portal hypertension, 247
Abscesses
    cholangitic, 132, 211
    fibrosis after healing, 119
    pylephlebitic, 247
Acetaminophen (tabulated), *18, 43, 64, 107, 139, 254*
Acetaminophen administration
    lipochrome deposition after, 193
    necrosis after, 104
Acetohexamide, *43, 139*
Acidophilic bodies, definition, 144
Acidophilic cytoplasmic inclusions, associated clinical conditions, 145

Acquired immune deficiency syndrome
　　bacillary peliosis hepatis in, 236
　　CMV cholangitis in, 224
　　CMV hepatitis in, 100
　　endotheliitis in, 27
　　lobular hepatitis in, 26, 27
　　other morphologic features, 236
　　tuberculosis in, 86, 87
Acute alcoholic cholestasis, morphologic features, 32
Acute cholangitis and cholangiolitis. See Neutrophilic cholangitis
Acute fatty liver of pregnancy, morphologic features, 56
Acute viral hepatitis. See Unresolved viral hepatitis
Acute viral hepatitis A
　　cholestasis in, 32, **33**
　　periportal hepatitis in, 10
Acute viral hepatitis A to E, 22
Acyl coenzyme A dehydrogenase deficiency and fatty changes, 60
Adenovirus hepatitis, morphologic features, 149
Adriamycin, 253
Adult polycystic liver disease. See Autosomal-dominant cystic disease of liver
Aflatoxin poisoning, morphologic features, 105, 252
Alagille's syndrome. See Paucity of intrahepatic bile ducts
Alanine aminotransferase, normal levels, 260
Albumin, normal levels, 260
Alcoholic cirrhosis
　　active, **124**
　　features of past disease, 124
　　in genetic hemochromatosis, 133
　　inactive, **125**
　　morphologic features, 123
Alcoholic fatty liver
　　morphologic features, 57
　　zonal distribution, **58**
Alcoholic foamy degeneration, morphologic features, 58
Alcoholic hepatitis
　　cholangitis in, 207
　　cholestasis in, 33, **34**
　　chronic, 113
　　features of past disease, 114, 175
　　Mallory bodies in, 70, **71**
　　other morphologic features, 33, 70
　　phlebitis and phlebosclerosis in, 70, **238**
　　veno-occlusive lesions in, 70
Alcoholic liver disease
　　and genetic hemochromatosis, 174-175

hemosiderosis in, 174
morphologic features, 33, 70, 123-124, 150
Alcoholic steatohepatitis. *See* Alcoholic hepatitis
Alkaline phosphatase, normal levels, 260
Allograft rejection. *See* also Hepatic allografts
    cholangitis in, 213, **214**
    cirrhosis in, 137
    vascular changes in, 243, **245**
Allopurinol, *43, 90, 107, 108*
Alpha-fetoprotein, normal levels, 260
Alpha-1-antichymotrypsin deficiency, morphologic features, 151
Alpha-1-antitrypsin
    in hepatocellular carcinoma, 160
    normal levels, 260
Alpha-1-antitrypsin deficiency
    and neonatal cholestatic jaundice, 190
    and periportal hepatitis, 10
    associated conditions, 151
    cirrhosis in, 124, **152, 153**
    copper in, 190
    globules in, 145
    globules in absence of alpha-1-antitrypsin deficiency, 152
    other morphologic features, 125, 152, 190
    serologic findings in, 152
Aluminum-containing granulomas, 83
Aminopurine administration and lipochrome deposition, 193
Aminosalicylic acid, *18, 28, 43*
Amiodarone (tabulated), *65, 76, 139*
Amiodarone administration
    Mallory bodies after, 157
    phospholipidosis after, 63, 157
    steatohepatitis after, 74
Amitriptyline hydrochloride, *28, 43, 108*
Amoxicillin-clavulanic acid, *43*
Ampicillin, *228*
Amyloid, definition, 183
Amyloidosis
    and cholestasis, 50
    in cystic fibrosis, 126
    morphologic features in, 190
    vascular involvement in, 237
Anemic infarcts, associated conditions and complications, 98
Anesthesia and lobular hepatitis, 26
Angioimmunoblastic lymphadenopathy, associated conditions, 238
Angiokeratoma corporis diffusum. *See* Fabry's disease

Angiosarcoma. *See* Hemangiosarcoma
Anthracosis and anthracosilicosis, morphologic features, 190
Anthracotic pigment, definition, 183
Antimitochondrial antibodies, interpretation, 261
Apoptotic bodies, definition, 144
Aprindine, *43*
Argininosuccinic aciduria, fibrosis in, 116
Argyria after silver administration, 187, 190
Arsenic poisoning, morphologic features, 119, 138, 252
Arterial changes induced by oral contraceptives, 242
Arteriohepatic dysplasia. *See* Paucity of intrahepatic bile ducts
Arteriosclerosis and nodular regenerative hyperplasia, 238
Arteritis. *See also* Polyarteritis nodosa
    in allograft rejection, 243
    in toxic shock syndrome, 251
    reactive vs systemic, 239
Artery to portal vein shunts in hereditary hemorrhagic telangiectasia, 126
Asparaginase, *64*
Aspartate aminotransferase, normal levels, 261
Aspergillosis, necrosis in 105
Aspirin, *18, 28, 65, 90*
Asteroid bodies in granulomas, 80, 85
Atenolol, *43*
Atransferrinemia, fibrosis in, 116
Atrophy. *See* Hepatic atrophy
Autoimmune CAH. *See also* CAH
    cholangitis in, 227
Autosomal-dominant cystic disease of the liver, histologic features, 210
Autosomal-recessive cystic disease of the liver, histologic features, 209
Azathioprine (tabulated), *43, 253, 254*
Azathioprine administration, induction cells after, 157
Azidothymidine (AZT), *64*

B

Bacillary peliosis hepatis in acquired immune deficiency syndrome, 236, 252
Bacterial endocarditis and peliosis hepatis, 239, 249
Bacterial toxins and fatty liver, 62
Ballooned hepatocytes in lobular hepatitis, 22
Ballooning degeneration, definition, 144
Barbiturates and induction cells, 157
Barium sulfate
    definition, 184
    embolization after radiographic studies, 198

BCG immunotherapy, granulomas after, 83
Benign postoperative intrahepatic cholestasis, morphologic features, 50
Bile. *See* also Cholestasis and Cholestatic hepatitis
    definition, 184
    periportal, and copper, 191
Bile duct abnormalities. *See* Abnormal bile ducts and Bile duct…
Bile duct adenomas, definition and morphologic features, 208
Bile duct obliteration in PSC, 3, 12, 35, 220
Bile duct obstruction
    cholestatic hepatitis after, **40**, 41, **41**
    cirrhosis after, 118, 132
    ductular proliferation after, **218**
    periductal fibrosis after, 118
    periportal hepatitis after, 14, **16**
    portal hepatitis after, 5
Bile ducts, postinflammatory states and degeneration, 205
Bile flow impairment, duct changes in, 218
Bile infarcts
    after bile duct obstruction, 41, **41**
    in obstructive biliary cirrhosis, 132
Bile lakes
    after bile duct obstruction, 41
    in obstructive biliary cirrhosis, 132
Bile leaks, neutrophilic cholangitis after, 217
Biliary atresia, hepatocellular giant cells in, **163**
Biliary cirrhosis. *See* also PBC
    after bile duct obstruction, 118, 132
    in chronic intrahepatic cholestasis of sarcoidosis, 211
    in cystic fibrosis, 126
    in graft-versus-host disease, 213
    in PSC, **35, 138**
    in toxic oil syndrome, 225
Biliary cystadenoma, definition and morphologic features, 207
Biliary fibrosis after bile duct obstruction, 118
Biliary microhamartomas, definition and morphologic features, 208, **209, 210**
Biliary piecemeal necrosis, definition, 94
Bilirubin, normal levels, 261
Blood transfusions, morphologic changes after, 180
Blood vessels in the liver, definition and terminology, 233
Bone marrow transplantation
    CMV cholangitis after, 224
    eosinophilic bodies after, 154
    fibrous-obliterative cholangitis after, 213
Bridging necrosis
    definition, 95

in lobular hepatitis, 27
in unresolved viral hepatitis, **99**
Brucellosis, granulomas in, 86
Budd-Chiari syndrome, clinical findings and morphologic features, 239-240, **241**
Budd-Chiari syndrome and veno-occlusive disease, drug-induced, 253
Burns, morphologic findings after, 165
Byler's disease. *See* Progressive intrahepatic cholestasis

C

CAH. *See* Chronic active hepatitis
Calcification
    associated conditions, 144, 184, 196
    in abscesses, 119
    in hepatic allografts, 160
    in hyperparathyroidism, 160, 245
    in idiopathic arterial calcification of infancy, 246
    in tumors, 200
Calcium oxalate in granulomas, 80, 85
Camphor and microvesicular fatty change, 63
Candidiasis, necrosis in, 105
Captopril, *18, 43, 108*
Carbamazepine, *43, 90, 108*
Carbarsone, *43*
Carbenicillin indanyl sodium, *28*
Carbimazole, *43*
Carbon tetrachloride poisoning
    steatohepatitis after, 72
    toxic hepatitis after, 104,105
Carcinoma. *See also* specific name of tumor
    granulomas associated with, 82
    of bile ducts in cystic fibrosis, 126
Cardiac cirrhosis in congestive heart failure, 240
Carisoprodol, *43*
Carmustine (BCNU), *253*
Caroli's disease, associated conditions, 116, 208-210, **211**
Cefadroxil monohydrate, *43*
Cefazolin sodium, *43*
Celiac disease, steatohepatitis in, 73
Cellulose, definition, 184
Centrilobular fibrosis. *See* Fibrosis
Centrilobular necrosis. *See also* Necrosis...
    definition and associated conditions, 95, 96
    in allograft rejection, 214
Cephalexin, *90*

Ceroid
    definition, 184
    in lobular (viral) hepatitis, 199
    in porphyria cutanea tarda, 178
Ceruloplasmin, normal levels, 261
Cessation of drinking, morphologic features after, 114, 175
Chaparral leaf and toxic hepatitis, 105
Chlorambucil, 43
Chlordiazepoxide, 43, 108
Chlorinated benzenes and toxic hepatitis, 105
Chlorothiazide, 18, 43, 139
Chlorpromazine (tabulated), 18, 43, 90, 139, 229
Chlorpromazine administration
    induction cells after, 157
    lipochrome deposition after, 193
Chlorpropamide, 44, 90
Chlortetracycline, 44, 65, 107
Chlorthalidone, 44
Cholangiectases and biliary cysts
    definition, 204
    in Caroli's disease, 208, 211
    in PSC, 220
Cholangiocarcinoma
    after thorotrast deposition, 198
    definition and morphologic features, 207
    in Caroli's disease, 208-210
    in fibropolycystic liver disease, 208
    in hepatolithiasis, 208
    in PSC, 208
Cholangiolar proliferation. See Proliferation of bile ductules
Cholangitic abscess
    in Caroli's disease, 210
    in obstructive biliary cirrhosis, 132
Cholangitis
    in acquired immune deficiency syndrome, 224
    in allograft rejection, 213, 214
    in bacterial infection, 223
    in obstructive biliary cirrhosis, 132
    in PBC, 223, 224, 225
    in PSC, 3, 12, 35, 220
    in viral hepatitis, 227, 228
    types and associated clinical conditions, 206
Cholangitis and cholangiolitis, definition, 204
Cholate stasis
    definition, 94

in PBC, 136, 144
in PSC, **35**
Choledochal cyst and fibropolycystic liver disease, 208
Choledocholithiasis, portal fibrosis in, **117**
Cholestasis
    and lymphoma, 51
    chronic copper accumulation in, 191
    drug-induced, 51, *53*
    in acute fatty liver of pregnancy, 56
    in acute viral hepatitis A, 10
    in acute viral hepatitis E, 22
    in alcoholic cirrhosis, 123
    in alcoholic foamy degeneration, 58
    in amyloidosis, 50
    in chronic lobular hepatitis, 36
    in CNDC, **36**, 37
    in copper storage disease, 191
    in cystic fibrosis, 126
    in heart disease and shock, 99
    in hepatocellular carcinoma, 51
    in Indian childhood cirrhosis, 196
    in liver cell adenoma, 51
Cholestatic hepatitis
    definition and associated clinical conditions, 31, *32*
    drug-induced, *43-45*
    feathery degeneration in, 144
    in allograft rejection, 214
    in CNDC, **36**
    in PSC, **35**
    in toxic oil syndrome, 225
Cholestatic steatohepatitis, alcoholic, **34**
Cholesterol, normal levels, 261
Cholesteryl ester storage disease, findings in, 63, 116, 154
Chronic active viral hepatitis. *See* Viral hepatitis
Chronic active hepatitis (CAH)
    cholestasis in, 34
    drug-induced, 14, *18*
    endotheliitis in, 237
    in remission, 2
    lobular hepatitis in, 22
    necrosis in, 98
    other morphologic features, 113
    periportal hepatitis in, 11
    piecemeal necrosis in, **100**
    steatohepatitis in, 71

Chronic active hepatitis B and posthepatitic cirrhosis, 134, **135**
Chronic active hepatitis C, histologic features, 11
Chronic alcoholic hepatitis. *See* Alcoholic hepatitis
Chronic congestion. *See* Congestion
Chronic granulomatous disease of childhood, lipofuscin in, 191
Chronic hemodialysis
    granulomas after, 83
    peliosis hepatis after, 250
Chronic intrahepatic cholestasis of sarcoidosis, clinical and morphologic features,
    42, 137, 211
Chronic lobular hepatitis
    cholestasis in, 36
    definition, 23
    in non-A, non-B infection, **25**
Chronic nonsuppurative destructive cholangitis (CNDC) and PBC
    cholestasis in, **36**, 37
    copper in, **192**
    granulomas in, **81, 82**
    other morphologic features, 80, 191
    periportal hepatitis in, 13, **13**
    portal hepatitis in, 3, **4**
Chronic persistent hepatitis, portal hepatitis in, 4
Cimetidine (tabulated), *44, 108*
Cimetidine hemochromatosis, morphologic features, 175
Circulatory failure, necrosis in, 99
Cirrhosis. *See* also under specific name such as Alcoholic cirrhosis
    after thorotrast deposition, 198
    and sideroblastic anemia, 179
    and thalassemia major, 179
    definition and associated clinical conditions, 121, *122-123*
    drug-induced, *139*
    in abetalipoproteinemia, 73
    in alpha-1-antichymotrypsin deficiency, 151
    in alpha-1-antitrypsin deficiency, 124, **152, 153**
    in chronic active hepatitis B, **135**
    in copper storage disease, 191
    reversibility in hemochromatosis, 177
Cisplatin, *44, 64*
Clometacine (tabulated), *18, 65*
Clometacine-induced multinucleated hepatocytes, 157
Clorazepate dipotassium, *44*
CMV. *See* Cytomegalovirus
CNDC. *See* Chronic nonsuppurative destructive cholangitis and PBC
Cocaine hepatitis, morphologic features in, 99
Common test abnormalities. *See* name of substance

Congenital atransferrinemia, morphologic features, 175
Congenital hepatic fibrosis
    and fibropolycystic liver disease, 208
    associated conditions and findings, 116, 210
    bile ducts in, **115**
    cholestasis in, 38
    portal hypertension in, 209
    portal vein hypoplasia in, 209, 240
Congestion
    cirrhosis in, 129
    fibrosis in, 114
    hyalin globules in, 154
    in Budd-Chiari syndrome, 239
    in heart failure, 240
    in heat stroke, 60
Contraceptive drugs, adverse effects, 53, 90, 253
Copper
    after total parenteral nutrition, 199
    histochemical characteristics, 184
    in CNDC, **192**
    in focal nodular hyperplasia, 200
    in hepatocellular carcinoma, 200
    in idiopathic adulthood ductopenia, 196
    in Indian childhood cirrhosis, 131, 196
    in infantile obstructive cholangiopathy, 197
    in nodular transformation of the liver, 200
    in paucity of intrahepatic bile ducts, 219
    in PBC, 136
    in PSC, 199
    in Wilson's disease, 18, 200
    normal levels, 262, 264
Copper poisoning, fibrosis in, 119
Copper storage disease, morphologic features, 191
Copper sulfate sprays, granulomas induced by, 81
Copper-associated protein, 131
Councilman bodies
    definition, 144
    in lobular hepatitis, 22
Corticosteroids, 65, 254
Cowdry type A inclusion bodies, associated clinical conditions, 103, 105
Coxsackie virus infection, necrosis in, 105
C-reactive protein in hepatocellular carcinoma, 160
Cromolyn sodium, 228
Cryptococcosis, necrosis in, 105
Cryptogenic cirrhosis, definition and features, 129

Cyanamide administration and groundglass hepatocytes, 157
Cyclosporin, *44*
Cystadenocarcinoma, definition and morphologic features, 207
Cysteamine, *253*
Cystic disease of the liver and fibropolycystic liver disease, 208-210
Cystic fibrosis
    biliary strictures in, 212
    cholestasis in, 38
    cirrhosis in, 126
    mucus plugging in, 38
    other morphologic features, 212
Cystine, definition, 185
Cystinosis, morphologic features, 192
CMV hepatitis
    associated clinical conditions, 224
    granulomas in, 88
    lobular hepatitis in, 26
    necrosis in, 100, **101**
    obliterative cholangitis in, 224
    other morphologic features, 155
    viral inclusions in, **155**
Cytosine arabinoside, *253*

D

Dacarbazine, *44, 108, 253*
Danazol, *254*
Danthron, *18*
Dantrolene sodium, *18, 28, 44, 65, 108, 139*
Dapsone, *90, 108*
Daunorubicin hydrochloride, *107, 253*
Delta antigen and sanded nuclei, 166
Desipramine hydrochloride, *107*
Diabetes mellitus
    and fatty liver, 62
    and peliosis hepatis, 249
    and steatohepatitis, 71
    nuclear glycogen in, 146
Diazepam, *44, 90, 107, 229*
Diclofenac, *18, 28, 44, 108*
Didanosine, *65*
Dietary iron ingestion, morphologic features, 175
Diethylstilbestrol diphosphate, *254*
Diltiazem hydrochloride, *76, 90*

Dimethylformamide-induced fatty change, 63
Dimethylnitrosamine poisoning, morphologic features in, 252
Disopyramide phosphate, 28, 44
Disseminated intravascular coagulation, morphologic features, 104, 241
Disulfiram (tabulated), 28, 107, 108
Disulfiram administration, groundglass hepatocytes after, 157
Diverticula of common bile duct and fibropolycystic liver disease, 208
Diverticulitis, suppurative pylephlebitis in, 247
Diverticulosis and steatohepatitis, 73
Drug-induced changes. See following and under generic names of drugs
Drug-induced cholangitis and cirrhosis, 137
Drug-induced cholestatic hepatitis, 38, 43-45
Drug-induced cirrhosis, 129, 139
Drug-induced fatty change, **59**, 64-65
Drug-induced hepatitis
    after nitrofurantoin administration, **26**
    after phenytoin sodium administration, **15**
    and bile duct abnormalities, 212, 229
    and granulomas, 80, 81, 90
    and lobular hepatitis, 24, **26**, 28
    and periportal hepatitis, 14, 18
    and portal hepatitis, 5
Drug-induced Mallory bodies, 76, 157
Drug-induced necrosis, 107, 108
Drug-induced steatohepatitis, 76
Drug-induced vascular changes, morphologic features, 242, 253, 254
Dubin-Johnson syndrome, morphologic features, 185, 193, **194**
Ductal obliteration. See Obliterative cholangitis
Ductal proliferation. See Proliferation of bile ducts
Ductopenia
    definition and associated clinical conditions, 205, 207
    drug-induced, 228
    in acquired immune deficiency syndrome, 224
    in allograft rejection, 214
    in bile duct obstruction, 42,132
    in CAH, 227
    in graft-versus-host disease, 213
    in idiopathic adulthood ductopenia, 215, **215**
    in infantile obstructive cholangiopathy, 40
    in lymphoproliferative disorders, 216
    in obstructive biliary cirrhosis, 132
    in paucity of intrahepatic bile ducts, 219
    in PBC, 13, **14**, 222
    in PSC, 3, 12
Ductular cholestasis in CNDC, **36**, 37

Ductular piecemeal necrosis, definition, 94
Ductular proliferation. *See* Proliferation of bile ductules
Dysplasia of hepatocytes, conditions with, 144

E

ECHO virus infection and necrosis, 105
Eclampsia and preeclampsia, morphologic features, 101, **102**, 249
Enalapril, *44*
Endotheliitis
    and phlebitis in acute fatty liver of pregnancy, 56
    and phlebitis in allograft rejection, 243
    and phlebitis in viral hepatitis, **237**
    in acquired immune deficiency syndrome, 27
    in alcoholic liver disease, 237
    in nonalcoholic steatohepatitis, 249
    in other clinical conditions, *234-235*
    in sarcoidosis, 250
Enflurane, *28, 107*
Epping jaundice. *See* Methylenediamine poisoning
Erythromycin, *18, 44, 108*
Erythrophagocytosis
    differential diagnosis, 150
    in benign postoperative intrahepatic cholestasis, 50
Erythropoietic disorders and hemochromatosis, 133
Erythropoietic protoporphyria, morphologic features, 126,194
Ethylene dichloride and toxic hepatitis, 105
Ethacrynic acid, *108*
Ethchlorvynol, *44, 53*
Ethinyl estradiol, *253*
Ethionamide, *44, 107*
Etretinate, 65
Extrahepatic biliary atresia and ductopenia, 40
Extrahepatic malignant tumors, granulomas in, 81, 82
Extramedullary hematopoiesis
    in acute fatty liver of pregnancy, 56
    in hepatic allografts, 160

F

Fabry's disease, morphologic features, 157
Familial intrahepatic cholestatic syndromes, histologic features, 52
Fasting and steatohepatitis, 73
Fatty changes, definitions and associated clinical conditions, 55-67

Fatty liver hepatitis. *See* Nonalcoholic steatohepatitis
Feathery degeneration
    features and associated clinical conditions, 144
    in allografts, **39**
Ferritin
    definition, 173
    in lobular (viral) hepatitis, 22, **180**
    in periportal (viral) hepatitis, 17
    in portal (viral) hepatitis, 8
    normal levels, 262
Ferrous fumarate (or other salts of iron), *139*
Ferrous sulfate poisoning, morphologic features, 105
Fibrin ring granulomas, possible causes, 88
Fibrin thrombi
    in disseminated intravascular coagulation, 104
    in eclampsia, 101, 250
Fibrinogen storage disease, morphologic features, 157
Fibropolycystic liver diseases
    cholangiocarcinoma in, 208
    cholestasis in, 38
    definition and morphologic features, 208
Fibrosing cholestatic viral hepatitis B, 38
Fibrosis
    definition and associated clinical conditions, 111, *112*
    in hypervitaminosis A, 246
    in sideroblastic anemia and thalassemia major, 179
Fibrous cholangitis. *See* Fibrous-obliterative cholangitis
    and periportal hepatitis, 12
    and portal hepatitis, 3
    as healing stage of nonsuppurative cholangitis, 212
    definition, 204
    in bile duct obstruction, 218
    in PBC, 222
    in PSC, 3, 12, 220, **220**
    in viral hepatitis and CAH, 227
Fibrous-obliterative cholangitis
    after bone marrow transplantation, 213
    and cholestatic hepatitis, 35
    definition, 204
    in PSC, 3, 12, 35, 220
Fibrous piecemeal necrosis, definition, 94
5-Fluoro-2'-deoxyuridine, *253*
Florid duct lesions. *See* Granulomatous cholangitis
Floxuridine, 65
Fluoxymesterone, *44, 53, 254*

Fluphenazine, *44*
Flurazepam hydrochloride, *44*, 65
Flutamide, *44*
Foam cell arteriopathy, intimal changes in, **246**
Focal biliary cirrhosis in cystic fibrosis of the liver, 212
Focal dilatation of intrahepatic bile ducts. *See* Caroli's disease
Focal fatty changes, morphologic features, 59, **60, 61,** 75
Focal necrosis, definition, 95
Focal nodular hyperplasia, morphologic features, 130, **130,** 200
Foreign body giant cells and granulomas
    after intravenous substance abuse, 196
    after long-term hemodialysis, 83
    after silicone administration, 82, 193
Formalin pigment, definition and morphologic features, 166, **168,** 185
Fructose intolerance and fatty change, 63
Fucosidosis, morphologic features, 158
Fulminant viral hepatitis, necrosis in, 97
Functional cholestasis in allografts, 39, **39**

G

Galactosemia
    and fatty changes, **62,** 63
    cirrhosis in, 126
Gamma globulin, normal levels, 262
Gamma-glutamyl transferase, normal levels, 262
Gastrointestinal and pancreatic disorders, fatty liver in, 62
Gastrointestinal disorders and steatohepatitis, 72
Gastroplasty and steatohepatitis, 73
Genetic hemochromatosis
    hepatic iron content in, 176
    hepatic iron index in, 176
    morphologic features, 133, **134, 176**
Genetic liver diseases. *See* also under specific disease name
    and fatty liver, 62
    and steatohepatitis, 73
    fibrosis in, 116
Giant cell transformation. *See* also Hepatocellular giant cells
    in galactosemia, 127
    in hereditary fructose intolerance, 127
    in neonatal liver disease, 163
    in paucity of intrahepatic bile ducts, 219
Giant lysosomes, morphologic features, 146, 150
Gilbert's syndrome, morphologic features, 194

Glycogen storage disease, morphologic features, 116, 159
Glycogen storage disease type I
    fatty changes in, 63
    liver cell adenoma in, 131
Glycogen storage disease type III, **158**
Glycogen storage disease type IV, cirrhosis in, 127
Glycogen storage in Mauriac's syndrome, 162
Glycogenated nuclei in Wilson's disease, 167
Glycogenic inclusions in nuclei, morphologic features, 146
Gold sodium thiomalate, *44, 53, 65, 90*
Graft-versus-host disease
    cirrhosis in, 137
    cholestatic hepatitis in, 38
    other morphologic features, 213, 242
    portal hepatitis in, 5
Granulomas and granulomatous hepatitis
    definition and associated clinical conditions, 79, 80
    drug-induced, 90
    in CNDC, **4**, 13, **13**, 80, **81, 82**
    in focal fatty change, 75
    in Hodgkin's disease, **83**
    in periportal hepatitis, 13, **13**
    in portal hepatitis, **4**
    in sarcoid cirrhosis, 136
    in tuberculosis and acquired immune deficiency syndrome, **86, 87**
    of unknown cause, **89**
    with giant cells, **13**
Granulomatous cholangitis
    definitions, 204
    in chronic intrahepatic cholestasis of sarcoidosis, 211
    in PBC, 80, **81, 82**, 222
    in toxic oil syndrome, 225
Granulomatous diseases, sinusoidal dilatation in, 242
Griseofulvin, *44*
Groundglass hepatocytes
    after cyanamide administration, 157
    after disulfiram administration, 157
    cytologic features, 145
    in fibrinogen storage disease, 157
    in hepatitis B, 165, **166**
    in hepatocellular carcinoma, 160

H

Haloperidol, *44, 229*

Halothane (tabulated), *18, 28, 44, 65, 90, 107, 108, 139*
Halothane administration, necrosis after, 102, **103**
Healed infarcts, associated conditions, 116
Health food and toxic hepatitis, 105
Heart diseases, necrosis in, 99
Heat stroke, morphologic features after, 59, 213
Hemangiomatosis after metoclopramide administration, 242
Hemangiosarcoma
    after thorotrast deposition, 198
    other etiologies and complications, 252
Hematoidin
    definition, 185
    in hemorrhages and infarcts, 197
Hematomas. *See* Hemorrhages
Hemochromatosis, primary (genetic), pigment cirrhosis in, 133
Hemochromatosis after portacaval shunting, morphologic features, 177
Hemochromatosis after venovenous shunts, cirrhosis in, 133
Hemochromatosis associated with alcoholism, cirrhosis in, 133
Hemochromatosis in erythropoietic disorders, cirrhosis in, 133
Hemodialysis. *See* Chronic hemodialysis
Hemolysis, morphologic features after, 43, 181
Hemolytic uremic syndrome, cholestasis in, 43
Hemorrhages
    after streptokinase administration, 250
    and hematoidin, 197
    in hemangiosarcomas, 252
    in liver cell adenomas, 242
    in preeclampsia and eclampsia, 250
Hemosiderin. *See also* Hemochromatosis… and Iron pigmentation…
    after phlebotomies, 133
    after total parenteral nutrition, 199
    definition, 174
    effects of phlebotomy therapy, 177
    in genetic hemochromatosis, 133, **176**
    in heat stroke, 59
    in leukemia and lymphoma, 6, 15
    in malaria, 197
    in periportal hepatitis, 6, 15
    in pigment cirrhosis, 133
    in posthepatitic cirrhosis, 134
    in thalassemia major, **178**
    in yellow fever hepatitis, 106
Hemozoin in malaria, 185, 197
Hepatic allografts
    and hepatitis B (fibrosing cholestatic hepatitis), 38

centrilobular fibrosis in, 116
CMV infection in, 100, 224
dysfunction and cholestasis, 39
necrosis in, 97
other morphologic features, 160
rejection in. *See* Allograft rejection
Hepatic atrophy, morphologic features, 195
Hepatic hypoperfusion and surgical hepatitis, 26
Hepatic venous outflow obstruction, findings and causes, 239, 244
Hepatitis. *See* etiologic designation such as Herpes simplex hepatitis
Hepatocellular carcinoma
abnormal cellular inclusions in, 160
after thorotrast deposition, 198
cholestasis in, 51
copper in, 200
in alpha-1-antitrypsin deficiency, 151
in genetic hemochromatosis, 177
in glycogen storage disease type Ia, 159
in tyrosinemia, 128
sinusoidal dilatation in, 247
with giant cells, **161**
Hepatocellular giant cells. *See* also Giant cell transformation
after vinyl chloride poisoning, 165
and infantile obstructive cholangiopathy, 40
drug-induced, *157*
in hepatic allografts, 160
in hepatocellular carcinoma, 160
in neonatal liver disease, 163, **163**
in syncytial giant cell hepatitis, 165
in viral hepatitis non-A, non-B, 166
Hepatocellular inclusions
definition and associated clinical conditions, 145-147, *147-148*
in porphyria cutanea tarda, 178
Hepatocellular necrosis, morphologic features, 195
Hepatocellular nodules, definition, 121
Hepatocellular rosettes and periportal hepatitis, **14**
Hepatocellular storage cells, definition, 145
Hepatolithiasis
cholangiocarcinoma in, 208
in Caroli's disease, 210
in cystic fibrosis, 126
Hepatoportal sclerosis in idiopathic portal hypertension, 117, 246, **247**
Hepatotoxic chemicals
and fatty changes, 62
and steatohepatitis, 72

Herbal hepatitis, necrosis in, 105
Hereditary fructose intolerance, morphologic features, 127
Hereditary hemorrhagic telangiectasia, morphologic features, 125, 126
Herpes simplex hepatitis, morphologic features, 102-103, 105, **156**
Hodgkin's disease, granulomas in, **83**, 88
Hornet stings, features of Reye's syndrome after, 64
Hunter's syndrome, fibrosis in, 127
Hurler's syndrome, fibrosis in, 127
Hyalin globules
    in congestion, 146, 154
    in hepatocellular carcinoma, 160
Hydralazine hydrochloride, 28, 90, *108*
Hydrochlorothiazide, 28
Hydroxyethyl starch administration, liver cell changes after, 157
Hyperparathyroidism, calcification in, 160, 245
Hypervitaminosis A, morphologic features, 116, 245
Hypoxia, morphologic features associated with, 62, 161

I

Ibuprofen, 65
I-cell disease, morphologic features, 161
Idiopathic adulthood ductopenia
    cirrhosis in, 137
    clinical findings and morphologic features, 214
    copper in, 196
Idiopathic arterial calcification of infancy, 246
Idiopathic CAH. *See* Viral hepatitis and idiopathic (autoimmune) CAH
Idiopathic copper toxicosis. *See* Copper storage disease and Indian childhood
    cirrhosis
Idiopathic granulomatous hepatitis, morphologic features, 89
Idiopathic perinatal hemochromatosis, morphologic features, 133, 177
Idiopathic portal hypertension, criteria and features, 117, 246, **247**
Imipramine, *44, 107, 229*
Immune diseases and granulomas, 83
Inclusion bodies. *See* Hepatocellular inclusions and Viral inclusion bodies
Indian childhood cirrhosis, morphologic features, 130, 196
Indomethacin, *44, 65, 107, 108*
Induction cells after drug administration, 157
Infantile obstructive cholangiopathy. *See also* Paucity of intrahepatic bile ducts
    cirrhosis in, 137
    copper in, 197
    in alpha-1-antitrypsin deficiency, 151
    other morphologic features, 40

Infantile polycystic liver disease. *See* Autosomal-recessive cystic disease of the liver
Infarctions
    after oral contraceptive administration, 242
    and liver cell adenomas, 242
    hematoidin in, 197
    in allografts, **98**
    in eclampsia and preeclampsia, 102, 250
Infarcts of Zahn, morphologic features, 247
Infectious mononucleosis
    granulomas in, 88
    lobular hepatitis in, 26, **76**
    necrosis in, 105
    portal hepatitis in, **6**
Infective intra-abdominal conditions, hepatic changes in, 216
Inspissated bile in congenital hepatic fibrosis, 209
Inspissated bile syndrome, morphologic features, 51
Interferon, *18*
Intravenous substance abuse, morphologic features after, 196
Iodipamide meglumine, *44, 107*
Iron, normal levels, 262-264
Iron index in genetic hemochromatosis, 176
Iron ingestion, morphologic features after, 175
Iron pigmentation, associated clinical conditions, 174-182
Iron-negative pigments, definition and associated clinical conditions, 183, *188-189*
Iron-positive pigments, definition and associated clinical conditions, 173, *174*
Isocarboxacid, *44*
Isoflurane, *108*
Isoniazid, *18, 28, 44, 65, 90, 107, 108, 139*
Ito cells in hypervitaminosis A, 116, 246

J

Jamaican vomiting sickness, microvesicular changes in, 60
Jejunoileal bypass surgery and steatohepatitis, 73, **74, 75**

K

Ketoconazole, *28, 108*
Ketoprofen, *65*
Kupffer cell hemosiderosis
    after blood transfusion, **179**
    in benign postoperative cholestasis, 50
Kwashiorkor and periportal fatty changes, 63

L

Labetalol (tabulated), *107, 108*
Labetalol hepatitis, necrosis in, 103
Labrea hepatitis. *See* Viral hepatitis D
Lactate dehydrogenase, normal levels, 263
Lafora bodies in progressive familial myoclonic epilepsy, 164
Lead poisoning, morphologic features, 162
Leishmaniasis and lobular hepatitis, 26
Leptospirosis and cholestasis, 43
Lergotrile mesylate, *28*
Leukemia
    simulating lobular hepatitis, 24
    simulating periportal hepatitis, 15
    simulating portal hepatitis, 6
Limb lipodystrophy and steatohepatitis, 73
Lipid inclusions in nuclei, 147
Lipochrome, definition, 185
Lipochrome deposition, drug-induced, 193
Lipocytes in hypervitaminosis A, 116, 246
Lipofuscin, definition and associated clinical conditions, 185, 189-199, **195**
Lipogranulomas
    after mineral oil ingestion, 84
    after weight-reducing surgery, 84
Lisinopril, *44, 107*
Listeriosis, necrosis in, 105
Liver cell adenoma
    associated clinical conditions and causes, 131
    cholestasis in, 51
    in galactosemia, 127
    in glycogen storage disease type Ia, 131, 159
    in toxic oil syndrome, 225
    in tyrosinosis, 131
    infarctions and hemorrhages in, 242
    other morphologic features, 131
    steatohepatitis in, 75
    vascular changes in, 247
Liver function abnormalities. *See* under name of substance
Lobular hepatitis
    ceroid deposition in, 199
    definition and associated clinical conditions, 21, *22*
    drug-induced, *28*
    necrosis in, 104
Loss of bile ducts. *See* Ductopenia
Lymphocytic cholangitis
    definition and associated clinical conditions, 204, 206

in PSC, 219
in viral hepatitis and idiopathic (autoimmune) CAH, 227
Lymphocytic piecemeal necrosis, definition and associated clinical conditions, 94, 96
Lymphoid follicles
    in CNDC, **81**
    in hepatitis C, 11-12
Lymphoma
    bile duct changes in, 216
    cholestasis associated with, 52
    granulomas associated with, 82, 88
    pseudoendotheliitis in, **249**
    simulating lobular hepatitis, 24
    simulating periportal hepatitis, 15
    simulating portal hepatitis, **5**, 6
    vascular changes in, 248
Lymphoproliferative disease. *See* Lymphoma

M

Macroregenerative nodules, definition, 131
Macrovesicular fatty changes, drug-induced, 64, 65
Malabsorption and malnutrition, fatty liver in, 62
Malabsorption and steatohepatitis, 73
Malaria, morphologic features, 26, 197
Malaria pigment, histochemical characteristics, 186
Malignancies, peliosis hepatis associated with, 248, 249
Malignancy-associated changes. *See* Tumor-associated changes
Malignant hepatocellular giant cells, **161**
Malignant lymphoma. *See* Lymphoma
Malignant melanoma, 197
Mallory bodies
    drug-induced, **76**, 157
    in alcoholic cirrhosis, 33, 70, 123
    in alcoholic hepatitis, 70, **71**, **150**
    in biliary cirrhosis, 123, 136
    in copper storage disease, 191
    in Indian childhood cirrhosis, 131, 196
    in liver cell adenoma, 75
    in nonalcoholic steatohepatitis, 71, **72**, **151**
    in PBC, 136
    in PSC, **35**
    in Wilson's disease, 18
    morphologic features, 146
    other associated clinical conditions, 148

Malnutrition and steatohepatitis, 73
Mannosidosis, morphologic features, 162
Marasmus, peliosis hepatis in, 248
Margosa oil and microvesicular fatty change, 63
Massive hepatic necrosis, possible causes, 104
Massive or submassive hepatic necrosis, cholestasis in, 41
Mauriac's syndrome, morphologic features, 162
Mediterranean-type chronic hepatitis, steatohepatitis in, 74
Megamitochondria
    in acute fatty liver of pregnancy, 56
    in alcoholic liver disease, 58, 150
    morphologic features, 150
Melanin, definition, 186
Melanin in malignant melanoma, 197
Melioidosis, necrosis in, 105
Mephobarbital, 108
Meprobamate, 44
Mercaptopurine (tabulated), 28, 44, 107, 139
Mercaptopurine-induced multinucleated hepatocytes, 157
Mestranol, 53, 90, 253
Methandrostenolone, 53, 254
Methimazole, 28, 65
Methotrexate (tabulated), 65, 76, 139
Methotrexate administration
    fatty changes after, 59
    multinucleated hepatocytes after, 157
Methoxsalen, 28
Methoxyflurane, 28, 107, 108
Methyldopa, 18, 28, 44, 65, 90, 107, 108, 139
Methylenediamine poisoning, bile duct damage after, 212
Methyltestosterone, 53, 139, 229, 253, 254
Metoclopramide administration, hemangiomatosis after, 242
Metolazone, 90
Microabscesses in systemic infections, 105
Microthrombi in disseminated intravascular coagulation, 241
Microvesicular fatty changes
    drug-induced, 65
    in acute fatty liver of pregnancy, 56, 57
    in cocaine hepatitis, 99
    in toxic shock syndrome, 224
    other associated clinical conditions, 56
Midzonal necrosis, definition and associated conditions, 95, 96, 106
Mineral oil granulomas, 84
Mitomycin, 108, 253
Mixed hamartoma, morphologic features, 131

Mixed-cell or pleomorphic cholangitis, definition and associated clinical
　　conditions, 204, 206, 219, 227
Morbid obesity. *See* Obesity
Mucocutaneous lymph node syndrome, cholangitis in, 217
Mucolipidosis, subtypes, 161, 162
Mucopolysaccharidosis, morphologic features, 116, 127
Mucoviscidosis. *See* Cystic fibrosis
Mucus in cystic fibrosis, 38
Multilobular biliary fibrosis in cystic fibrosis of the liver, 212
Multilobular (confluent) necrosis, definition, 95
Multilobular necrosis, associated clinical conditions, 96
Multilobular necrosis and lobular hepatitis, 27
Multinucleated giant cells. *See* Hepatocellular giant cells and Giant cell
　　transformation
Multiple myeloma, peliosis hepatis in, 252
Mushroom poisoning, necrosis in, 104
Myeloproliferative disease. *See* Leukemia
Myoclonic epilepsy. *See* Progressive familial myoclonic epilepsy

N

Naproxen, 76
Necrosis
　　and postnecrotic states, associated clinical conditions, 96
　　definition, 93
　　drug-induced, *107, 108*
　　in allografts, 97, **97**
　　in halothane hepatitis, **103**
Necrosis of liver cells, morphologic features, 195
Necrotizing vasculitis and peliosis hepatis, 249
Neonatal hemochromatosis. *See* Idiopathic perinatal hemochromatosis
Neonatal hepatitis
　　and idiopathic perinatal hemochromatosis, 177
　　morphologic features, 163
Neutrophilic cholangiolitis
　　in periportal hepatitis, **16**
　　in septicemia, **226**
Neutrophilic cholangitis
　　after bile duct obstruction, **216, 217**
　　and cholangiolitis, definition and associated clinical conditions, 204, 206
　　as tumor-associated change, 226, 252
　　in alcoholic hepatitis, 207
　　in Caroli's disease, 116, **210**, 211
　　in heat stroke, 60, 213

in infective intra-abdominal conditions, 216
in PSC, 220
in toxic shock syndrome, 64, 224
Neutrophils in surgery-associated hepatitis, 25
Nicardipine, 76
Nicotinic acid, *18, 28, 44, 108*
Niemann-Pick disease, morphologic features, 164
Nifedipine (tabulated), *44, 76*
Nifedipine-induced steatohepatitis, 75
Nitrofurantoin, *18, 28, 44, 65, 90, 108, 139*
Nodular regenerative hyperplasia
    and portal vein obliteration, 251
    copper in, 200
    in angioimmunoblastic lymphadenopathy, 238
    in hereditary hemorrhagic telangiectasia, 126
    in idiopathic portal hypertension, 246
    in toxic oil syndrome, 225
    other morphologic features, 131, **132**
Nonalcoholic fatty liver, associated clinical conditions and morphologic features,
    62, 164
Nonalcoholic steatohepatitis
    associated clinical conditions, 71-73
    cirrhosis in, 128
    endotheliitis in, 249
    fibrosis in, 115
    other morphologic features, **72, 74, 75**, 164
Nonspecific reactive hepatitis
    lobular hepatitis in, 25
    periportal hepatitis in, 16
    portal hepatitis in, 6
Nonsuppurative cholangitis
    definition, 204
    drug-induced, *228*
    in acquired immune deficiency syndrome, 27
    periductal fibrosis after, 118
Norethindrone, *53, 90, 253*
Norethynodrel, *53, 90*
Norfloxacin, *107*
Norgestrel, *53, 90*
North American Indian cholestasis, classification, 52
Norwegian cholestasis, classification, 52

O

Obesity
    fatty liver in, 62

lipogranulomas in, 84
    steatohepatitis in, 73, **74, 75**
Obliterative cholangitis
    after CMV infection, 224
    after graft-versus-host disease, 213
    in PSC, 220, **221, 222**
Obstruction of bile ducts. *See* Bile duct obstruction
Omphalitis, pylephlebitic abscesses in, 247
Oncocytes
    etiology and morphologic features, 150-151
    in alcoholic liver disease, 150
    in PBC, **167**
Oral contraceptive administration. *See* also specific names of drugs
    arterial changes after, 104, 242
    necrosis after, 104, 242
Oxacillin, *18, 44, 76, 90*
Oxymetholone, *254*
Oxyphenbutazone, *18*

P

Pale bodies in hepatocellular carcinoma, 160
Pancreatic disorders and steatohepatitis, 72
Papaverine hydrochloride, *18, 28, 44, 90, 139*
Para-aminosalicylic acid–induced multinucleated hepatocytes, 157
Paraneoplastic cholestasis, 52
Paraneoplastic granulomas, 82, **83**
Paraquat poisoning and bile duct damage, 212
Partial nodular transformation, morphologic features, 133
Paucity of intrahepatic bile ducts, definition, and morphologic features, 218-219
PBC. *See* Primary biliary cirrhosis
Peliosis hepatis
    associated clinical conditions, *235-236*
    drug-induced, *254*
Pemoline, *108*
Penicillamine, *44*
Penicillin, *18, 28, 44, 90*
Perhexiline maleate (tabulated), *76, 139*
Perhexiline maleate–induced steatohepatitis, 75
Pericholangitis, associated clinical conditions, 137, 220
Periductal fibrosis. *See* also Fibrous cholangitis
    in nonsuppurative cholangitis, 118
    near hepatic tumors, 218
    unknown causes, 119

Periportal hepatitis
    definition and associated clinical conditions, 9, *10*
    drug-induced, **15**, *18*
    in drug addicts, 17
Periportal necrosis
    after phosphorus and ferrous sulfate poisoning, 105
    definition, 95
    in viral hepatitis A, 10
Perphenazine, *18, 44*
Phagosomes in congestion, 155
Phenacetin administration, lipochrome deposition after, 193
Phenazopyridine hydrochloride, 28
Phenelzine sulfate, *108*
Phenobarbital, *44, 108*
Phenylbutazone, *28, 45, 90, 108, 139, 229*
Phenytoin sodium, *18, 28, 45, 90, 108*
Phlebitis and phlebosclerosis in alcoholic liver disease, 33, 70, 237, **238**
Phlebitis in lobular hepatitis, 22, **25**
Phlebosclerosis
    in alcoholic hepatitis, 70, **238**
    in hypervitaminosis A, 116
    in idiopathic portal hypertension, 117, 246
Phospholipidosis
    drug-induced, 63, 157
    in Niemann-Pick disease, 63
Phosphorus poisoning, morphologic features, 105
Piecemeal necrosis. *See also* Periportal hepatitis and Lobular hepatitis
    definition, 94
    in CAH, **100**
    in obstructive biliary cirrhosis, 153
    in PBC, 136, **136**, **137**
Pigment cirrhosis in primary hemochromatosis, 133, **134**
Pigmented macrophages
    in lobular hepatitis, 22
    in periportal hepatitis, 17
    in portal hepatitis, 8
Pigments. *See* Iron pigmentation and Iron-negative pigments
Piperazine preparations, *45*
Pipestem fibrosis in schistosomiasis, 119
Piroxicam, *45, 53, 108*
Pirprofen, *107*
Pizotyline, *45*
Polyarteritis nodosa, morphologic features, 83, 239, **239**
Polythiazide, *45*
Porphyria cutanea tarda, morphologic features, 63, 128, 178, 198

Portal edema
    after bile duct obstruction, 15, **40, 41, 216**
    as tumor-associated change, 7
Portal fibrosis
    in choledocholithiasis, **117**
    in idiopathic portal hypertension, 117, 246, **247**
Portal hepatitis
    definition and associated clinical conditions, 1, *2*
    in chronic persistent hepatitis, *3*
Portal vein changes in schistosomiasis, 119
Portal vein hypoplasia in congenital hepatic fibrosis, 209, 240
Portal vein obliteration in idiopathic portal hypertension, 117
Portal vein thrombosis
    in idiopathic portal hypertension, 117
    in infectious intra-abdominal processes, 247
    in toxic shock syndrome, 224
Posthepatitic cirrhosis, morphologic features, 134
Postnecrotic states, definition, 93
Postshunt hemochromatosis, definition, 133
Povidone, definition, 186
Povidone administration, morphologic features after, 198
Preeclampsia. *See* Eclampsia
Primary biliary cirrhosis (PBC). *See* also CNDC
    cholangitis in, **223, 224, 225**
    cholestasis in, **36**
    copper in, **192**
    endotheliitis in, 237
    feathery degeneration in, 144
    oncocytes in, **167**
    other morphologic features, 135, 222
    piecemeal necrosis in, **136, 137**
Primary hemochromatosis. *See* Genetic hemochromatosis
Primary portal hypertension. *See* Idiopathic portal hypertension
Primary sclerosing cholangitis (PSC)
    cholangiectases and bile duct obliteration in, **221, 222**
    cholangiocarcinoma in, 208
    cholestatic hepatitis in, 35
    cirrhosis in, 35, **138**
    endotheliitis in, 237
    fibrosis in, 118
    fibrous cholangitis in, **220**
    fibrous-obliterative cholangitis in, 3, 12, 35, 220
    granulomas in, 89
    other morphologic features, 88, 199, 219-220
    periportal hepatitis in, 12, **12**

portal hepatitis in, 2
Probenecid, *108*
Procainamide hydrochloride, *90*
Procarbazine hydrochloride, *90*
Prochlorperazine, *45, 53, 108, 229*
Progressive familial myoclonic epilepsy, morphologic features, 164
Progressive intrahepatic cholestasis, morphologic features, 52, 128
Proliferation of bile ducts
    definition, 203
    in bile duct obstruction, 41, **216**
Proliferation of bile ductules
    definition, 204
    in bile duct obstruction, **16**, 41
Propoxyphene hydrochloride, *45*
Propranolol, *28, 107*
Propylthiouracil, *18, 108*
Prothrombin time, normal levels, 262
Protoporphyrin
    histochemical characteristics, 186
    in erythropoietic protoporphyria, 194
PSC. *See* Primary sclerosing cholangitis
Pseudoendotheliitis in malignant lymphoma, 248, **249**
Pseudoinclusions in nuclei, 147
Pure cholestasis
    definition and associated clinical conditions, 49, 50
    drug-induced, 53
Pylephlebitic abscesses in infectious intra-abdominal processes, 247
Pylephlebitis after extrahepatic infections, 247, 251

Q

Q fever, granulomas in, 88
Quinethazone, *45*
Quinidine, *90, 107*
Quinine sulfate, *90*

R

Ranitidine hydrochloride, *90*
Recurrent intrahepatic cholestasis, morphologic features, 42, **52**
Recurrent pyogenic cholangitis, clinical findings and morphologic features, 220
Rejection. *See* Allograft rejection

Renal cell carcinoma
    sinusoidal dilatation associated with, 251
    Stauffer's syndrome in, 226, 251
Renal transplantation, peliosis hepatis in, 250
Rendu-Osler-Weber disease. See Hereditary hemorrhagic telangiectasia
Retinol. See Vitamin A
Reye's syndrome, clinical findings and morphologic features, 64
Rheumatoid arthritis, sinusoidal dilatation associated with, 250
Rifampin, 45, 65, 107
Rubella hepatitis, necrosis in, 105
Rupture of liver. See Hemorrhages

S

Salmonellosis, necrosis in, 105
Sanded nuclei in hepatitis B and D, 147, 166
Sanfilippo's syndrome, fibrosis in, 127
Sarcoidosis
    chronic intrahepatic cholestasis in, 42, 137, 211
    cirrhosis in, 136
    endotheliitis in, 250
    granulomas in, 84, **84**, 85, **85**
    other morphologic features, 85
Schaumann's bodies in granulomas, 80, 85
Schistosomiasis
    fibrosis in, 119
    other morphologic features, 199
    pigment in, 186
    portal vein changes in, 119, 250
Sclerosing cholangitis in acquired immune deficiency syndrome, 224
Secondary biliary cirrhosis. See Bile duct obstruction
Sepsis, hemolysis, and shock, morphologic findings in, **42**, 43, 64, 216, 251
Serologic findings in viral hepatitis, 265-266
Shock, morphologic features, 43, 99
Sideroblastic anemia, associated conditions and morphologic features in, 179
Silica, definition, 186
Silicone
    appearance after embolization, 193
    definition, 187
Silicosis. See Anthracosis and anthracosilicosis
Silver. See Argyria
Sinusoidal dilatation, associated clinical conditions, 234-235
Small-duct biliary cirrhosis, associated clinical conditions, 137
Smooth muscle antibodies, interpretation, 262

Solitary hepatic cyst, histologic features, 221
Spironolactone, 76
Spotty necroses
    definition, 95
    in lobular hepatitis, 22
    in portal hepatitis, 8
Sprue and peliosis hepatis, 249
Starch, definition and postsurgical deposition, 187, 198
Stauffer's syndrome. See Renal cell carcinoma
Steatohepatitis
    definition and associated clinical conditions, 69, 70
    drug-induced, 76
    in focal fatty change, 59
    morphologic features, 73-75
    obesity-related, Mallory bodies in, **151**
Streptokinase administration, hematomas after, 250
Submassive hepatic necrosis
    associated clinical conditions, 104
    endotheliitis in, 237
    possible causes, 104
Sudden childhood death, microvesicular fatty changes in, 64
Sulfadoxine, 90
Sulfamethizole, *18*
Sulfamethoxazole, *45, 90, 108*
Sulfanilamide, 90
Sulfasalazine, *28, 45, 76, 90, 107*
Sulfathiazole, 90
Sulfonamide(s), type unspecified, *18, 28, 45, 90, 108*
Sulindac (tabulated), *45, 65, 107*
Sulindac administration, neutrophilic cholangitis after, 212
Surgery, talc and starch deposition after, 198
Surgery-associated hepatitis, lobular changes in, 25
Syncytial giant cell hepatitis, morphologic features, 165
Syphilitic hepatitis, fibrosis in, 119
Systemic bacterial infections, hepatic changes in, 223
Systemic diseases and infections. See also Neutrophilic cholangitis and Pylephlebitis...
    lobular hepatitis in, 26
    necrosis in, 105
    periportal hepatitis in, 16
    portal hepatitis in, 7
Systemic viral diseases, hepatic changes in, 223

T

Talc, definition and postsurgical deposition, 187, 198

Tamoxifen, 65, 254
Tetracycline, 65
Thalassemia major, morphologic features in, **178**, 179
Thermal injury. See Burns and Heat stroke
Thiabendazole, 45, 139, 229
6-Thioguanine, 253, 254
Thiopental sodium, 45
Thioridazine, 45
Thorotrast, histologic and physical characteristics, 187
Thorotrast administration, hepatic changes after, 198, 251, 252
Thrombi and emboli, associated conditions, 251
Tocainide hydrochloride, 90
Tolazamide, 18, 45, 107
Tolbutamide, 45, 90, 229
Torres bodies in yellow fever hepatitis, 106
Total iron-binding capacity, normal levels, 263
Total parenteral nutrition
    cholestasis after, 51
    cholestatic hepatitis after, 34
    cirrhosis after, 126
    fatty liver after, 62
    other morphologic features after, 199
    steatohepatitis after, 34, 73
Toxemia of pregnancy. See Eclampsia
Toxic cirrhosis, associated conditions, 137
Toxic hepatitis. See Toxic cirrhosis
    bile duct abnormalities in, 212
    granulomas in, 80-81
    necrosis in, 105
    other morphologic features, 165
Toxic oil syndrome, bile duct changes in, 212, 225
Toxic shock syndrome, morphologic features, 64, 223, 251
Toxoplasmosis, morphologic features, 26, 88, 105
Transfusions. See Blood transfusions
Tranylcypromine sulfate, 28, 45
Trauma, morphologic findings in, 251
Triazolam, 45
Trichlormethiazide, 90
Trifluoperazine hydrochloride, 45, 229
Trimethadione, 28
Trimethobenzamide hydrochloride, 45
Trimethoprim, 45
Trimethoprim-sulfamethoxazole administration and phospholipidosis, 157
Tripelennamine, 45
Troleandomycin, 45

Tropical splenomegaly syndrome and lobular hepatitis, 26
Tuberculosis, granulomas in, 86, **86**, 87, **87**
Tumor necrosis, morphologic features, 105-106
Tumor-associated changes, 7, **7**, 226, 248, 251
Tyrosinemia
    and idiopathic perinatal hemochromatosis, 177
    fatty changes in, 63
    liver cell adenoma in, 131
    other morphologic features and associated conditions, 128

U

Unresolved viral hepatitis
    cholestatic hepatitis in, 33
    lobular hepatitis in, 27
    other morphologic features, 113
    periportal hepatitis in, 16
    portal hepatitis in, 7
    prognostic features, 27
    with bridging necrosis, **99**
Uric acid, normal levels, 263
Uroporphyrin
    histochemical characteristics, 187
    in porphyria cutanea tarda, 198

V

Vacuolated nuclei in Wilson's disease, 18
Valproic acid, *45, 65, 107, 108, 139, 253*
Vanishing bile duct syndrome in allograft rejection, 214
Varicella zoster infections, necrosis in, 105
Vascular tumors and pseudotumors, etiologies, 252
Veno-occlusive disease
    after thorotrast deposition, 198
    and obliterative venopathy, 240
    in alcoholic hepatitis, 70
    in hypervitaminosis A, 246
    other etiologies and findings, 252
Verapamil hydrochloride, *45*
Vinblastine sulfate, *253*
Vineyard workers, toxic hepatitis in, 81
Vinyl chloride poisoning
    angiosarcoma and other vascular changes after, 165, 252

multinucleated hepatocytes after, 157, 165
Viral hepatitis
    ceroid in, 199
    cholangitis in, 227, **227**, **228**
    endotheliitis and phlebitis in, 237
    ferritin deposition in, **180**, 181
    necrosis in, 97
    serologic findings in, 265-266
Viral hepatitis A, special morphologic features, 10, 32, 88
Viral hepatitis B
    and fibrosing cholestatic allograft hepatitis, 38
    core antigen in, 166
    surface antigen in, 165, **166**
    prognostic features, 28
Viral hepatitis B and D, sanded nuclei in, 147, 166
Viral hepatitis B and non-A, non-B (C,D), morphologic features, 165-167
Viral hepatitis C, prognostic features, 28
Viral hepatitis D, fatty changes in, 64, 71
Viral inclusion bodies
    in adenovirus hepatitis, 149
    in CMV hepatitis, **155**
    in herpes simplex hepatitis, **156**
Visceral bacillary epithelioid angiomatosis, morphologic findings in, 236, 252
Visceral leishmaniasis, 88
Vitamin A, normal levels, 263
Vitamin D (25-hydroxy vitamin D), normal levels, 264
Vitamin E, normal levels, 264
von Meyenburg complex. *See* Biliary microhamartomas

W

Waldenström's macroglobulinemia and peliosis hepatis, 252
Warfarin sodium, 53
Weber-Christian disease, steatohepatitis in, 73, 75
Weight-reducing surgery, steatohepatitis after, 73
Whipple's disease, granulomas in, 86
Wilson's disease
    cholestasis in, 43
    cirrhosis in, 128
    copper in, 18, 200
    other morphologic features, 167
    periportal hepatitis in, 17
    steatohepatitis in, 74
Wolman's disease, morphologic features, 63, 128

Y

Yellow fever hepatitis, morphologic features, 105, 106, **106**

Z

Zieve's syndrome and alcoholic fatty liver, 57
Zonal necrosis, definition and associated clinical conditions, 95, 96